DIFFERENTIAL DIAGNOSIS IN DERMATOPATHOLOGY

I

Differential Diagnosis in Dermatopathology I

Second Edition

A. Bernard Ackerman, M.D.
Professor of Dermatology and Pathology
Director of Dermatopathology
New York University School of Medicine
Consultant Dermatopathologist, Department of Pathology
Memorial Sloan-Kettering Cancer Center
New York, New York

ANA MARIA N. MENDONÇA, M.D.
Visiting Fellow in Dermatopathology
New York University School of Medicine
New York, New York

YING GUO, M.D.
Visiting Fellow in Dermatopathology
New York University School of Medicine
New York, New York

LEA & FEBIGER PHILADELPHIA/LONDON
1992

Lea & Febiger
200 Chester Field Parkway
Malvern, PA 19355
U.S.A.

First edition, 1982

Library of Congress Cataloging-in-Publication Data

Ackerman, A. Bernard, 1936–
Differential diagnosis in dermatopathology I/A. Bernard Ackerman, Ana Maria Mendonça, Ying Guo.—2nd ed.

p. cm.
ISBN 0-8121-1383-7
1. Skin—Diseases—Diagnosis. 2. Diagnosis, Differential. 3. Skin—Histopathology—Atlases. I. Mendonça, Ana Maria, 1947–. II. Ying, Guo. III. Title. IV. Title: Differential diagnosis in dermatopathology.
[DNLM: 1. Diagnosis, Differential. 2. Skin Diseases—diagnosis. WR 140 A182o]
RL105.A25 1992
616.5′075—dc20
DLC
for Library of Congress 91-8881
CIP

PRINTED IN THE UNITED STATES OF AMERICA
Print Number 5 4 3 2 1

To

RUDOLF BAER

whose magnificent spirit helped make
this book possible
—and so much more

Preface to the First Edition

Although there are now several textbooks of dermatopathology in English, none is especially designed to help pathologists and dermatologists to differentiate by microscopy between skin diseases that are similar histologically but are different clinically and in biologic course. Probably no other organ has as many diseases that histologically look alike as does the skin. Among these are an ever-increasing number of benign inflammatory diseases that masquerade microscopically as malignant neoplasms (pseudomalignancies) and, in reverse, malignant neoplasms that histologically simulate benign conditions (pseudobenignancies). In addition, within the categories of hamartomatous malformations, abnormal autochthonous deposits, alopecias, vesicular and bullous disease, and neoplasias in general, there are many problems in differential diagnosis that may be resolved if only one attends to subtle histologic distinctions. Many of the major problems of histologic differential diagnosis in dermatopathology, as we perceive them, are listed in the Contents.

In this work, apparent histologic similarities are contrasted in a manner that establishes criteria for differentiating them. These distinctions are presented in capsule and table form by emphatic telegraphic statements. Photomicrographs of contrasted diseases that differentiate strikingly the histologic features are reproduced in low and high magnification. Clinical photographs permit the reader, particularly the pathologist, to visualize the pathologic condition in the gross.

The discussions that follow the tabulated points and counterpoints expatiate first on the histologic features that each pair of contrasted diseases have in common, and then on the correlations between their histologic and clinical appearances, their usual clinical courses and, lastly, their histologic differential diagnoses. For simplification and teaching purposes, we have tended to use the classical presentation of fully developed lesions as our models.

We derived criteria by laboriously examining tens, scores, and sometimes hundreds of histologic examples of the contrasted diseases. We were not swayed by traditional interpretations, although we did not deliberately and completely disregard them. No bibliography accompanies any of the 45 sections because the data presented here are our own.

During the years in which this book was evolving, I was fortunate to collaborate with two energetic Fellows in dermatopathology, Drs. John Niven and Jane Grant-Kels. Dr. Niven collected the slides for histologic study and helped to prepare the first of many drafts of the manuscript. Dr. Grant-Kels collated the clinical pictures and was responsible for the photomicrography. As has been the case for virtually all of my writings during the past eight years, Dr. Morris Leider kindly, carefully, and critically edited this manuscript from Preface to Glossary. A special word of thanks is also due Drs. Helmut Kerl and Hans Kresbach of the Department of Dermatology at the University of Graz for kindly permitting us to use some of their clinical photographs, and to Dr. James Rasmussen of the Department of Dermatology at the University of Michigan for the clinical photograph of staphylococcal scalded skin syndrome, Dr. William Mahoney for the clinical photograph of hidradenoma papilliferum, Dr. George Popkin for the clinical photograph of trichoepitheliomas, and Dr. Phillip Frost for the clinical photograph of bullous congenital ichthyosiform erythroderma. I also appreciate the efforts of Tom Colaiezzi and Ken Bussy of Lea & Febiger, who shepherded the work from manuscript to bound book—a book designed by the incomparable Howard King, painstakingly and lovingly.

We hope that this book will be a useful adjunct to Sherlockian solving of histologic puzzles in dermatopathology and will enable differential diagnosis to become specific diagnosis.

A. Bernard Ackerman
New York, New York

Preface

It has been more than 15 years since work commenced on the first edition of the first in a series of volumes about differential diagnosis in dermatopathology. In the interim, my thinking about each of the paired subjects has been affected profoundly as a consequence of having "read out" sections from more than 750,000 histopathologic specimens, worked closely on various papers and books with more than 200 Fellows in dermatopathology, and exchanged ideas with them and with countless colleagues in dermatology and pathology the world over through correspondence, courses and symposia, and exchanges of visits to sites where professional lives are lived. In short, I have learned much more since I and my co-workers completed the first edition of this volume than I knew before that first edition was undertaken. It is fitting, proper, and socially conscionable, therefore, that this book be made contemporaneous with my current knowledge, concepts, and perspectives. Toward that end, I began a second edition with the collaboration of two outstanding Fellows in dermatopathology, namely, Dr. Ana Mendonça from Brazil and Dr. Ying Guo from China. Ana collected the histopathologic sections and Ying "shot" the superb photomicrographs that grace the pages that follow. Not only has the text been updated and rewritten, but photomicrographs that we consider to be more instructive or more esthetic have replaced most of the original ones. The glossary, too, has been enlarged and enriched. In this way, the second edition of *Differential Diagnosis in Dermatopathology I* is an expression of our own intellectual growth in dermatopathology and a vehicle through which we can share that development with colleagues. We hope that readers delight in it.

A. Bernard Ackerman
New York, New York

Contents

DIFFERENTIAL DIAGNOSIS IN DERMATOPATHOLOGY

I

1. Psoriasis *vs.* Nummular Dermatitis

Psoriasis	*Nummular Dermatitis*
1. Confluent parakeratosis	1. Focal scale-crust
2. Granular zone mostly absent	2. Granular zone mostly present
3. Psoriasiform hyperplasia (rete ridges of even lengths); some rete ridges thinned, and some of those markedly	3. Irregular psoriasiform hyperplasia (rete ridges of unequal lengths); rete ridges not thinned
4. Suprapapillary plates thinned	4. Suprapapillary plates not thinned
5. Pallor of keratinocytes in uppermost spinous zone	5. No pallor of epidermal keratinocytes
6. Spongiosis, when present, early and mostly in suprapapillary plates; no vesicles	6. Spongiosis mostly in rete ridges; vesicles often
7. Neutrophils within the epidermis, especially in parakeratotic foci	7. No neutrophils within the epidermis (unless eroded and impetiginized)
8. Increased number of mitotic figures above the basal layer	8. Few, if any, mitotic figures above the basal layer
9. Capillaries in the papillary dermis markedly tortuous (i.e., seemingly increased in number) and very near the epidermis	9. Capillaries in the papillary dermis dilated but not tortuous, and not very near the epidermis
10. Sparse superficial perivascular mostly lymphocytic infiltrate with few neutrophils; no eosinophils usually	10. Moderately dense superficial perivascular and interstitial lymphocytic infiltrate with many eosinophils often; no neutrophils usually

Psoriasis | *Nummular Dermatitis*

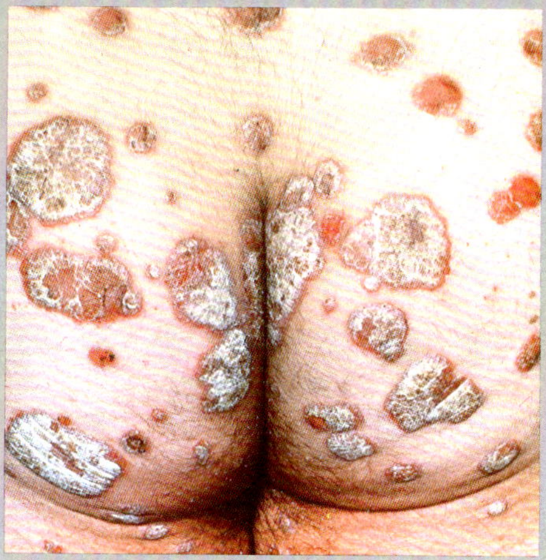

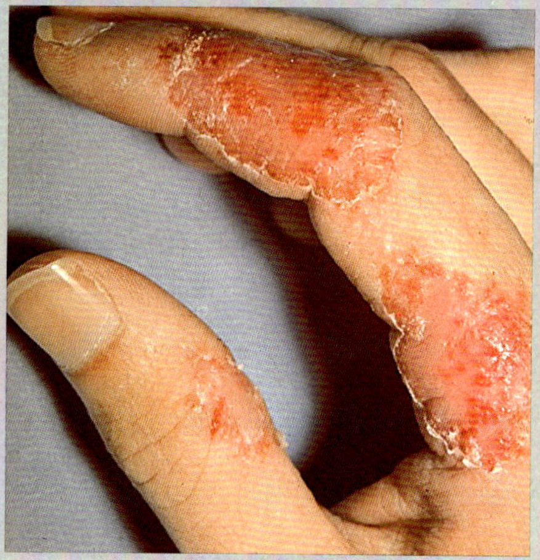

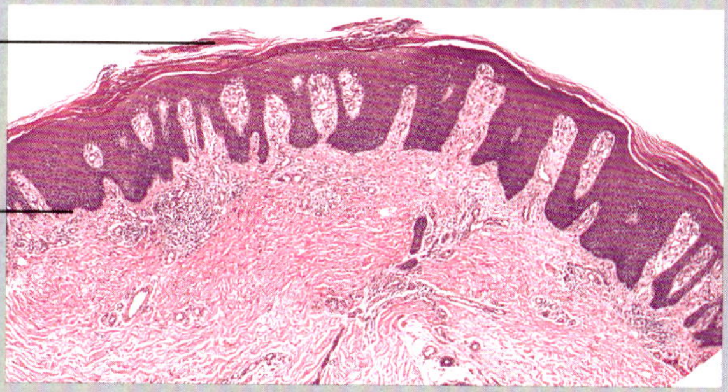

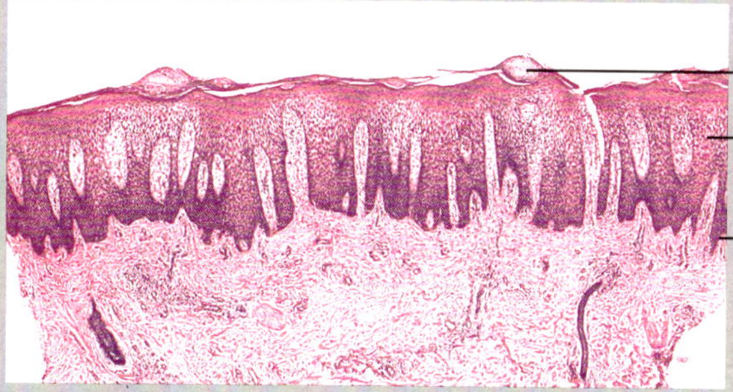

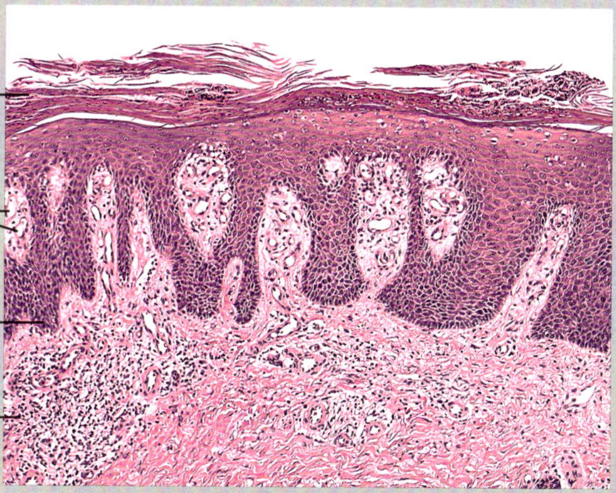

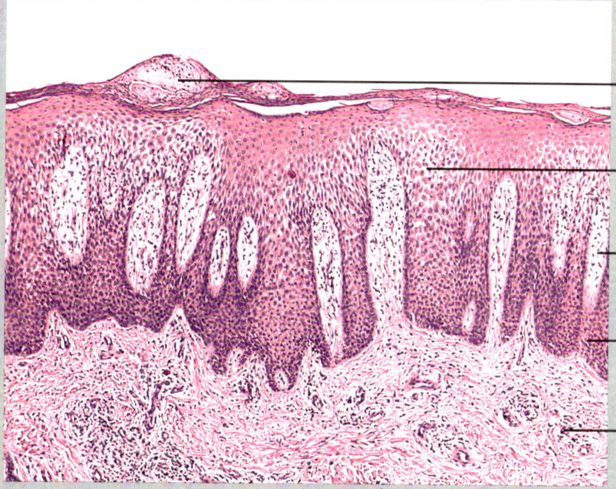

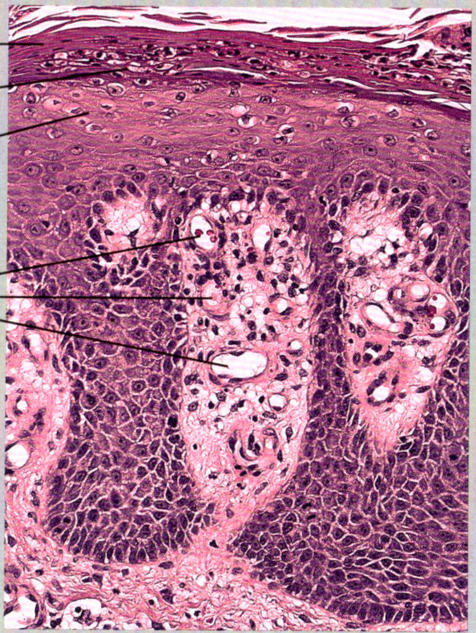

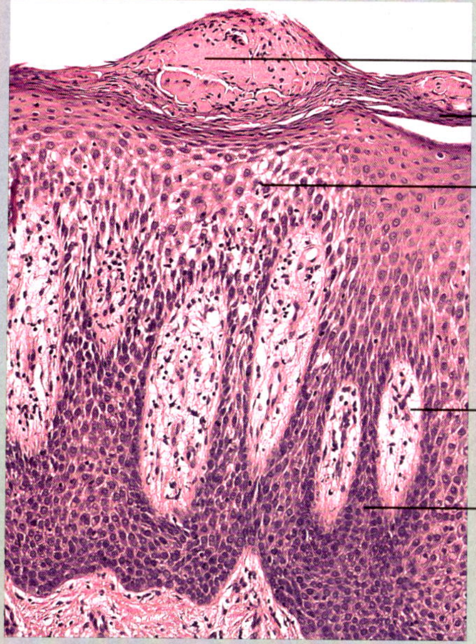

PSORIASIS and nummular dermatitis share several histopathologic features, namely, some parakeratosis, psoriasiform hyperplasia, edema of the papillary dermis, and an infiltrate of inflammatory cells around dilated blood vessels of the superficial plexus. Evolving lesions of psoriasis, like those of nummular dermatitis, are even marked by spongiosis.

The histopathologic changes enumerated here apply only to fully developed, active lesions of psoriasis and nummular dermatitis, i.e., scaly, reddish plaques in the case of psoriasis and papulovesicles in reddish, crusted, coin-shaped plaques in the case of nummular dermatitis. Both diseases have a wide spectrum of pathologic features, grossly and microscopically, as would be expected for conditions whose lesions last for weeks or months (and even years in the case of some lesions of psoriasis).

Clinically, psoriasis begins as tiny, reddish macules that soon enlarge to become slightly elevated and scaly. Early guttate (drop-sized) psoriatic lesions gradually enlarge centrifugally and, in time, may become extensive. Nummular dermatitis starts as reddish macules that soon become scratched because of intense pruritus that accompanies them. In time, papules that are eroded and crusted develop into coin-shaped plaques. When rubbed persistently, lesions of nummular dermatitis become lichenified (by superimposition of lichen simplex chronicus). When lesions of both psoriasis and nummular dermatitis resolve, hyperpigmentation tends to be residual. In some patients, hyperpigmentation remains.

Salient histopathologic features of early guttate lesions of psoriasis are:

1. Mounds of parakeratosis that contain neutrophils at their summits
2. Neutrophils in intra- and subcorneal (Munro) or spongiform (Kogoj) pustules
3. Normal granular zone, except beneath parakeratotic foci
4. Normal suprapapillary plates
5. Slight epidermal hyperplasia
6. Slight spongiosis
7. Marked edema of the papillary dermis
8. Superficial perivascular infiltrate of lymphocytes, neutrophils, and extravasated erythrocytes around widely dilated capillaries and venules, and scatter of neutrophils in dermal papillae; a few erythrocytes are present focally within the epidermis in some lesions.

The early lesions of nummular dermatitis are characterized histopathologically by:

1. Normal or focally parakeratotic cornified layer
2. Focal spongiosis, sometimes diffuse

3. Slight epidermal hyperplasia
4. Edema of the papillary dermis
5. Superficial infiltrate of lymphocytes and often numerous eosinophils perivascularly and interstitially; cells also in the papillary dermis.

A biopsy specimen from the center of a long-standing resolving plaque of psoriasis shows histopathologically:

1. Confluent compact orthokeratosis with only focal parakeratosis
2. Granular zone mostly of normal thickness
3. Supra-papillary plates of normal thickness
4. Psoriasiform hyperplasia with rete ridges of approximately equal length and breadth
5. Tortuous capillaries in dermal papillae
6. Sparse to moderately dense superficial perivascular lymphocytic infiltrate.

Late lesions of nummular dermatitis are marked histopathologically by:

1. Compact orthokeratosis with focal parakeratosis
2. Irregular psoriasiform hyperplasia
3. Papillary dermis thickened by coarse bundles of collagen arranged in vertical streaks parallel to elongated rete ridges, i.e., signs of lichen simplex chronicus
4. Moderately dense superficial perivascular mixed inflammatory-cell infiltrate of lymphocytes, histiocytes (including melanophages), plasma cells, and eosinophils.

Lichen simplex chronicus often is superimposed upon long-standing lesions of nummular dermatitis and less often upon those of psoriasis. In those instances, the histopathologic evidence of persistent rubbing, namely, a papillary dermis thickened markedly by coarse bundles of collagen arrayed in vertical streaks, may obscure the underlying nummular dermatitis or psoriasis. Helpful clues to recognizing the underlying process as nummular dermatitis are slight spongiosis within the psoriasiform epidermis, crusts as well as scales, and some eosinophils within the infiltrate in the upper part of the dermis. Clues to the psoriatic nature of the underlying process are neutrophils within parakeratotic foci, tortuous capillaries in the papillary dermis, and some thin rete ridges.

A few lines should be devoted to two interesting morphologic expressions of psoriasis, namely, the pustular and the erythrodermic. Pustular psoriasis is merely explosive psoriasis in which the process is so accelerated that it bypasses guttate macules and papules and proceeds directly to pustules. Erythrodermic psoriasis is universal, or nearly so, and exhibits generalized redness and scaling. The histopathologic findings are just like those of fully developed lesions of psoriasis, except that there is little, if any, scale as a consequence of exfoliation.

2. Pityriasis Rosea *vs.* Guttate Parapsoriasis

Pityriasis Rosea	*Guttate Parapsoriasis*
1. Parakeratosis in dome-shaped mounds	1. Scale-crusts in elongated mounds
2. Spongiosis prominent usually	2. Spongiosis slight or absent
3. Epidermal hyperplasia	3. Little or no epidermal hyperplasia
4. No lymphocytes aligned as solitary units in the basal layer focally	4. Lymphocytes sometimes aligned as solitary units in the basal layer focally.
5. No cluster of lymphocytes in the epidermis in the near absence of spongiosis.	5. Cluster(s) of lymphocytes in the epidermis in concert with scant spongiosis sometimes.
6. Marked edema of the papillary dermis often	6. Little or no edema of the papillary dermis
7. Few or many extravasated erythrocytes in the dermal papillae (and sometimes in the epidermis)	7. No or very few extravasated erythrocytes
8. Moderately dense superficial perivascular lymphocytic infiltrate; eosinophils present episodically	8. Sparse superficial perivascular lymphocytic infiltrate without eosinophils
9. Melanophages occasionally	9. Melanophages rarely

Pityriasis Rosea | *Guttate Parapsoriasis*

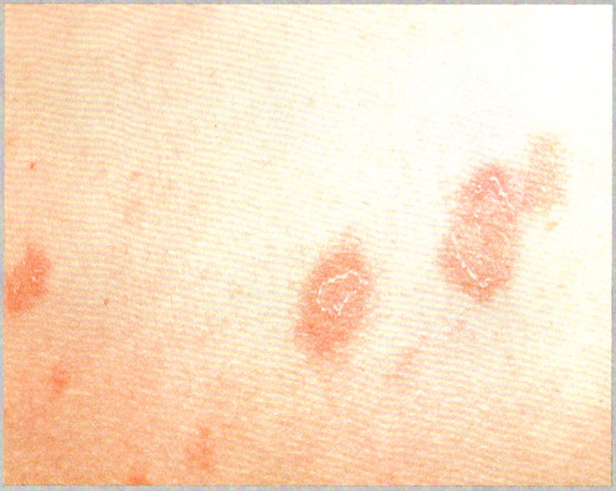

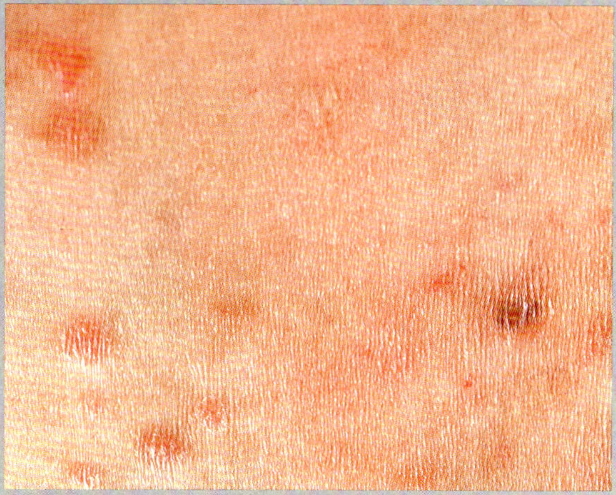

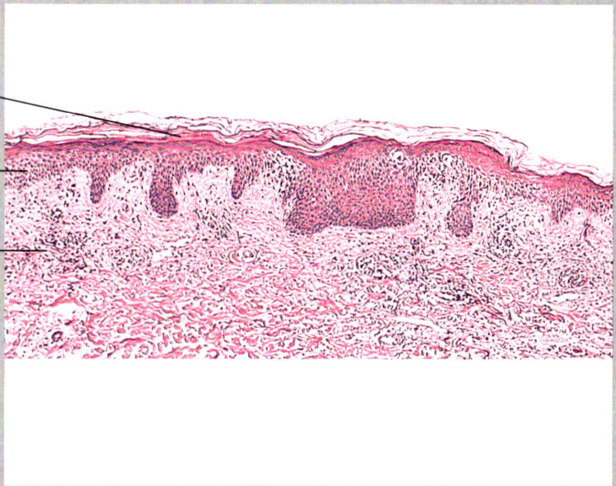

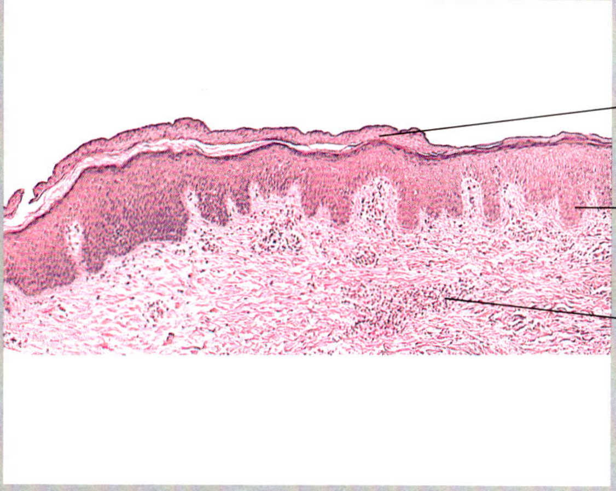

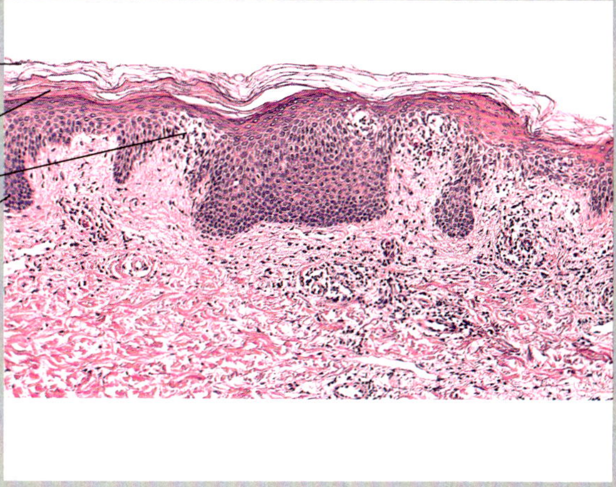

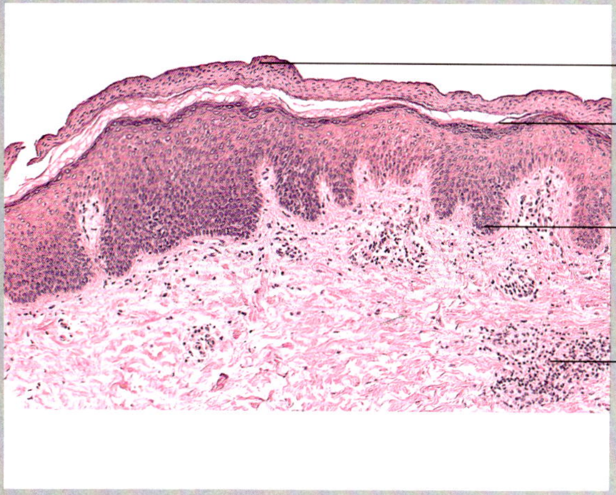

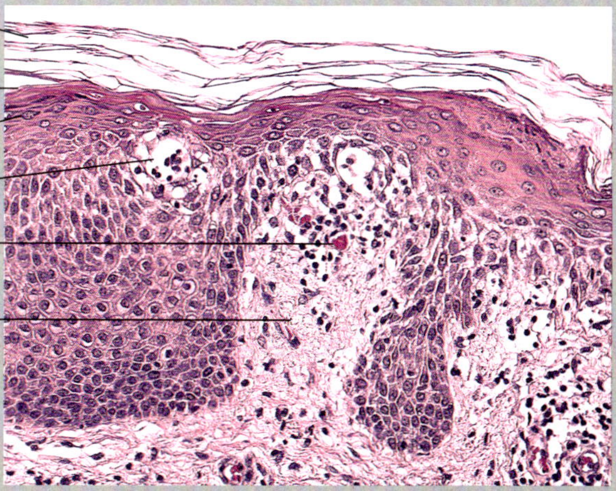

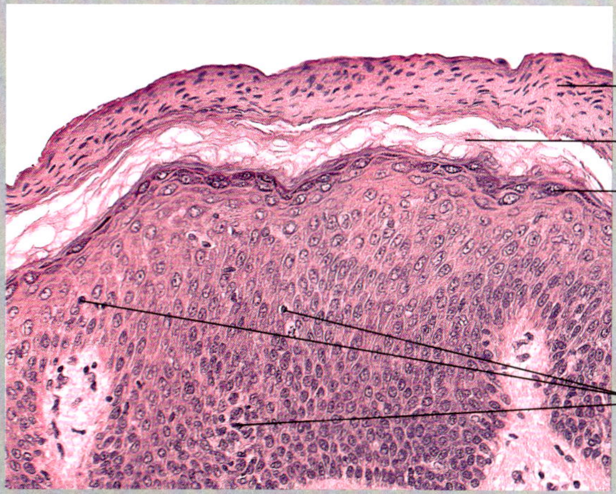

PITYRIASIS rosea and guttate parapsoriasis, at first glance, seem to have more histopathologic features in common than they have differences. Both have a superficial perivascular predominantly lymphocytic infiltrate, spongiosis, and parakeratosis. They differ primarily in that pityriasis rosea has a somewhat denser infiltrate, extravasated erythrocytes, more noticeable spongiosis, and epidermal hyperplasia. Another difference is a greater tendency toward formation of scale-crusts in guttate parapsoriasis, and those scale-crusts usually are very elongated. Last, some lesions of guttate parapsoriasis exhibit tiny clusters of lymphocytes within epidermal foci poor in spongiosis, and lymphocytes aligned as solitary units in foci in the basal layer. In some instances, however, it may be extremely difficult to differentiate between the two diseases histopathologically.

Pityriasis rosea tends to involve the torso from the neck to the knees and to consist of oval to round, salmon-pink papules and plaques with delicate scales that form collarettes. On the trunk, the lesions align themselves along lines of cleavage of the skin (Langer's lines). Days or a week or two before the appearance of the eruption, a larger scaly lesion ("mother" or "herald" patch) had become manifest. Biopsy of this larger lesion reveals histopathologic changes similar to those in the later smaller lesions of pityriasis rosea, but the perivascular infiltrate of lymphocytes often is both superficial and deep, there is less spongiosis, and epidermal hyperplasia is more psoriasiform. Pityriasis rosea usually resolves without treatment in about six to nine weeks.

Clinically, guttate parapsoriasis consists of widespread, drop-sized pink or tan papules covered by fine, wafer-like scales. The lesions are not pruritic, but they persist indefinitely and are refractory to treatment. Histopathologically, guttate parapsoriasis shows little or no spongiosis within the epidermis in a routine section. The finding of plasma in scale-crusts, however, implies that spongiosis must have been present in the epidermis previously.

We consider digitate dermatosis to be a variant of guttate parapsoriasis. Clinically, it consists of large, ovoid, scaly patches situated mostly on or near the trunk that persist despite treatments of various kinds, and histopathologically, it is indistinguishable from guttate parapsoriasis. Lesions of guttate parapsoriasis and digitate dermatosis may be present together in the same patient. Even more important is the observation that some patients with typical patches and plaques of mycosis fungoides, confirmed histopathologically, also may have typical lesions of guttate parapsoriasis and digitate dermatosis, the latter pattern verified histopathologically, too.

Careful study of lesions of guttate parapsoriasis-digitate dermatosis reveals subtle signs of mycosis fungoides in many lesions, namely, lymphocytes aligned as solitary units in the basal layer focally, one or two tiny clusters of lymphocytes within the spinous zone in the presence of but a tad of spongiosis, a few lymphocytes within the epidermis larger than those in the dermis, and one or two foci of wiry bundles of collagen arranged haphazardly in the papillary dermis where they are accompanied by lymphocytes, sometimes in patchy array. In sum, we now conclude that guttate parapsoriasis-digitate dermatosis (small plaque parapsoriasis), like parapsoriasis en plaque, parapsoriasis variegata, xanthoerythroderma perstans, and poikiloderma vasculare atrophicans (large plaque parapsoriasis), is a distinctive morphologic macular/patch expression of mycosis fungoides.

Superficial types of figurate erythemas (e.g., erythema annulare centrifugum) also must be considered in the histopathologic differential diagnosis of pityriasis rosea. Both diseases are characterized by a superficial perivascular lymphocytic infiltrate, edema of the papillary dermis, spongiosis, and focal parakeratosis. Although histopathologically it is impossible to distinguish between pityriasis rosea and superficial figurate erythemas, those two conditions are differentiated readily from guttate parapsoriasis, clinically and histopathologically. Lesions of pityriasis rosea and erythema annulare centrifugum both are characterized clinically by oval shapes and collarettes of scales at their peripheries. Clinically, a lesion of erythema annulare centrifigum seems to be a caricature of a lesion of pityriasis rosea. The rare vesicular variant of pityriasis rosea, which occurs mostly in blacks, must be differentiated histopathologically from fully developed lesions of allergic contact dermatitis, nummular dermatitis, and "id" reactions. Although this differentiation is not always possible, vesicular lesions of pityriasis rosea tend to have less epidermal hyperplasia and fewer eosinophils than those three diseases that tend to eventuate in vesicles.

3. Lichen Planus *vs.* Lichen Planus-like Keratosis

Lichen Planus	*Lichen Planus-like Keratosis*
1. Compact orthokeratosis; no parakeratosis usually	1. Compact orthokeratosis and focal parakeratosis
2. Granular zone thickened focally in wedge shape	2. Granular zone thickened and thinned focally; wedge shapes not present consistently
3. Irregular, jagged epidermal hyperplasia	3. Variably hyperplastic, sometimes thinned epidermis; not necessarily jagged hyperplasia
4. Keratinocytic nuclei not atypical	4. Keratinocytic nuclei in lower part of epidermis may be atypical
5. Dense band-like lymphocytic infiltrate in the upper part of the dermis	5. Dense band-like lymphocytic infiltrate with occasional plasma cells and/or eosinophils in the upper part of the dermis
6. Infiltrate of lymphocytes obscures dermo-epidermal interface along the entire length of the lesion	6. Infiltrate of inflammatory cells obscures dermo-epidermal interface intermittently
7. Solar elastosis not present usually	7. Solar elastosis invariable
8. No solar lentigo or thin seborrheic keratosis contiguous to the lesion	8. Solar lentigo or thin seborrheic keratosis contiguous to the lesion commonly

Lichen Planus | *Lichen Planus-Like Keratosis*

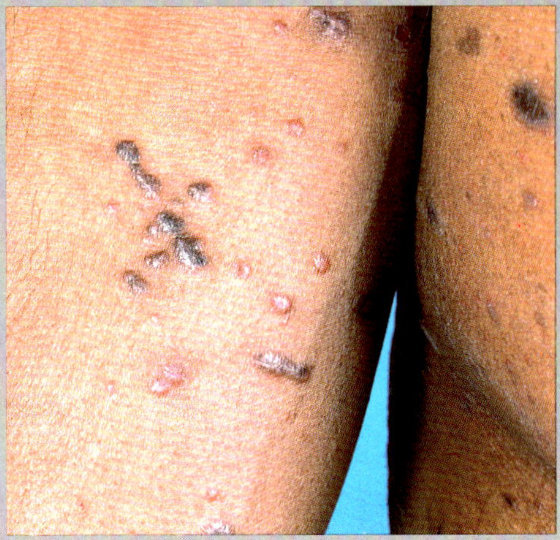

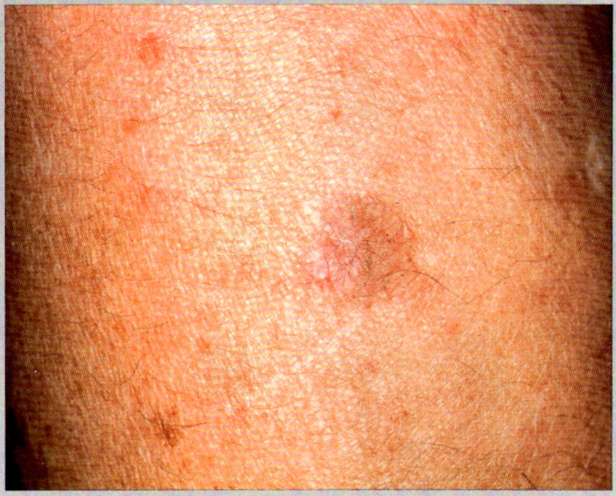

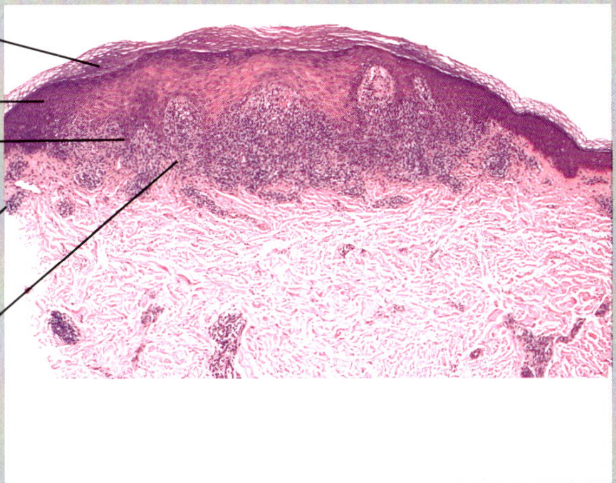

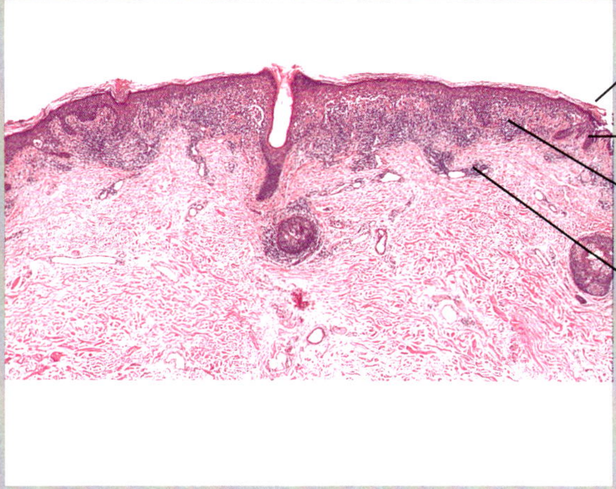

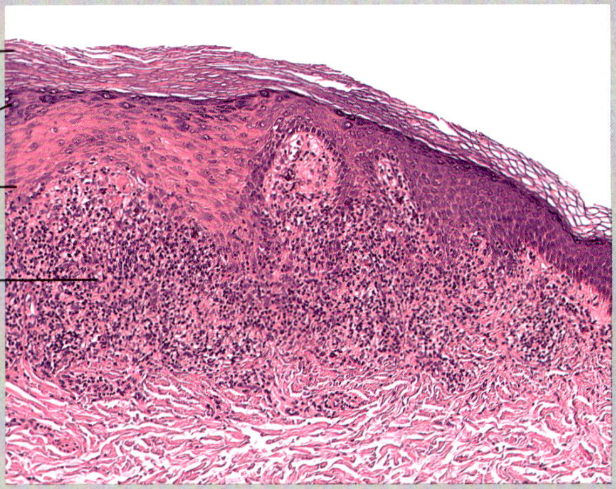

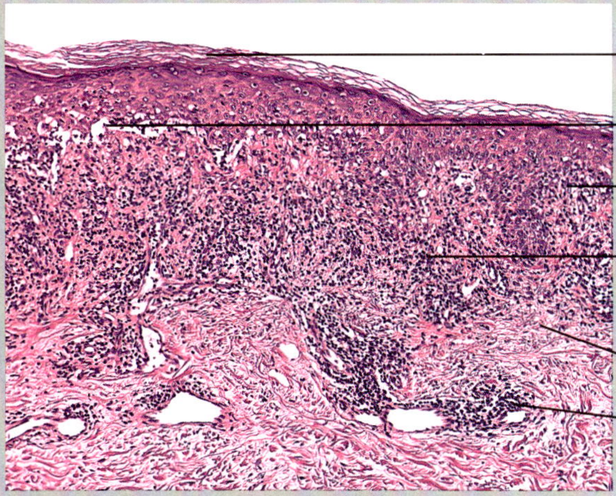

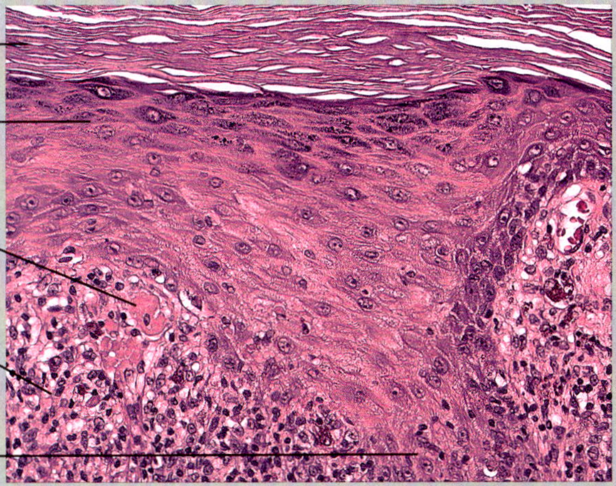

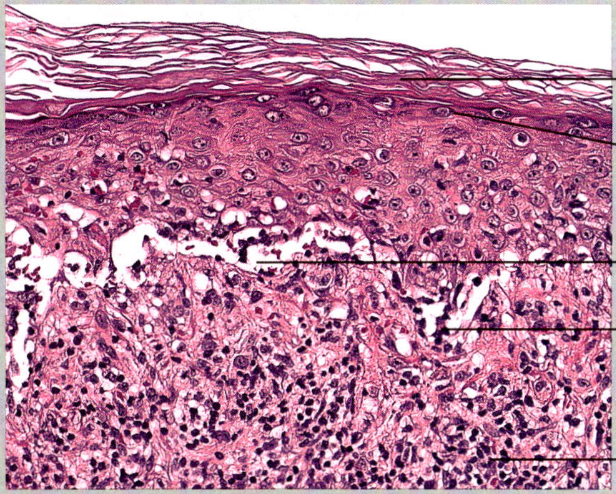

LICHEN planus-like keratosis may be confused easily with lichen planus histopathologically, especially in specimens taken by punch technique. Ostensibly, both are superficial perivascular dermatitides with lichenoid, mostly lymphocytic infiltrates that obscure the dermo-epidermal junction where there are vacuolar alteration and necrotic keratinocytes (interface dermatitides, lichenoid type). Lichen planus-like keratosis begins as a solar lentigo or reticulated seborrheic keratosis that, in time, is associated with a dense lichenoid infiltrate composed mostly of lymphocytes. The keratosis usually is removed by shave excision technique, and the lesion generally extends broadly from one end of the histopathologic section to the other, or nearly so. In contrast, lichen planus is idiopathic. A lesion of it usually is biopsied by punch excision technique and, more often than not, the lesion does not extend across the width of even a 4-mm specimen.

Clinically, a lichen planus-like keratosis usually develops as a solitary, reddish-brown, scaly lesion, predilectively on sun-exposed skin, especially of the chest and arms of older persons. The lesion often is misdiagnosed clinically as basal-cell carcinoma. In time, lichen planus-like keratosis tends to regress with residual changes that may be indistinguishable from those in regression of primary cutaneous malignant melanoma. Those findings are a thinned epidermis and a papillary dermis "thickened" by delicate fibroplasia, melanophages, a sprinkling of lymphocytes, necrotic keratinocytes, and telangiectases. In fact, the papillary dermis in resolved lesions of lichen planus-like keratosis (and primary melanoma) and in atrophic lesions of lichen planus is reduced in volume because of the loss of dermal papillae that ordinarily account for much of the volume of the skin above the reticular dermis.

Lichen planus presents itself as a pruritic, widespread eruption of flat-topped, shiny, violaceous, polygonal papules. The disease may involve mucous membranes, nail units, and hair follicles (lichen plano-pilaris). Although there are many variants of lichen planus (e.g., atrophic, hypertrophic, bullous), most have in common the following histopathologic features:

1. Compact orthokeratosis
2. Focal hypergranulosis in wedge shape
3. Jagged epidermal hyperplasia
4. Necrotic keratinocytes (Civatte bodies, colloid bodies) at the dermo-epidermal junction and above it
5. Vacuolar alteration at the dermo-epidermal junction

6. Dense, band-like lymphocytic infiltrates with melanophages in the thickened papillary dermis and that obscure the interface between epidermis and dermis
7. Coarse bundles of collagen in the thickened papillary dermis.

In atrophic (resolving or resolved) lichen planus, the epidermis is thinned, the cellular infiltrate in the upper part of the dermis is relatively scant, and the usual undulations between rete ridges and dermal papillae are muted as a result of subtle fibroplasia. In hypertrophic lichen planus, both the epidermis and papillary dermis are thickened markedly by superimposition of features of lichen simplex chronicus (the result of persistent rubbing). Bullous lichen planus usually does not show the band-like infiltrate of lymphocytes characteristic of papular lichen planus because the blister forms so quickly that the lesion has no chance to become fully developed, i.e., lichenoid as a consequence of a band of lymphocytes.

Other lichenoid inflammatory-cell infiltrates that must be differentiated from lichen planus and lichen planus-like keratosis are:

1. Lichenoid photodermatitis (such as may be induced by thiazides) in which the infiltrate often is deep as well as superficial
2. Lichenoid drug eruptions (such as caused by gold) in which there may be eosinophils in the dermal infiltrate, many necrotic keratinocytes in a focally thinned epidermis, focal hypogranulosis, and parakeratosis
3. Lichenoid discoid lupus erythematosus in which the epidermal basement membrane frequently is thickened
4. The lichenoid form of persistent pigmented purpuric dermatitis (Gougerot and Blum) in which there usually are numerous extravasated erythrocytes and siderophages.

Why an apparently banal solar lentigo calls forth a lichenoid inflammatory-cell infiltrate and, in the process, becomes a lichen planus-like keratosis which then is destroyed by that same infiltrate remains an enigma.

4. Allergic Contact Dermatitis *vs.* Irritant Contact Dermatitis

Allergic Contact Dermatitis	*Irritant Contact Dermatitis*
1. No erosions or ulcerations usually	1. Erosions or ulcerations not unusual
2. Lower portion of epidermis altered early in the course	2. Upper portion of epidermis altered early in the course
3. Marked spongiosis leads to intra-epidermal spongiotic vesicles	3. Slight spongiosis early; no spongiotic vesicles
4. Slight ballooning	4. Marked ballooning leads to intra-epidermal ballooning vesicles
5. No necrotic keratinocytes	5. Necrotic keratinocytes range from individual units in variable numbers to necrosis of the entire epidermis
6. Lymphocytes or eosinophils in foci of spongiosis	6. Neutrophils in foci of ballooning and necrosis
7. Superficial perivascular lymphocytic infiltrate with variable numbers of eosinophils;neutrophils	7. Superficial perivascular lymphocytic infiltrate with variable numbers of neutrophils;eosinophils

Allergic Contact Dermatitis	Irritant Contact Dermatitis

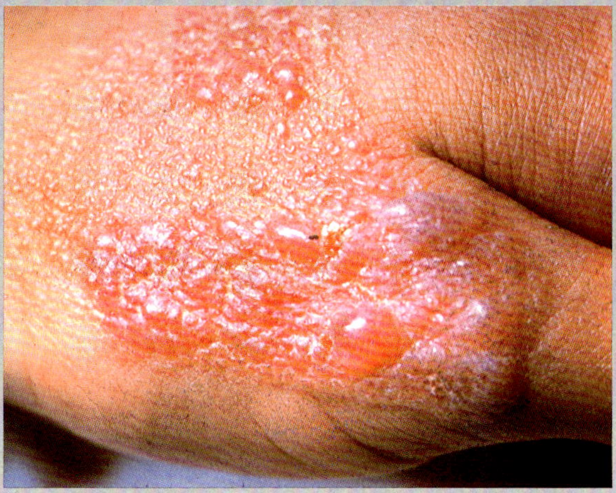

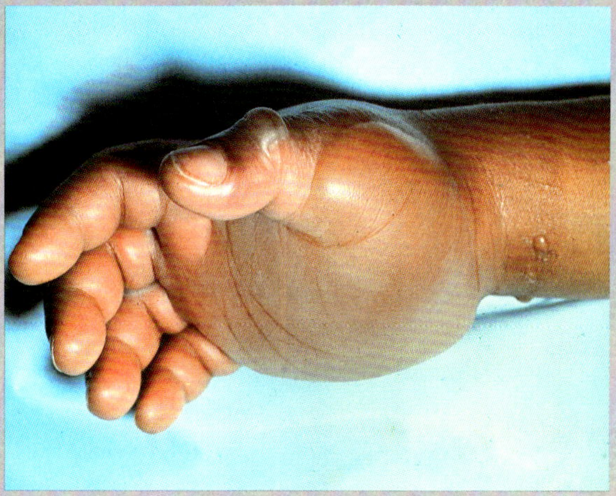

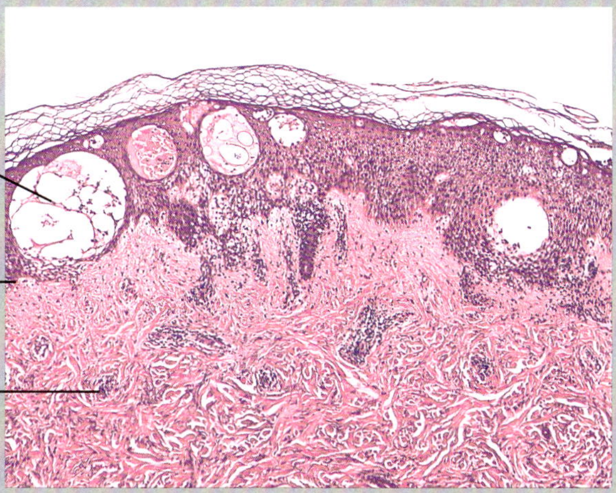

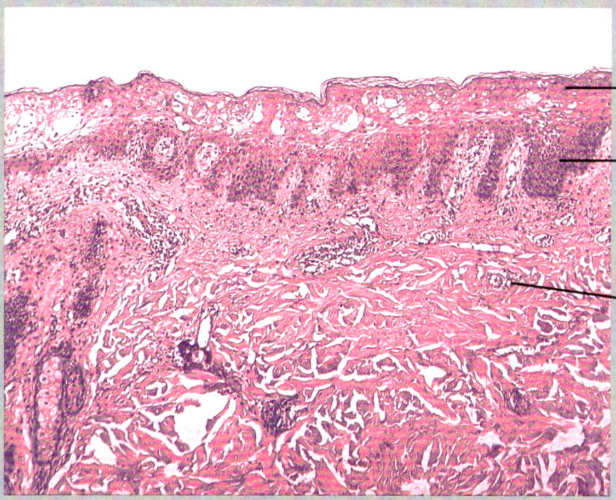

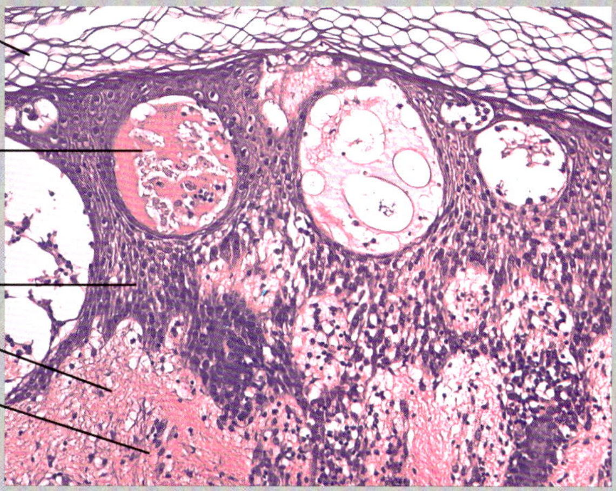

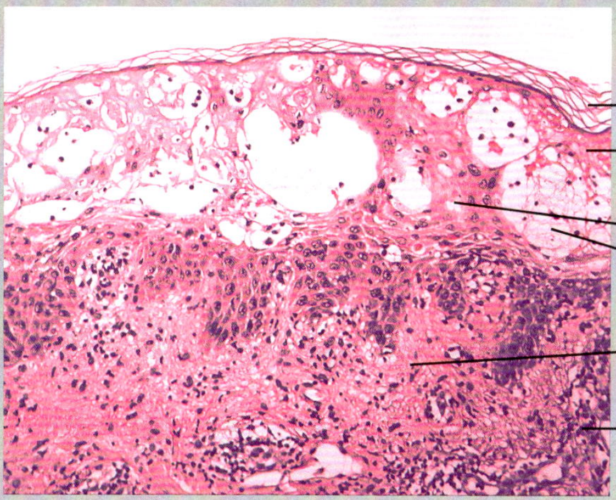

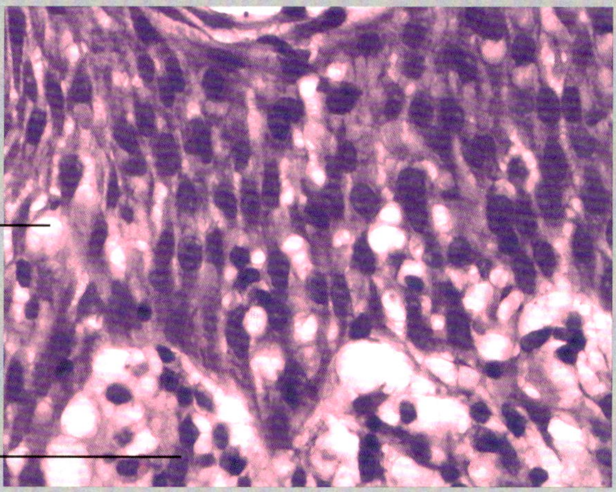

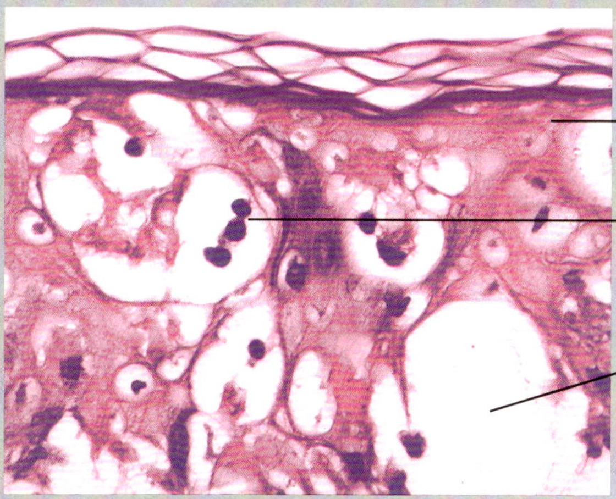

In their fully developed form, allergic contact dermatitis and irritant contact dermatitis are both intra-epidermal vesicular dermatitides that appear after exposure to different kinds of contactants, namely, allergens in the former and irritant substances in the latter.

Histopathologically, allergic and irritant contact dermatitides have in common intra- and intercellular edema, edema of the papillary dermis, and superficial perivascular mixed inflammatory-cell infiltrates. Both also may be associated with subepidermal vesiculation. In allergic contact dermatitis, that occurrence is secondary to either bursting of intra-epidermal spongiotic vesicles or extensive edema of the papillary dermis. In irritant contact dermatitis, that phenomenon comes about as a consequence of rupture of intra-epidermal ballooning vesicles or of severe epidermal necrosis with subsequent dermo-epidermal separation.

Allergic contact dermatitis results from exposure of previously sensitized persons to contact allergens. It is a delayed type of hypersensitivity reaction, in contrast to irritant contact dermatitis, which is not a hypersensitivity reaction at all. Irritant contact dermatitis results from direct injury to the skin by a variety of agents such as strong acids and alkalis, and by less irritating substances such as croton oil and sodium lauryl sulfate.

Clinically, allergic contact dermatitis appears as edematous pink papules that soon become papulovesicles. That these are actually vesicles often can be appreciated better by gentle palpation than by observation. With progression, the vesicles become discernible clearly and, in severe cases, huge bullae may form. Biopsy specimens taken serially reveal the early stage of allergic contact dermatitis to consist of spongiosis that becomes decidedly focal (spongiotic dermatitis), a fully developed stage that shows epidermal hyperplasia in addition to spongiotic vesicles (spongiotic psoriasiform dermatitis), and a late stage in which there is psoriasiform hyperplasia (psoriasiform dermatitis) devoid of spongiosis. In long-enduring lesions of allergic contact dermatitis, there usually are histopathologic evidences of persistent rubbing (i.e., lichen simplex chronicus) in the form of a papillary dermis thickened by coarse bundles of collagen arranged in vertical streaks and of compact orthokeratosis.

The histopathologic differential diagnosis of allergic contact dermatitis at all stages of the process involves consideration of early nummular dermatitis, dyshidrotic dermatitis, "id" reactions, and vesicular dermatophytic infections, all of which may show the same histopathologic features in sections stained by hematoxylin and eosin. The presence of hyphae within the cornified layer establishes the diagnosis of dermatophytosis. The other four conditions cannot be differentiated histopathologically from one another. Some patients may present themselves with widespread papulovesicular, vesicular, and even bullous eruptions that on the hands and feet may be interpreted as dyshidrotic dermatitis and "id" reactions, on other areas of the integument as allergic contact dermatitis, and on other sites as nummular dermatitis. Given this circumstance clinically and the identity of these four conditions histopathologically, these four spongiotic dermatitides seem to be related to one another.

Photo-allergic contact dermatitis, such as to salicylanilides, and photo-allergic dermatitis, such as to systemically administered chlorpromazine, are similar histopathologically to allergic contact dermatitis, except that in the photodermatitides the infiltrate of inflammatory cells tends to be both deep as well as superficial, and the epidermis tends to harbor a few necrotic keratinocytes. Clinically, photo-allergic contact dermatitis and photo-allergic dermatitis usually are confined to regions of the skin that ordinarily are exposed to sunlight.

Irritant contact dermatitis may range clinically from slight erythema and scaling to severe blisters and ulcerations. Like allergic contact dermatitis, irritant contact dermatitis has a photo-related counterpart, namely, phototoxic contact dermatitis caused by substances that become irritants only after photo-activation. Phototoxic dermatitis may result from systemically administered chemicals such as psoralens, and phototoxic contact dermatitis may result from chemicals such as psoralens applied topically. The phototoxic lesions are similar to irritant contact dermatitis clinically and histopathologically, and they, too, occur only on areas exposed to ultraviolet light.

Some contactants, such as turpentine, may be both sensitizing and irritating.

5. Dermatitis Herpetiformis *vs.* Bullous Pemphigoid

Dermatitis Herpetiformis	*Bullous Pemphigoid*
1. Subepidermal blister that contains mostly neutrophils; variable numbers of eosinophils present about three days after onset	1. Subepidermal blister that contains mostly eosinophils; variable numbers of neutrophils may be present from near the onset
2. Acantholytic cells, singly and in clumps, within the blister occasionally	2. No acantholytic cells within the blister
3. No spongiosis as a rule	3. Spongiosis associated with eosinophils at the sides of the blister often
4. Normal pattern of epidermal rete ridges and dermal papillae not preserved usually	4. Normal pattern of epidermal rete ridges and dermal papillae preserved usually
5. Neutrophils in collections, neutrophilic nuclear "dust," basophilic alteration of collagen bundles, and fibrin at tips of dermal papillae are present beneath and at the sides of a blister	5. No neutrophils or altered collagen bundles at tips of dermal papillae at the sides of a blister; sometimes eosinophils in collections in dermal papillae beneath a blister
6. Little edema of the papillary dermis	6. Marked edema of the papillary dermis
7. Superficial perivascular mixed-cell infiltrate of lymphocytes, neutrophils, and a few eosinophils	7. Superficial, and sometimes deep, perivascular mixed-cell infiltrate of lymphocytes and numerous eosinophils; neutrophils and plasma cells are uncommon and usually few

Dermatitis Herpetiformis | *Bullous Pemphigoid*

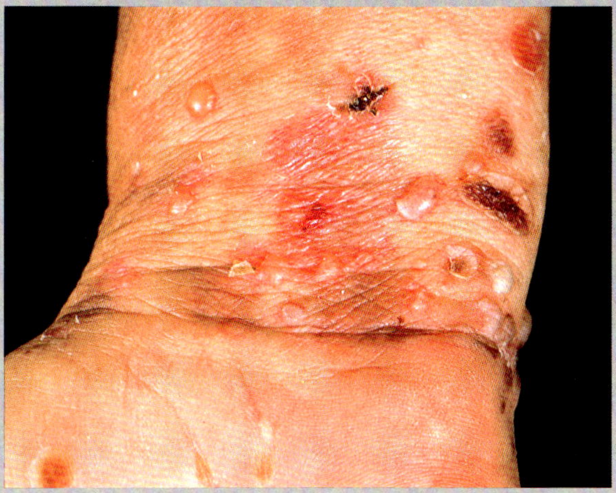

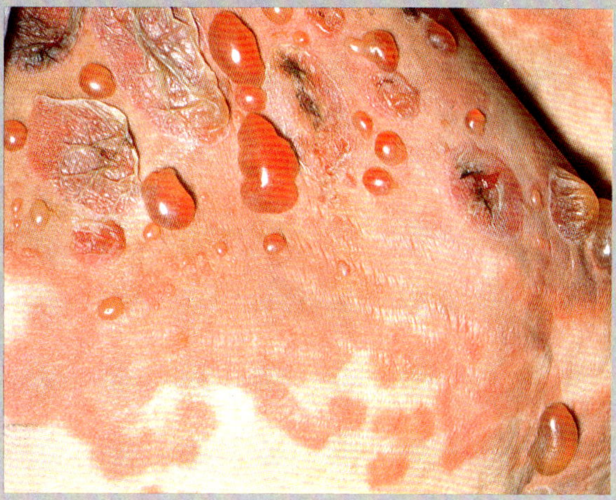

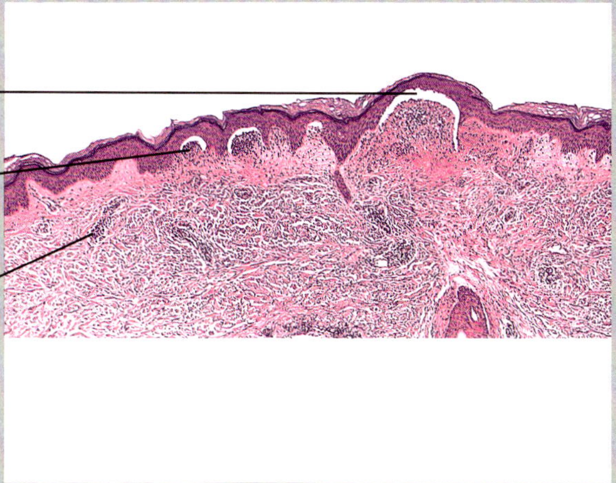

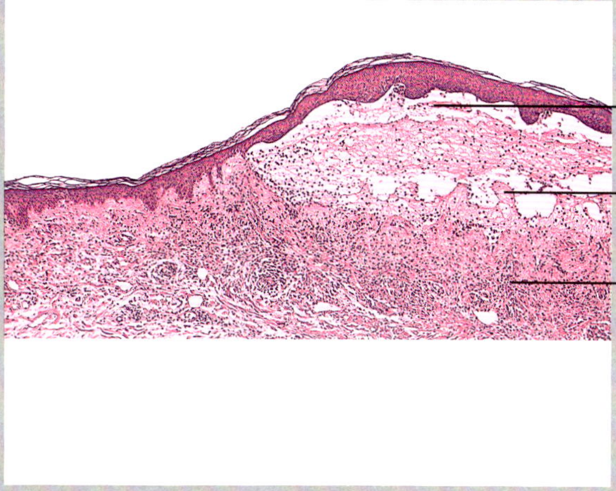

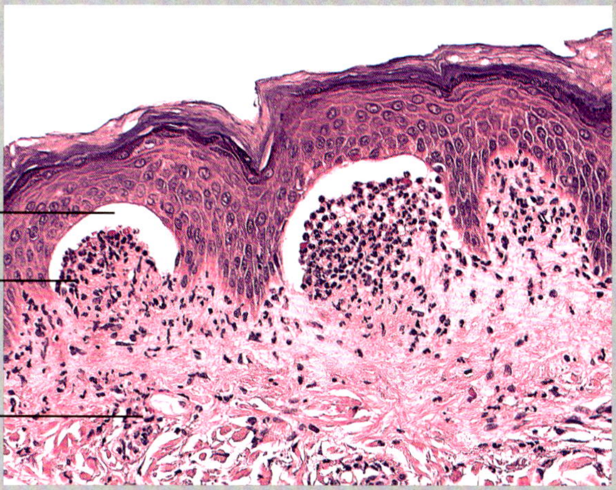

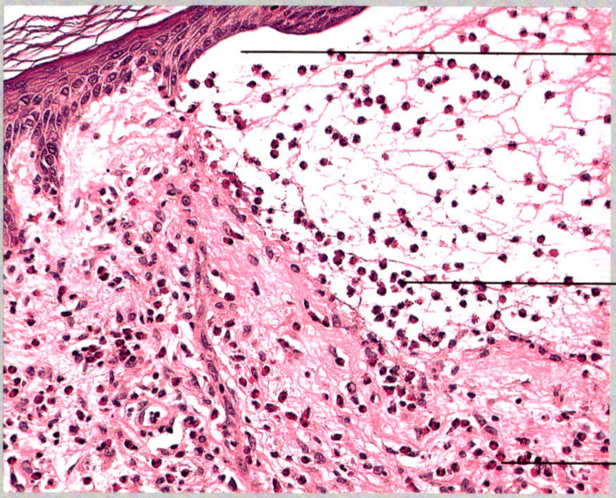

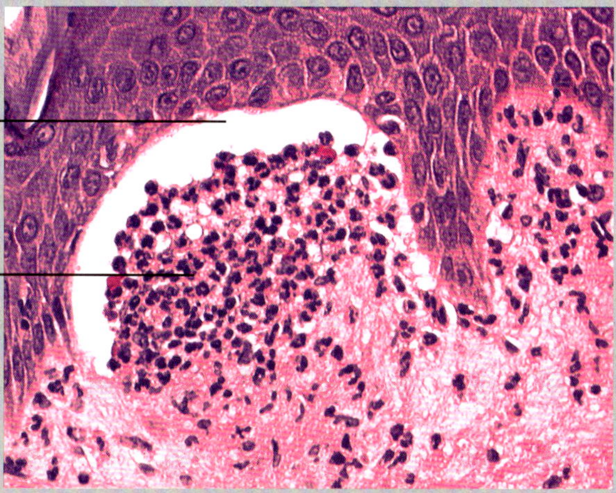

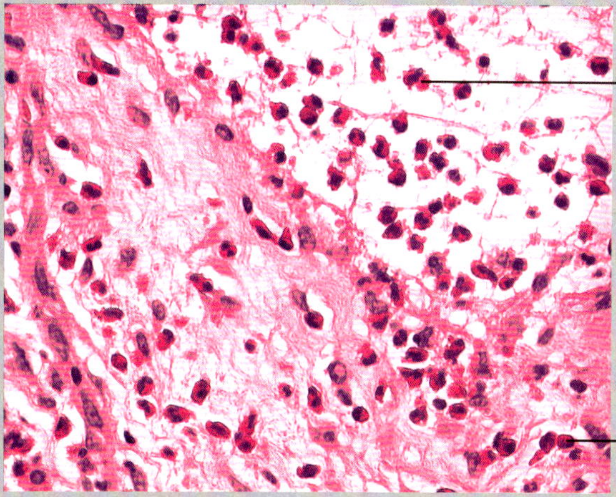

DERMATITIS herpetiformis and bullous pemphigoid share several features, namely, subepidermal vesiculation, fibrin in subepidermal spaces, and a mixture of inflammatory cells, among them some neutrophils and eosinophils.

The histopathologic changes enumerated at the outset of this chapter occur in the earliest blisters of dermatitis herpetiformis and the cell-rich type of pemphigoid. A less common cell-poor type of pemphigoid is typified by a sparse infiltrate of inflammatory cells but, in other respects, resembles pemphigoid as described here.

As in all inflammatory diseases of the skin, pathologic changes in dermatitis herpetiformis (a disease that begins in young adults usually) unfold over time. Early edematous erythematous papules evolve into papulovesicles that become discrete vesicles. Rarely is there progression to bullae. Erosions and ulcerations are common features in dermatitis herpetiformis, typically as a consequence of excoriations induced by severe pruritus. The lesions of dermatitis herpetiformis commonly involve the scalp and are distributed symmetrically over the scapulae, sacrum, buttocks, and extensor surfaces of the arms and legs. In contrast, bullous pemphigoid (a disease of older persons) begins with widespread edematous erythematous papules and plaques that often have arcuate, annular, and other configurations. Tense vesicles and, eventually, bullae arise on the urticarial bases. Excoriations of the pruritic lesions also result in erosions and ulcerations. Lesions of both dermatitis herpetiformis and pemphigoid resolve with hyperpigmentation.

Early edematous erythematous papules of dermatitis herpetiformis (urticarial stage) show the following histopathologic findings:

1. Discrete vacuolar alteration and subepidermal clefts
2. Neutrophils, including band forms, sprinkled along and beneath the dermo-epidermal junction
3. Variable edema of the papillary dermis
4. Dilation of capillaries in dermal papillae
5. Sparse to moderately dense superficial, mostly perivascular, lymphocytic infiltrate associated with neutrophils.

Early edematous erythematous papules of bullous pemphigoid (urticarial stage) exhibit:

1. Vacuolar alteration and scattered eosinophils along the dermo-epidermal interface
2. Eosinophils, singly and in tiny clusters, within the epidermis where spongiosis is concurrent
3. Prominent edema of the papillary dermis

4. Superficial perivascular and interstitial infiltrate of lymphocytes, eosinophils, and rare neutrophils.

Late vesicular lesions of dermatitis herpetiformis are characterized by:

1. Confluence of tiny subepidermal vesicles
2. Dense collections of neutrophils and eosinophils within dermal papillae
3. Edema of the papillary dermis
4. Moderately dense superficial perivascular mixed-cell infiltrate of lymphocytes, eosinophils, and neutrophils
5. Epidermal necrosis to variable degree.

Late bullous lesions of pemphigoid exhibit:

1. Focal or confluent epidermal necrosis above the blister
2. Superficial and mid-dermal mixed-cell infiltrate of lymphocytes and eosinophils, joined occasionally by neutrophils and plasma cells
3. Marked edema of the papillary dermis.

It may be difficult to differentiate with certainty some late vesicular lesions of bullous pemphigoid from those of dermatitis herpetiformis because both may show subepidermal vesiculation with numerous eosinophils and neutrophils in the upper part of the dermis and necrosis of the epidermis. However, there usually are more neutrophils in dermatitis herpetiformis, especially in collections at the tips of papillae to the sides of the blister. It is advisable, therefore, to perform a biopsy on an early papule or papulovesicle of these diseases and, if only a blister is available, the biopsy specimen should include it and the skin immediately contiguous to it.

The histopathologic changes in dermatitis herpetiformis are similar, if not identical, to those of linear IgA bullous dermatosis. Dermatitis herpetiformis also must be differentiated histopathologically from bullous systemic lupus erythematosus (in which abundant mucin is found frequently in the reticular dermis), cicatricial pemphigoid (in which fibrosis often is present at a site where blisters have recurred), and rare drug eruptions that may simulate it. The histopathologic changes in bullous pemphigoid are identical to those of herpes gestationis.

6. Erythema Multiforme *vs.* Pityriasis Lichenoides et Varioliformis Acuta (Mucha-Habermann Disease)

Erythema Multiforme	*Pityriasis Lichenoides et Varioliformis Acuta*
1. In early lesions, basket-weave pattern of the cornified layer; in later lesions, slight parakeratosis	1. In early lesions, focal or confluent parakeratosis within which are neutrophils; in later lesions, scale-crusts
2. Epidermis not hyperplastic	2. Epidermis hyperplastic occasionally
3. In early lesions, many necrotic keratinocytes scattered as solitary units in the epidermis	3. In early lesions, few necrotic keratinocytes scattered in the epidermis
4. In late lesions, confluent necrosis throughout the entire thickness of the epidermis	4. In late lesions, well-circumscribed wedge-shaped necrosis, especially in the upper half of the epidermis
5. Neutrophils present only in zones of epidermal necrosis	5. Neutrophils in zones of epidermal necrosis, in parakeratosis, and scale-crusts
6. Vesiculation common	6. Vesiculation uncommon
7. Subepidermal vesiculation more common	7. Intra-epidermal vesiculation more common
8. Few extravasated erythrocytes in the papillary dermis	8. Many extravasated erythrocytes in the papillary dermis and often within the epidermis
9. Sparse infiltrate of lymphocytes and vacuolar alteration obscure the dermo-epidermal junction	9. Moderately dense infiltrate of lymphocytes and vacuolar alteration obscure the dermo-epidermal junction
10. No lichenoid infiltrate of lymphocytes in the papillary dermis	10. Lichenoid infiltrate of lymphocytes in the papillary dermis often
11. Sparse to moderately dense superficial perivascular lymphocytic infiltrate	11. Moderately dense superficial and deep (sometimes only superficial) perivascular and interstitial lymphocytic infiltrate, often in V-shape

Erythema Multiforme

Pityriasis Lichenoides et Varioliformis Acuta (Mucha-Habermann Disease)

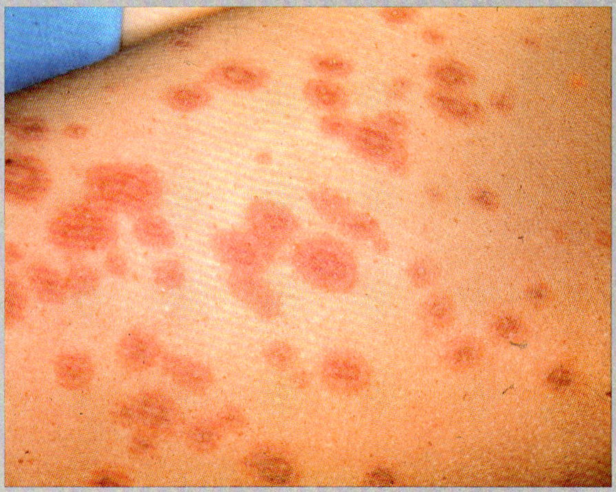

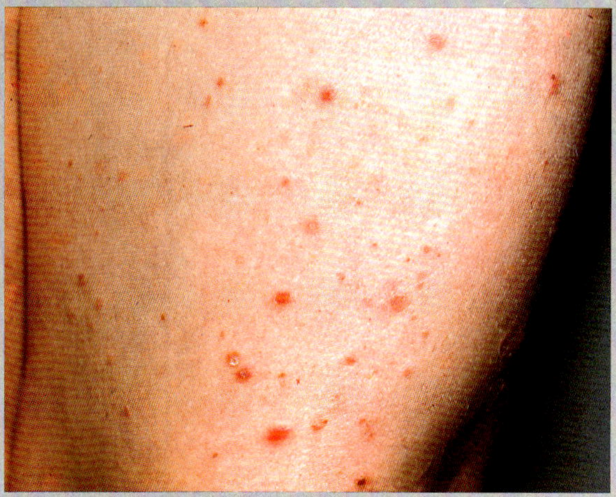

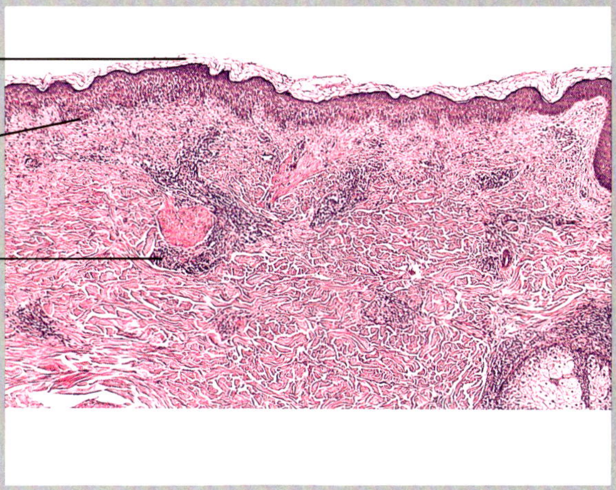

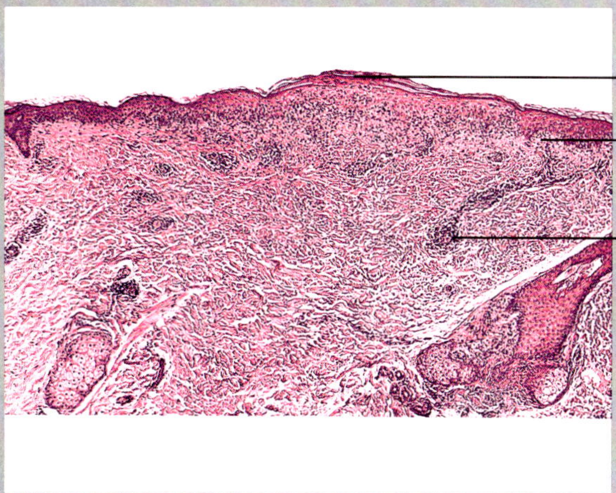

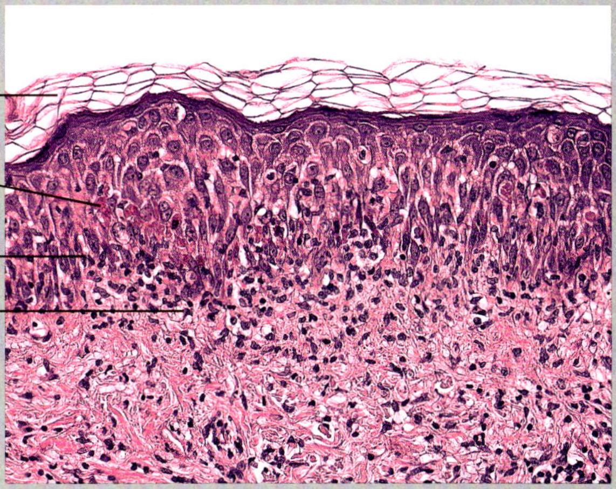

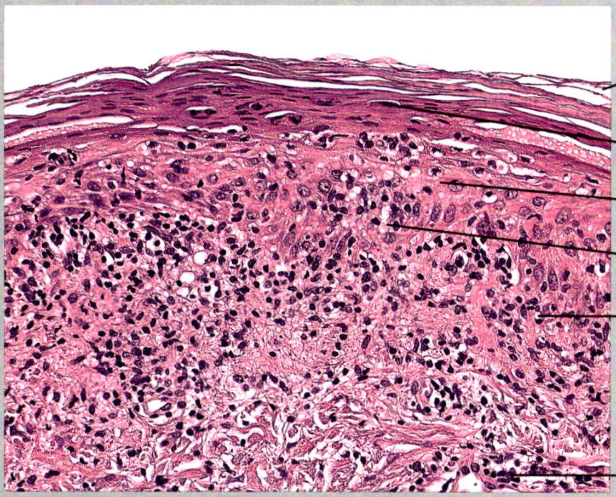

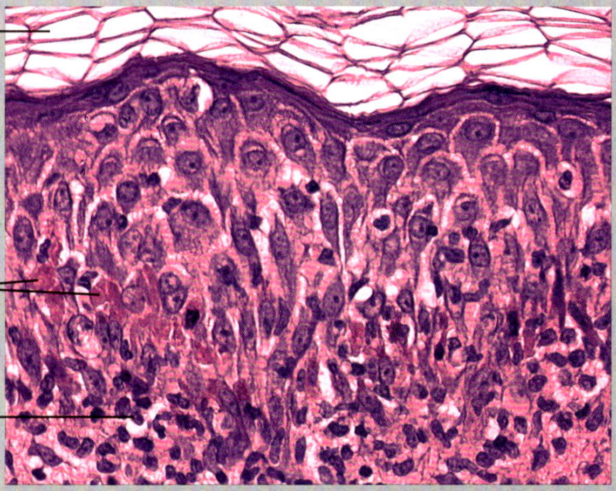

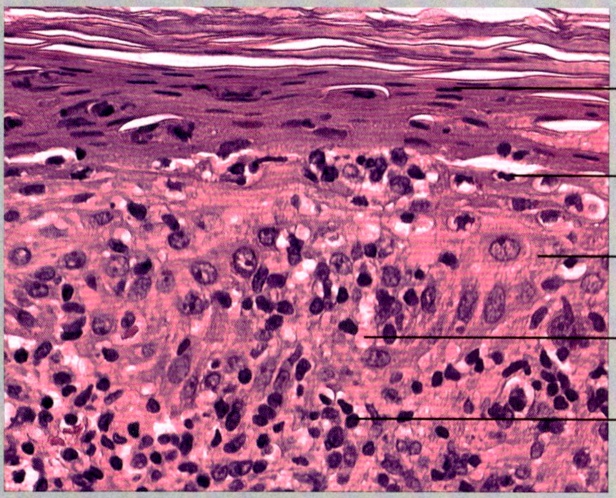

It may be difficult or impossible to differentiate the histopathologic changes in the lower portion of the epidermis and at the dermo-epidermal interface of erythema multiforme from those of Mucha-Habermann disease. In both diseases there may be intra- and intercellular edema, necrotic keratinocytes arranged as solitary units, and vacuolar alteration and a sprinkling of lymphocytes along the dermo-epidermal junction. In most instances, however, the differential features just outlined enable a histopathologist to render a specific and precise diagnosis.

The early clinical lesions of erythema multiforme are edematous papules that soon become slightly purpuric plaques upon which blisters form. When a papule or plaque is ring-shaped with a central purpuric punctum, the lesion is termed an iris (after Iris, the Greek goddess of the rainbow for whom the structure of the eye also was named), and when concentric rings develop, the lesion is called a target (after a marksman's target). The lesions of erythema multiforme have a predilection for acral parts of the skin and for mucous membranes.

The blisters of erythema multiforme may develop beneath the epidermis, in part as a consequence of extensive vacuolar alteration, or within the epidermis secondary to spongiosis and to marked ballooning. Intra- and subepidermal blisters may be present together in the same section. The gray color of the roof of a blister reflects confluent necrosis of epidermal keratinocytes.

A cause for erythema multiforme cannot be determined with certainty in most cases; drugs and infectious agents (viruses, bacteria, and mycoplasmata) have been implicated. The most common association is with infection by herpesvirus, both types of lesions recurring together, the viral ones coming first. Erythema multiforme usually is short-lived, waning without treatment and vanishing completely in a few weeks, or less if systemic corticosteroids are administered in sufficiently high dosage.

The histopathologic differential diagnosis of erythema multiforme, besides Mucha-Habermann disease, includes fixed drug eruption and graft-vs.-host reaction during the acute phase of those diseases. Those processes may have epidermal features indistinguishable from those of erythema multiforme. Fixed drug eruption, however, unlike erythema multiforme, usually shows mixed-cell infiltrates composed of many eosinophils and neutrophils, as well as of lymphocytes, and the infiltrate is deep as well as superficial, interstitial as well as perivascular. Some acute graft-vs.-host reactions are accompanied by lesions in the skin that closely resemble those of erythema multiforme histopathologically. The features that help to differentiate them from erythema multiforme are absence of ballooning and confluent necrosis and presence of an abnormal usually parakeratotic, cornified layer and nuclear atypica of keratinocytes in graft-vs.-host reactions.

Although a very few eosinophils may be spied episodically in lesions of erythema multiforme, for practical purposes they are irrelevant to diagnosis and differential diagnosis of it. Eosinophils are practically never spotted in Mucha-Habermann disease.

Clinically, Mucha-Habermann disease is a remarkably polymorphous eruption of widespread small lesions with no propensity for acral parts or mucous membranes. The lesions are papules surmounted by brawny scales (pityriasis), flat-topped (lichenoid) papules, purpuric, necrotic, and ulcerated papules, vesicles, and scars (varioliformis). The disease tends to occur in adolescents and young adults, but may erupt at any age, to have a protracted course that usually lasts for months, and to respond poorly, if at all, to treatment. The purpuric, vesicular, necrotic, and ulcerated lesions of Mucha-Habermann disease sometimes are misinterpreted clinically as representing vasculitis, but true vasculitis hardly ever is seen histopathologically in those lesions. Mucha-Habermann disease is not related in any way to lymphomatoid papulosis.

Erythema multiforme and Mucha-Habermann disease involve both the dermis and the epidermis throughout the entire course of their lesions. Just as there is no "epidermal type" and "dermal type" of Mucha-Habermann disease, so, too, there is no authentic subdivision in that fashion of erythema multiforme. All lesions of erythema multiforme, at all stages of their evolution and devolution, involve both the epidermis and the dermis.

7. Staphylococcal Scalded Skin Syndrome *vs.* Toxic Epidermal Necrolysis

Staphylococcal Scalded Skin Syndrome	*Toxic Epidermal Necrolysis*
1. Intra-epidermal blister (situated approximately in the granular zone or upper part of the spinous zone)	1. Subepidermal blister
2. Subcorneal pustules common	2. No subcorneal pustules
3. No notable number of necrotic epidermal cells	3. Necrotic keratinocytes scattered individually along the dermo-epidermal interface and throughout the epidermis in early lesions; confluent necrosis of epidermis in later lesions
4. Acantholytic cells within the blister usually	4. No acantholytic cells
5. Moderately dense superficial perivascular mixed-cell infiltrate that contains neutrophils	5. Scant superficial perivascular lymphocytic infiltrate that is devoid of neutrophils usually

Staphyloccal Scalded Skin Syndrome

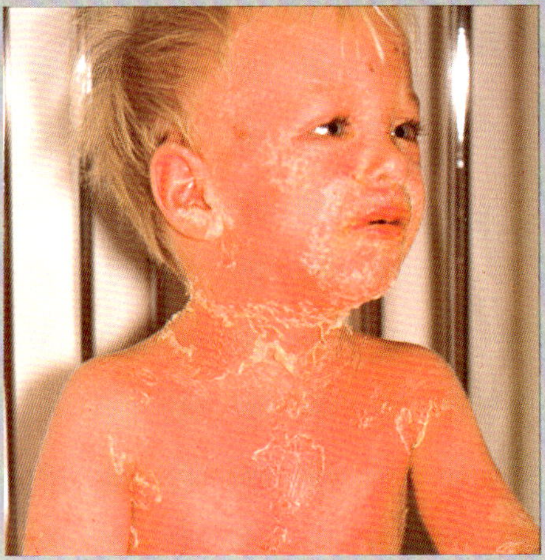

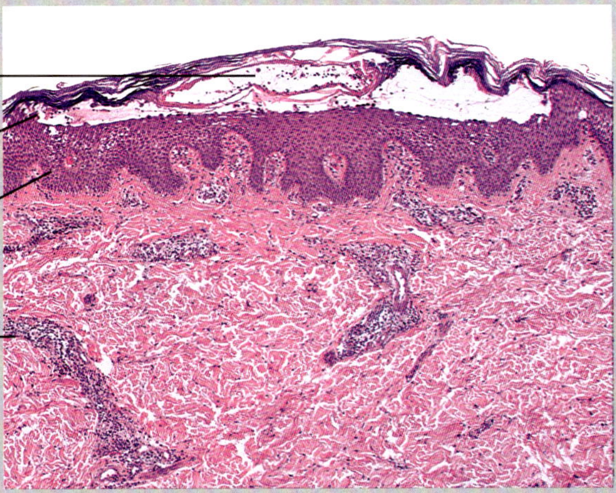

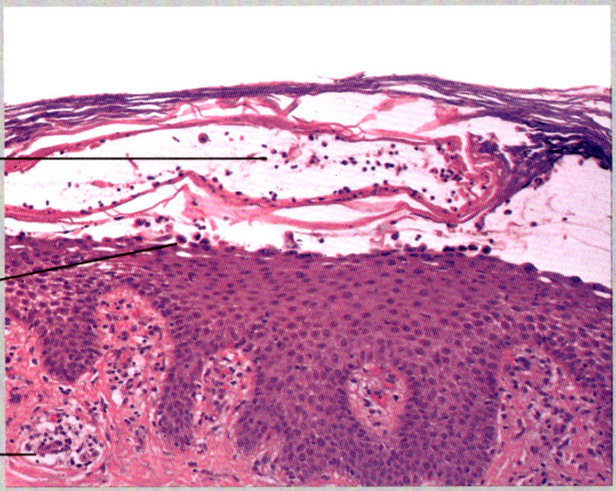

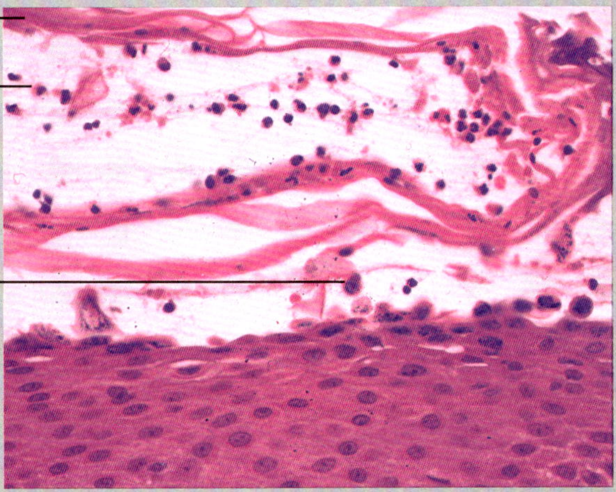

Toxic Epidermal Necrolysis (Severe Widespread Erythema Multiforme)

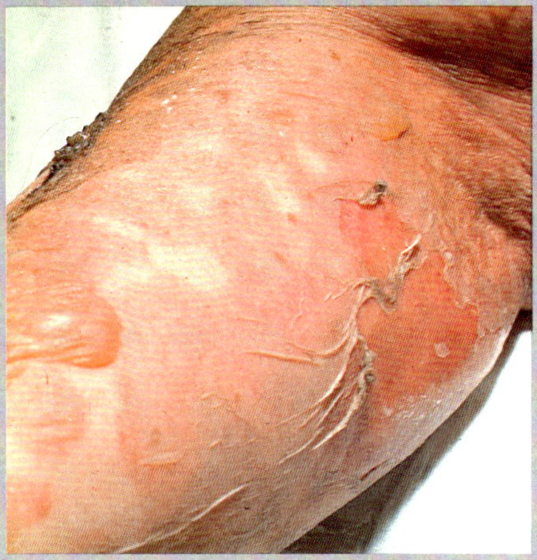

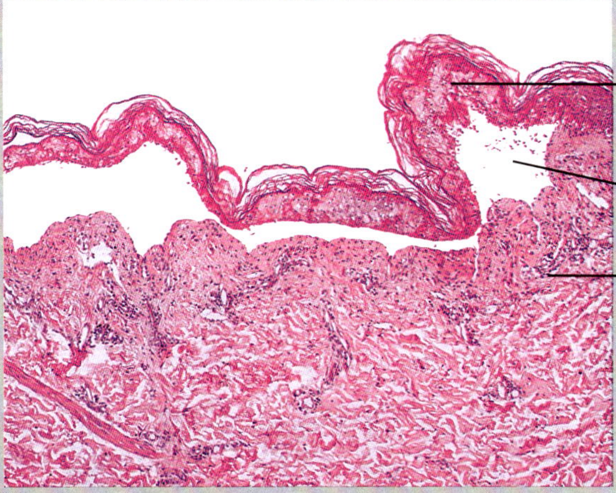

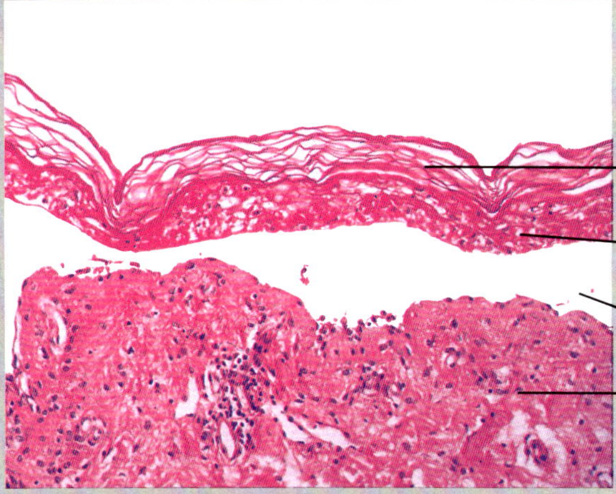

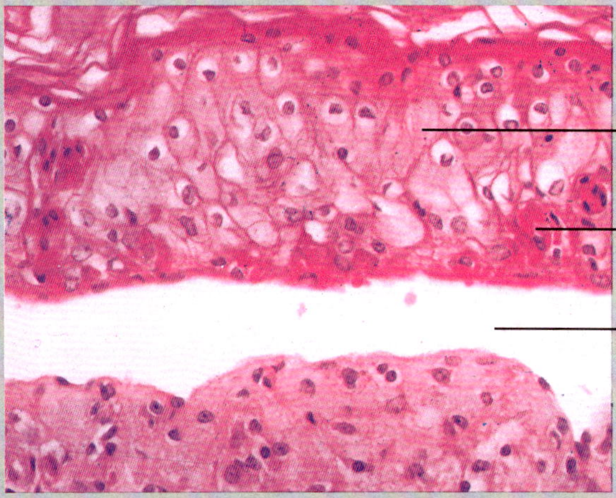

Toxic epidermal necrolysis and staphylococcal scalded skin syndrome are blistering dermatitides that, in the past, were considered to be one disease because they both resemble scalded skin clinically. In fact, they are completely different diseases histolopathologically, biologically, causally, and in response to therapy. Pemphigus vulgaris and extensive thermal burns at times may resemble scalded skin clinically, but each of them, like staphylococcal scalded skin syndrome, is a distinctive pathologic process, unrelated to one another.

We use the term "toxic epidermal necrolysis" here to refer strictly and specifically to a widespread subepidermal blistering expression of erythema multiforme that afflicts adults (children rarely) and, in most instances, is idiopathic, although on occasion it seems to be connected circumstantially to administration of drugs or exposure to chemicals. An example of the latter is inhalation of fumes, such as fumigants. Staphylococci cannot be cultured from the blisters or from the surrounding skin. Clinically, toxic epidermal necrolysis is characterized by sudden appearance of areas of redness and tenderness that evolve into large flaccid bullae. Mucous membranes often are affected, too. Nikolsky's sign, i.e., induction of a lesion by firm oblique pressure against apparently normal skin, is elicitable readily. Because the blisters develop at the dermo-epidermal junction and are huge, excessive loss of fluids and electrolytes is a serious complication, as it is in severe burns. Indeed, toxic epidermal necrolysis should be managed like an extensive burn. Even with meticulous treatment and administration of large doses of corticosteroids systemically, mortality from the disease is about 25%.

Toxic epidermal necrolysis, as just described, is a severe widespread expression of erythema multiforme, with which it has in common, in addition to blisters, several clinical features ("iris" and "target" lesions in the skin of some patients and involvement of mucous membranes) and many histopathologic characteristics (superficial perivascular lymphocytic infiltrate, vacuolar alteration along with dermo-epidermal junction, and necrotic epidermal and adnexal keratinocytes). Lyell, who introduced the term "toxic epidermal necrolysis," initially grouped staphylococcal scalded skin syndrome of children and severe widespread erythema multiforme in adults together under that formidable title. Toxic epidermal necrolysis, as Lyell employed it, is not a specific disease, but an umbrella for two entirely different diseases, namely, the staphylococcal scalded skin syndrome and a severe, often fatal, widespread form of erythema multiforme. For that reason, the term "toxic epidermal necrolysis" is antiquated and confusing, just as is

"Stevens-Johnson syndrome," which is simply a severe, often fatal, widespread expression of erythema multiforme in children.

In contrast to severe widespread erythema multiforme, the staphylococcal scalded skin syndrome is a specific intra-epidermal blistering disease that mainly affects children (adults rarely) and is caused, in every instance, by an epidermolytic toxin produced by a virally lysogenized staphylococcus. The presence of acantholytic cells in a blister high within the epidermis imparts to this condition histopathologic similarities to bullous impetigo and superficial forms of pemphigus (foliaceus, erythematosus, and fogo selvagem). Unlike bullous impetigo, in which staphylococci are culturable readily from blister fluid, no bacteria can be cultured from blisters of staphylococcal scalded skin syndrome; a toxin produced by the bacteria does the damage.

The staphylococcal scalded skin syndrome evolves clinically in a sequence that begins with erythematous macules on the face and neck and in the axillae and groin, progresses to extensive formation of bullae, and eventuates in "potato-chip" exfoliation. During the blistering phase, the Nikolsky sign may be elicited with ease. Unlike severe widespread erythema multiforme, the prognosis is very good; the condition responds promptly and completely to specific antibiotics.

In conclusion, because the term "toxic epidermal necrolysis" means different things to different dermatologists, pathologists, and pediatricians, it is preferable to avoid the term completely and to refer directly to either staphylococcal scalded skin syndrome or severe widespread erythema multiforme.

8. Pemphigus Vulgaris *vs.* Benign Familial Chronic Pemphigus (Hailey-Hailey Disease)

Pemphigus Vulgaris	*Benign Familial Chronic Pemphigus (Hailey-Hailey Disease)*
1. Epidermis mostly intact above a suprabasal separation	1. Epidermis altered markedly by acantholysis above a suprabasal separation
2. Few acantholytic cells above the suprabasal separation	2. Many acantholytic cells above the suprabasal separation
3. Acantholytic cells limited to a zone immediately above the basal layer	3. Acantholytic cells present at least throughout the lower half of the epidermis in some rete ridges, sometimes in the upper half
4. No notable changes in the stratum corneum	4. Stratum corneum often altered by ortho- and parakeratosis, crusts, and scale-crusts
5. Epidermal hyperplasia rare	5. Epidermal hyperplasia usual
6. Suprabasal separation usually confluent within a 4-mm punch biopsy specimen	6. Multiple, discrete foci of suprabasal separation within a 4-mm punch biopsy specimen usually
7. Epithelium of adnexa affected commonly by suprabasal separation and acantholytic cells	7. Epithelium of adnexa not affected by suprabasal separation and acantholytic cells as a rule
8. Acantholytic cells associated almost always with suprabasal separation	8. Acantholytic cells sometimes discernible in the absence of suprabasal separation
9. No dyskeratotic cells within the epidermis	9. Many dyskeratotic cells with pyknotic nuclei and eosinophilic cytoplasm within the epidermis of fully developed lesions
10. No mitotic figures above the basal layer	10. Mitotic figures above the basal layer commonly
11. Eosinophils may be present in addition to lymphocytes in the dermal infiltrate	11. Neutrophils may be present in addition to lymphocytes in the dermal infiltrate

Pemphigus Vulgaris

Benign Familial Chronic Pemphigus (Hailey-Hailey Disease)

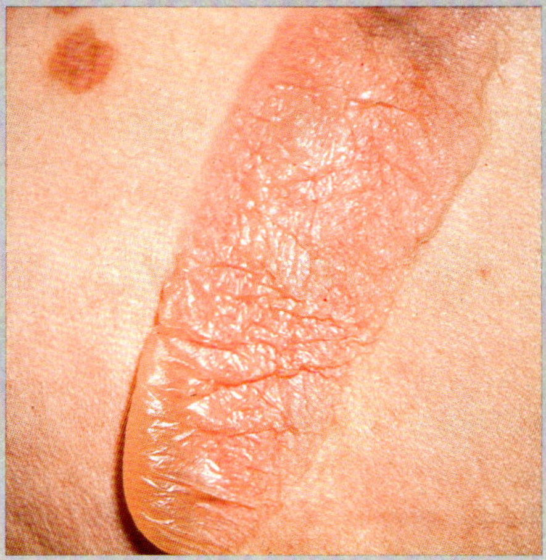

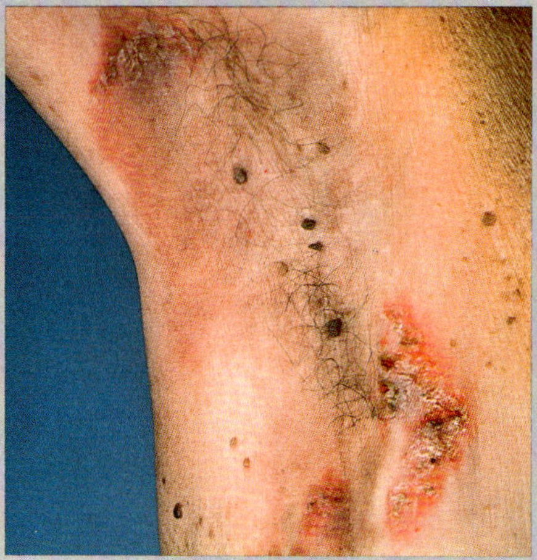

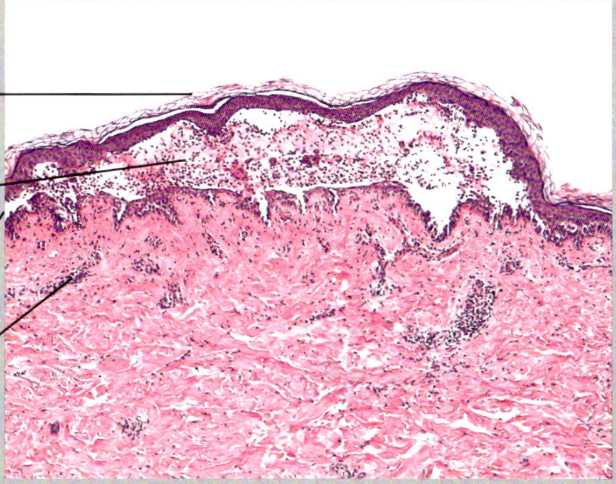

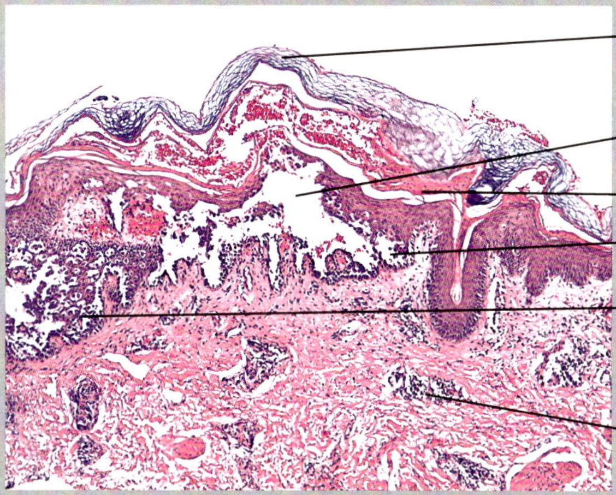

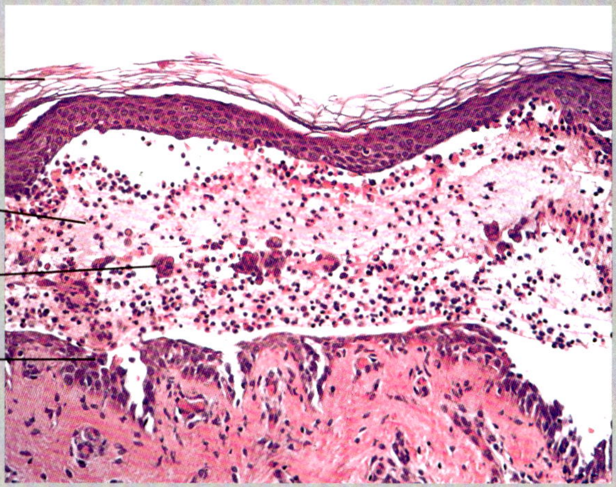

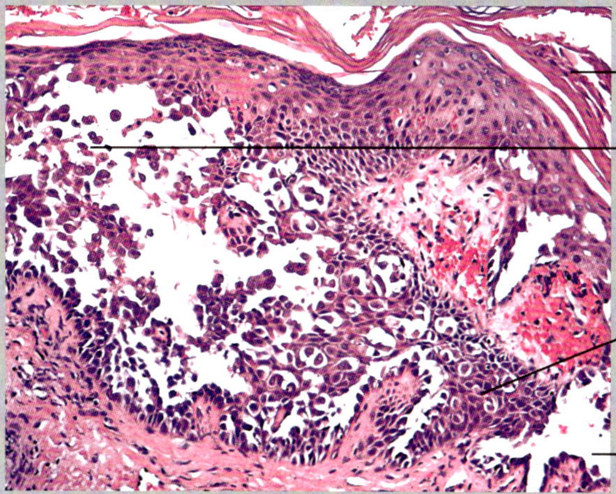

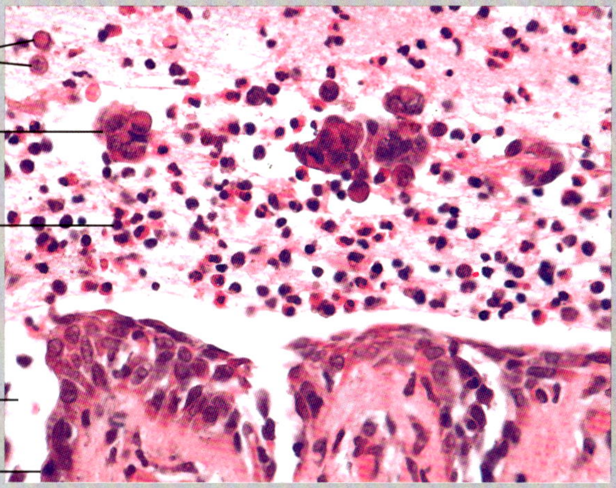

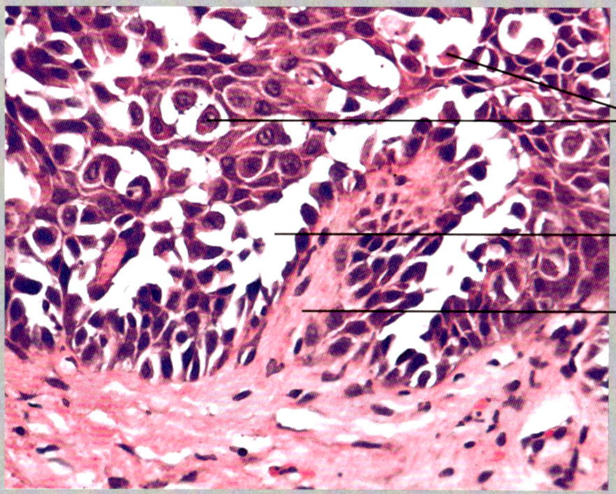

PEMPHIGUS vulgaris and benign familial chronic pemphigus are both acantholytic vesiculo-bullous dermatitides that in some instances may be impossible to differentiate from each other histopathologically. This is especially true of very early lesions in which there are only a few acantholytic cells within an epidermis otherwise apparently normal, except for just a hint of suprabasal separation and subtle vacuoles between suprabasal spinous cells. In these difficult cases, deeper sections through the specimen may reveal a focus of acantholytic cells that extends throughout much of the epidermis and that serves as a clue to the diagnosis of Hailey-Hailey disease. Such acantholytic changes may be confined to a single rete ridge. Deeper sections might show that epithelia of adnexa are involved prominently by the acantholytic process, a finding that favors a diagnosis of pemphigus vulgaris. Unfortunately, neither extensive involvement of rete ridges nor involvement of adnexal epithelium alone is decisive for diagnosis.

Typical clinical lesions of pemphigus vulgaris are flaccid bullae that arise on normal-appearing skin and mucous membranes. The blisters eventually break and leave a weeping base that on histopathologic examination is covered by only a single layer of basal cells. The blisters of pemphigus vulgaris may be broadened markedly by downward pressure upon them, and fresh blisters often may be induced by firm, oblique pressure upon apparently normal skin (Nikolsky's sign). Uncomplicated lesions of pemphigus vulgaris heal without scarring because the blistering process is wholly intra-epidermal.

The blisters of Hailey-Hailey disease vary from smooth-surfaced, flaccid vesicles and bullae to vesiculopustules, vegetating plaques, or grayish zones of maceration. They occur predilectively in intertriginous regions and only rarely on mucosae. Scarring does not result unless complications supravene. A familial history of the condition can be elicited commonly.

Immunofluorescent studies, both direct and indirect, reveal intercellular deposits of antibodies and complement in most specimens of pemphigus vulgaris, but not in those of Hailey-Hailey disease.

Pemphigus vulgaris-like changes in the epidermis may be induced by penicillamine and, rarely, by other drugs. Histopathologic features of pemphigus vulgaris also may be encountered, along with features of superficial pemphigus, in some biopsy specimens from patients with pemphigus foliaceus, pemphigus erythematosus, and fogo selvagem. Foci like those of pemphigus vulgaris are characteristic of one variant of transient acantholytic dermatosis (Grover's disease). Pemphigus vulgaris-like changes also may occur in the epidermis of severely anoxic limbs, particularly gangrenous ones. Powerful chemicals, such as cantharidin and sodium hydroxide, induce changes similar to those in pemphigus vulgaris but, in the instance of caustics, the acantholytic cells are elongated rather than round. Last, discrete foci with histopathologic features like those of pemphigus vulgaris may be found, as an incidental finding, confined to one or a few epidermal rete ridges, analogous to isolated foci of acantholytic dyskeratosis, epidermolytic hyperkeratosis, cornoid lamellation, and pale-cell acanthosis, distinctive patterns of cutaneous epithelium all.

In the years following the original description of benign familial chronic pemphigus by the brothers Hailey, many pathologists considered the condition to be indistinguishable histopathologically from keratosis follicularis (Darier's disease). In fact, they are entirely different diseases. Darier's disease is not a blistering disease; vesicles and bullae are not seen on clinical inspection, and plasma is not seen in clefts within the epidermis on histopathologic examination. Furthermore, Darier's disease differs histopathologically from Hailey-Hailey disease by having changes that are more focal, parakeratosis that is more prominent, and dyskeratosis that is more extensive in the granular and cornified layers.

In sum, the vast majority of biospy specimens of pemphigus vulgaris can be differentiated from those of Hailey-Hailey disease if the histopathologic criteria set forth in this chapter are applied scrupulously. It can be stated with equal conviction, however, that some specimens thought to fulfill criteria for Hailey-Hailey disease will prove to have come from a patient with indubitable pemphigus vulgaris, and vice versa.

9. Keratosis Follicularis (Darier's Disease) *vs.* Transient Acantholytic Dermatosis (Grover's Disease)

Keratosis Follicularis (Darier's Disease)	*Transient Acantholytic Dermatosis (Grover's Disease)*
1. No evidence of excoriation usually	1. Erosions, ulcerations, and scale-crusts, i.e., evidences of excoriation, present often
2. Focal parakeratosis in vertical columns	2. Little parakeratosis as a rule (except in the purely Darier type) and that little is not usually in distinct columns
3. Intra-epidermal clefts; no vesicles	3. Intra-epidermal vesicles as well as clefts
4. No spongiosis	4. Spongiosis and acantholysis in the same focus (spongiotic-acantholytic type of Grover's disease) sometimes
5. Features of focal acantholytic dyskeratosis are the sole manifestations	5. Features sometimes of pemphigus (superficial and deep types), familial benign chronic pemphigus (Hailey-Hailey disease), spongiosis with acantholysis, and focal acantholytic dyskeratosis in the same biopsy specimen
6. Several foci of acantholytic cells and dyskeratotic cells per 4-mm specimen usually	6. Only one or two foci of acantholytic cells and dyskeratotic cells per 4-mm specimen usually
7. Clefts and acantholytic cells obvious in most instances	7. Clefts and acantholytic cells exceedingly subtle often
8. No edema of the papillary dermis	8. Edema of the papillary dermis sometimes
9. No eosinophils in the dermis	9. Eosinophils in the upper part of the dermis often

Keratosis Follicularis (Darier's Disease)

Transient Acantholytic Dermatosis (Grover's Disease)

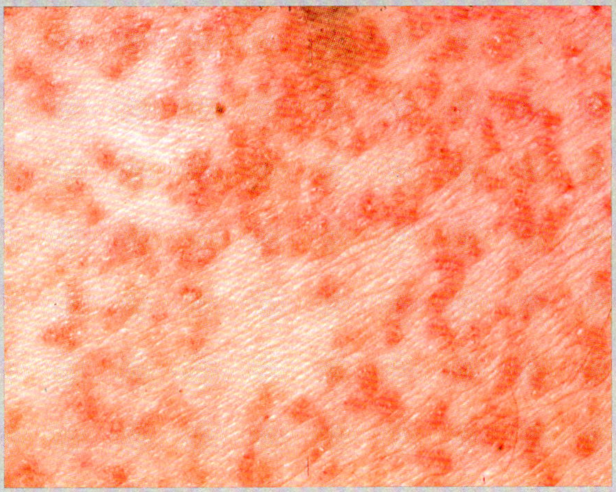

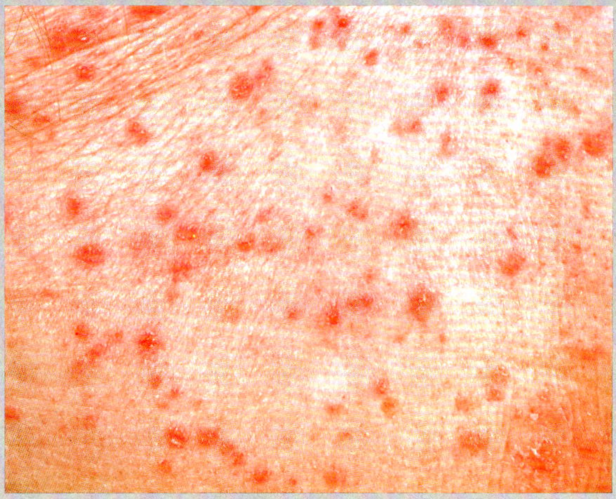

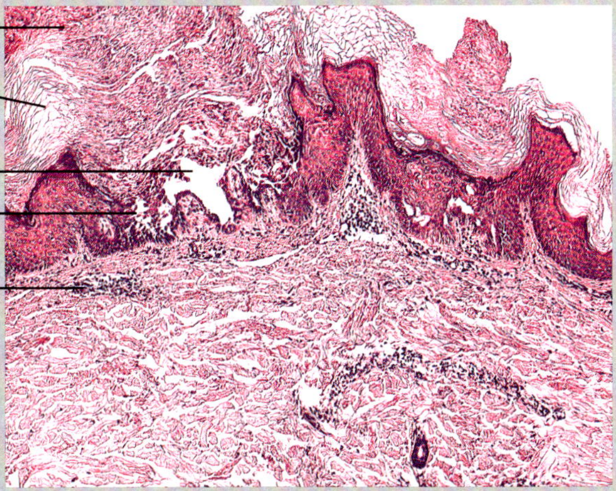

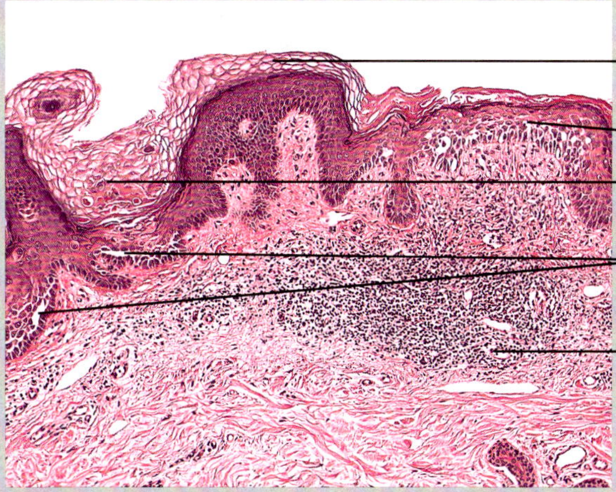

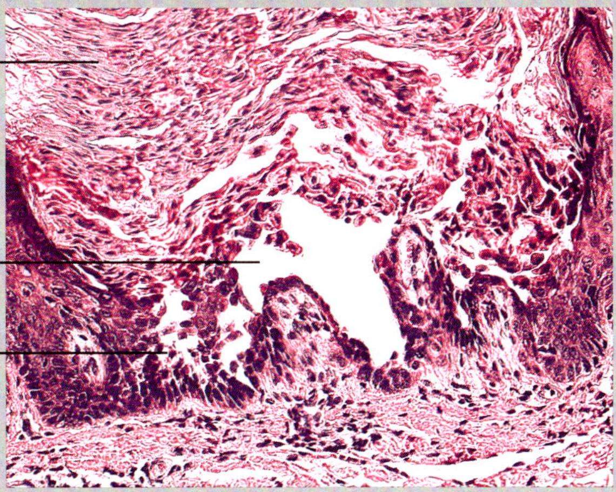

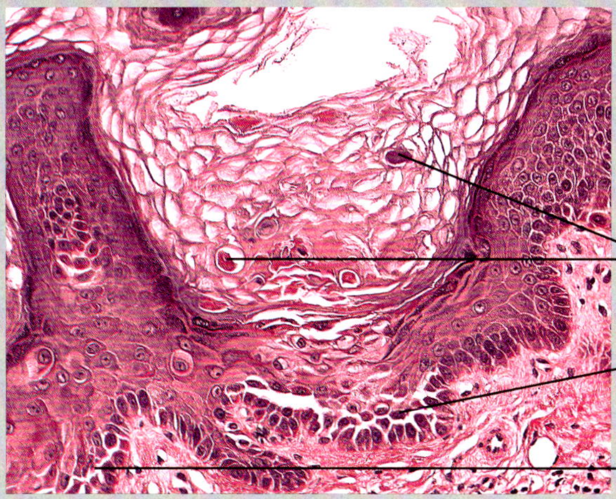

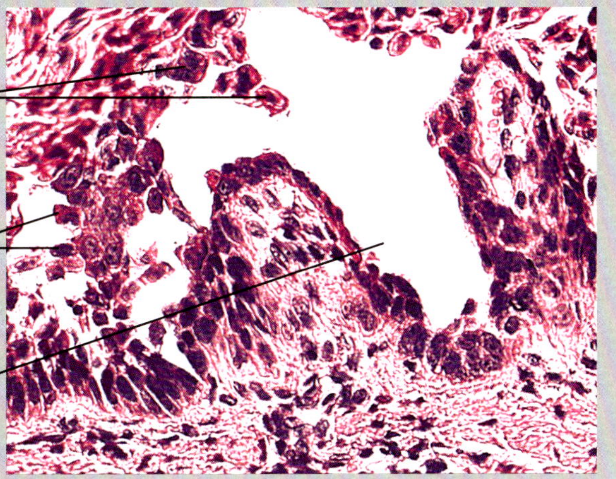

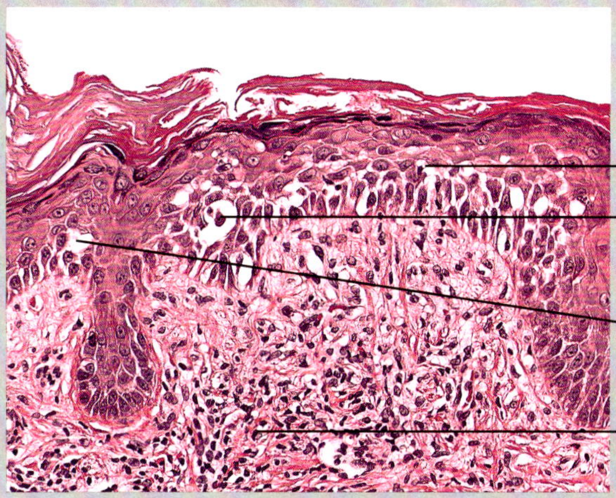

DARIER'S disease and Grover's disease have several histopathologic features in common, among them foci of acantholytic cells and dyskeratotic cells within the epidermis, and a superficial perivascular infiltrate of inflammatory cells within the dermis. One variant of Grover's disease may be indistinguishable histopathologically from Darier's disease and, for that reason, it is termed the Darier variant of Grover's disease.

Keratosis follicularis (Darier's disease) is a genodermatosis inherited in autosomal-dominant fashion. The lesions usually appear during the second decade of life as widespread, rough-surfaced, dirty brown, keratotic papules. On the skin there is some predilection of Darier's disease for "seborrheic areas" and extensor surfaces, but the disease also may affect mucous membranes and nail units. Darier's disease does not exhibit vesicles clinically or histopathologically. The condition generally waxes and wanes throughout life. Prior to the use of retinoids, Darier's disease usually was refractory to treatment. The term "keratosis follicularis" is a misnomer as a synonym for Darier's disease because the critical histopathologic findings, namely, those of focal acantholytic dyskeratosis, spare follicles rather than involve them.

In contrast to Darier's disease, transient acantholytic dermatosis (Grover's disease) almost always occurs in adults over 40 years of age and especially in those over 60. Except for the type of transient acantholytic dermatosis that resembles Darier's disease in which discrete, gray, small papules are keratotic, lesions of Grover's disease are smooth-surfaced papules and, less often, papulovesicles. They have a predilection for the V of the chest, trunk, flanks, and thighs. There is no involvement of mucous membranes or nail units. The lesions, frequently maddeningly pruritic, are evanescent and the condition ordinarily disappears within weeks or months without treatment. Rarely, it persists for years. Histopathologically, Grover's disease often consists of vesicles, rather than simply clefts like Darier's disease.

In times past, i.e., before the observations of Grover were published under the title "transient acantholytic dermatosis," there were a few reports of evanescent cases of Darier's disease that developed in adults. Almost certainly those represented examples of Grover's disease that resembled Darier's disease in histopathologic features.

The histopathologic constituents of focal acantholytic dyskeratosis are common not only to classic Darier's disease and the variant of Grover's disease that resembles it, but to some epidermal nevi, some solitary keratoses and uncommon infundibular cysts (warty dyskeratomas). These histopathologic findings occur also as an incidental finding confined to a single rete ridge or an infundibulum of a biopsy specimen that was taken for an unrelated pathologic process.

There are five basic histopathologic patterns of acantholysis in Grover's disease. In addition to the variant that resembles Darier's disease, there are forms that simulate superficial pemphigus (i.e., foliaceus and erythematosus), deep pemphigus (i.e., vulgaris), and familial benign chronic pemphigus (Hailey-Hailey disease), and there is the form in which acantholytic cells are accompanied by signs of spongiosis. Acantholytic cells are the histopathologic mark of each of the variants of Grover's disease. In some biopsy specimens, two or more of these patterns may be found concurrently.

Although most biopsy specimens of Grover's disease may be differentiated from Darier's disease if the aforementioned criteria are employed, the Darier-like variant of Grover's disease may be indistinguishable histopathologically from authentic Darier's disease. In such instances, the two diseases usually can be differentiated from one another by the utilization of clinical criteria, namely, age of the patient, duration and distribution of the lesions, and the presence or absence of severe pruritus.

10. Discoid Lupus Erythematosus *vs.* Polymorphous Light Eruption

Discoid Lupus Erythematosus	*Polymorphous Light Eruption*
1. Compact orthokeratosis of epidermis	1. Normal basket-weave cornified layer usually
2. Follicular infundibula plugged by orthokeratotic cells sometimes; acrosyringia less often	2. No plugs of cornified cells in follicular infundibula or acrosyringia
3. Epidermis usually thinned, at least focally; sometimes hyperplastic focally	3. Epidermis not thinned; normal usually
4. No preservation of normal undulating pattern of epidermal rete ridges and dermal papillae	4. Normal pattern of epidermal rete ridges and dermal papillae preserved
5. Necrotic keratinocytes in the epidermis occasionally	5. No necrotic keratinocytes in the epidermis usually
6. No spongiosis and no scale-crusts	6. Spongiosis occasionally and scale-crusts sometimes
7. Vacuolar alteration at the dermo-epidermal junction	7. No vacuolar alteration at the dermo-epidermal junction
8. Basement membrane thickened at the dermo-epidermal junction	8. Basement membrane not thickened
9. Little, if any, edema of the papillary dermis	9. Marked edema of the papillary dermis; when edema is severe, subepidermal vesiculation results
10. Few extravasated erythrocytes	10. Many extravasated erythrocytes when edema is extensive
11. Melanophages and siderophages in the papillary dermis	11. No melanophages and siderophages in the papillary dermis as a rule
12. Stellate fibrocytes, some multinucleated, in the upper part of the dermis	12. No stellate or multinucleated fibrocytes
13. Mucin, in variable amounts, in the reticular dermis often	13. No increased mucin in the dermis
14. Perivascular infiltrate of lymphocytes with peri-adnexal inclination	14. Perivascular lymphocytic infiltrate with no peri-adnexal proclivity

Discoid Lupus Erythematosus, Fully-Developed Lesion

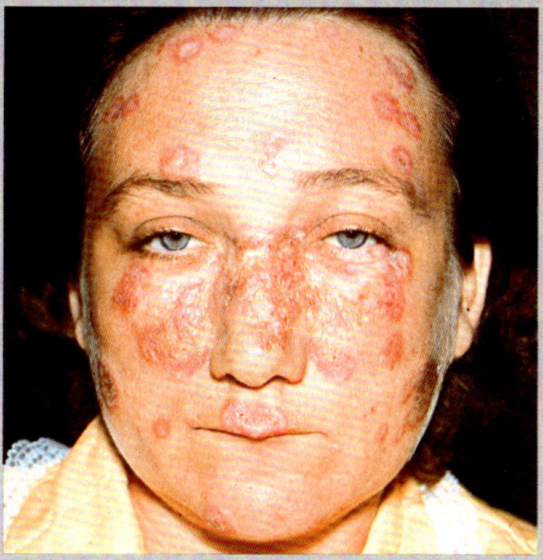

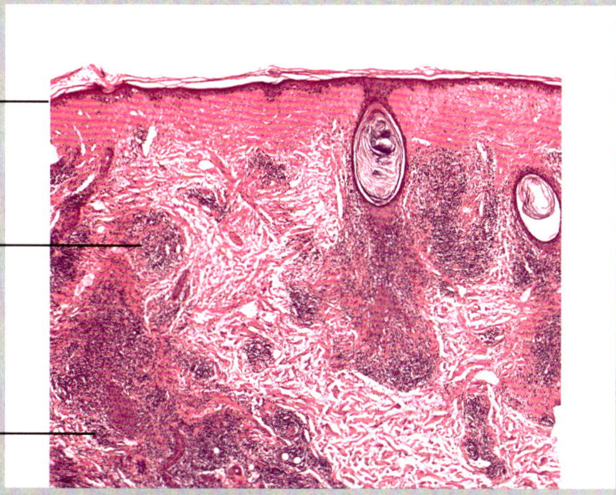

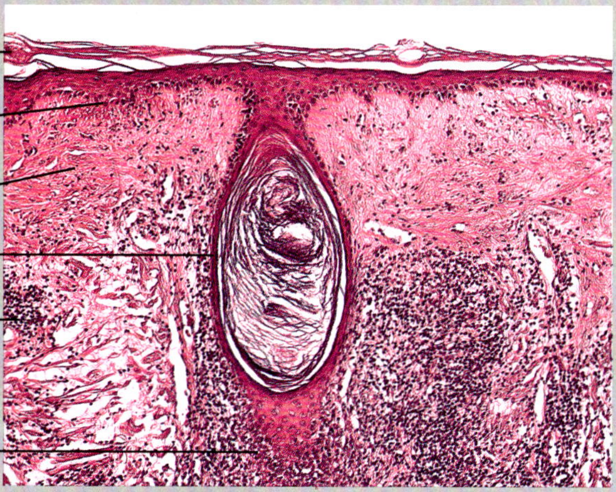

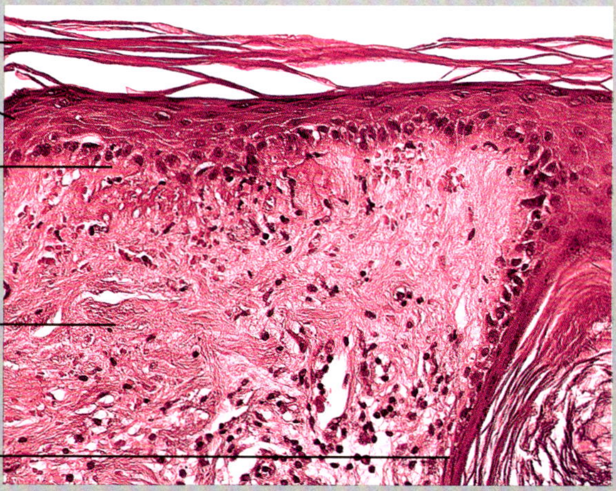

Polymorphous Light Eruption

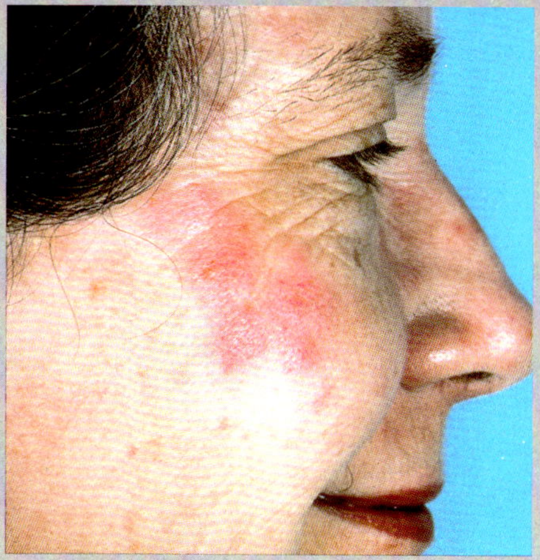

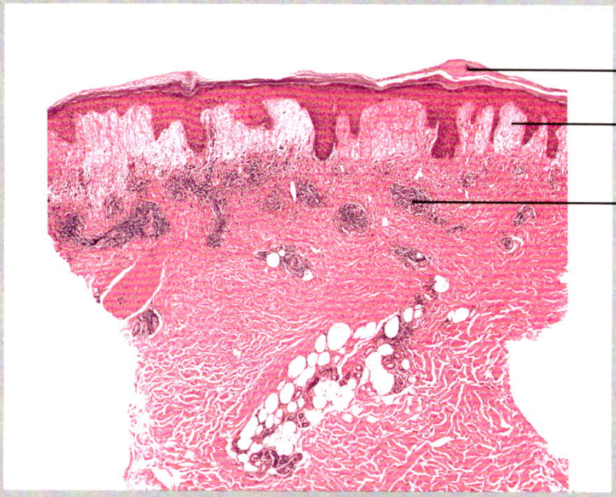

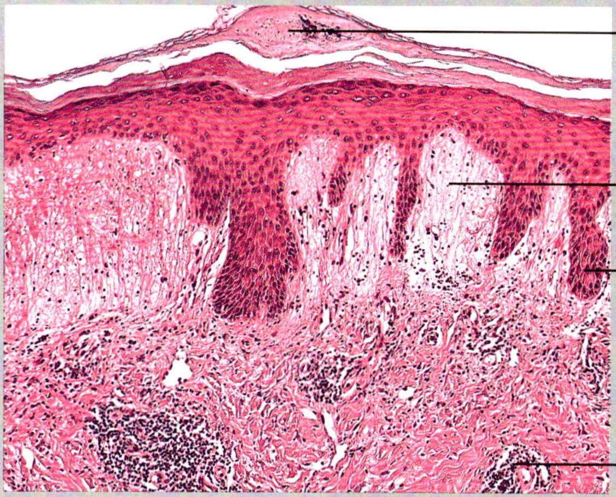

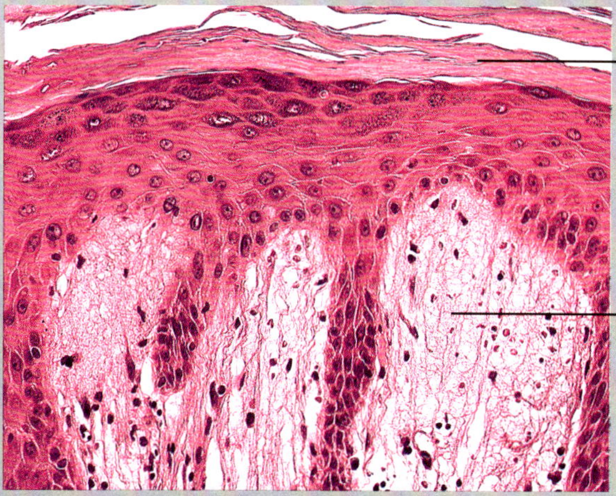

HISTOPATHOLOGICALLY, fully developed lesions of discoid lupus erythematosus and polymorphous light eruption have in common the presence of moderately dense, predominantly lymphocytic infiltrates around blood vessels of the superficial and deep vascular plexuses. Clinically, both diseases occur on sun-exposed parts of the body. In fact, polymorphous light eruption always is induced by sunlight and discoid lupus erythematosus often is.

Discoid lupus erythematosus is a specific skin disease that often proceeds through stages of redness, scaling (including follicular plugs of cornified cells), induration, hyper- and hypopigmentation, atrophy, and telangiectasia. Each of these clinical stages has a histopathologic equivalent. The clinical and histopathologic features of discoid lupus erythematosus are as recognizable as those of psoriasis and lichen planus. However, those distinctive morphologic features of discoid lupus erythematosus, clinically and histopathologically, give no clue to whether a patient affected by it has concurrent disease of internal organs, i.e., systemic lupus erythematosus. As a rule, if lesions of discoid lupus erythematosus are widespread, there is greater likelihood that a patient has or will have systemic lupus erythematosus. Studies for antinuclear antibodies and L.E. preparations are far more reliable indicators of systemic lupus erythematosus than are histopathologic findings. The only skin disease that is utterly specific histopathologically for systemic lupus erythematosus is bullous systemic lupus erythematosus, a subepidermal bullous dermatitis in which neutrophils predominate overwhelmingly.

Lesions of discoid lupus erythematosus may be one manifestation of systemic lupus erythematosus (just as may be leukocytoclastic [allergic] vasculitis, deep ulcers in the vicinity of the internal malleoli, periungual telangiectases, and diffuse alopecia, for example). In most instances, however, patients with discoid lupus erythematosus never develop signs or symptoms of systemic lupus erythematosus. The clinical spectrum of discoid lupus erythematosus ranges from early reddish macules and patches to late forms characterized by atrophic scars. The histopathologic findings along this spectrum parallel the clinical changes. The histopathologic features of fully developed lesions of discoid lupus erythematosus, as noted previously, are a combination of those found in early and late lesions of discoid lupus erythematosus.

At an early stage, sections of discoid lupus erythematosus show:

1. Predominantly lymphocytic infiltrates confined to the upper part of the dermis; a few neutrophils and neutrophilic nuclear "dust" in

dermal papillae; no or few melanophages
2. Dilated venules
3. Edema of the papillary dermis
4. Vacuolar alteration along the dermo-epidermal junction
5. Individual necrotic keratinocytes; confluent necrosis rare
6. Focally thinned epidermis.

There is neither a thickened basement membrane nor dermal sclerosis in early lesions of discoid lupus erythematosus.

Late lesions of discoid lupus erythematosus have the following histopathologic features:

1. Sclerosis in the upper part of the dermis, sometimes obliterating epithelial structures of adnexa (when hair follicles are destroyed, permanent alopecia results)
2. Telangiectases
3. Melanophages in the upper part of the dermis
4. Vacuolar alteration, variable in extent
5. Marked thickening of the basement membrane at the junction between dermis and epidermis, between dermis and adnexal epithelium, and sometimes around telangiectatic superficial blood vessels
6. Relatively sparse lymphocytic infiltrate in the lower and/or upper part of the dermis
7. Epidermal atrophy with occasional atypical keratinocytes (sometimes simulating a solar keratosis).

Abundant acid mucosubstances and dilated follicular infundibula plugged by compact orthokeratosis may be seen in late, as well as in early, lesions of discoid lupus erythematosus.

It may be difficult, even impossible, to differentiate histopathologically between some lesions of discoid lupus erythematosus and dermatomyositis.

Polymorphous light eruption is characterized clinically by edematous, erythematous, smooth-surfaced papules that often coalesce to form plaques on sun-exposed skin, especially of the dorsal surfaces of the arms and hands, and of the face. In rare instances, the edema becomes so severe that vesicles develop. All the lesions of polymorphous light eruption show, upon biopsy, variations on a single histopathologic theme, namely, a superficial and deep perivascular infiltrate of lymphocytes in association with variable degrees of edema in the upper part of the dermis.

The histopathologic differential diagnosis of polymorphous light eruption, in addition to discoid lupus erythematosus, is figurate erythema of the deep type. In some instances the two diseases may be indistinguishable, but if edema is noticeable in the upper part of the dermis, the diagnosis must be polymorphous light eruption.

11. Urticarial Reactions to Arthropod Assaults *vs.* Urticaria

Urticarial Reactions to Arthropod Assaults	*Urticaria*
1. Marked edema of the papillary dermis sometimes	1. Slight edema of the papillary dermis
2. Subepidermal vesicles sometimes secondary to marked edema of the papillary dermis	2. No subepidermal vesiculation
3. Many extravasated erythrocytes in the upper part of the dermis commonly	3. Few extravasated erythrocytes in the upper part of the dermis as a rule
4. Moderately dense superficial and deep, perivascular and interstitial, mixed inflammatory-cell infiltrate; sometimes just superficial	4. Sparse superficial, predominantly interstitial, mixed inflammatory-cell infiltrate; sometimes deep as well as superficial
5. V-shaped infiltrate with the base of the V in the direction of the subcutaneous fat	5. Infiltrate not V-shaped
6. Eosinophils and lymphocytes predominate; no neutrophils usually	6. Neutrophils and eosinophils predominate; some lymphocytes around venules
7. Blood vessels have thick walls and plump endothelial cells often	7. Blood vessels dilated, but not otherwise abnormal
8. Thrombi in capillaries and venules sometimes; in larger vessels of the deep reticular dermis occasionally	8. No signs of vasculitis
9. Perifollicular orientation of dermal infiltrate in the center of a lesion sometimes	9. No perifollicular orientation of dermal infiltrate
10. Infiltrate extends into the subcutaneous fat occasionally	10. Infiltrate confined to the dermis as a rule

Reactions to Arthropod Assaults | *Urticaria*

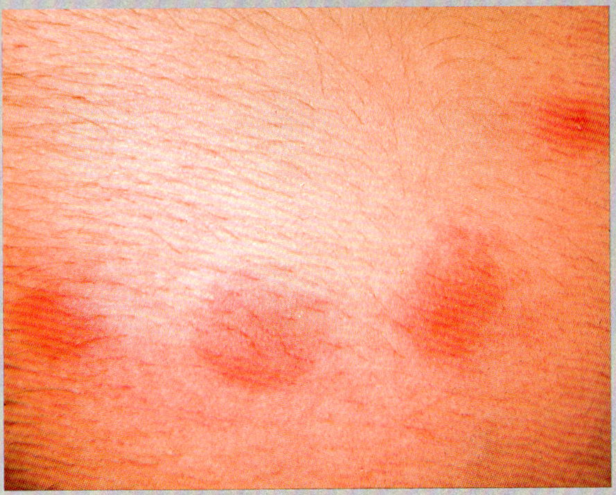

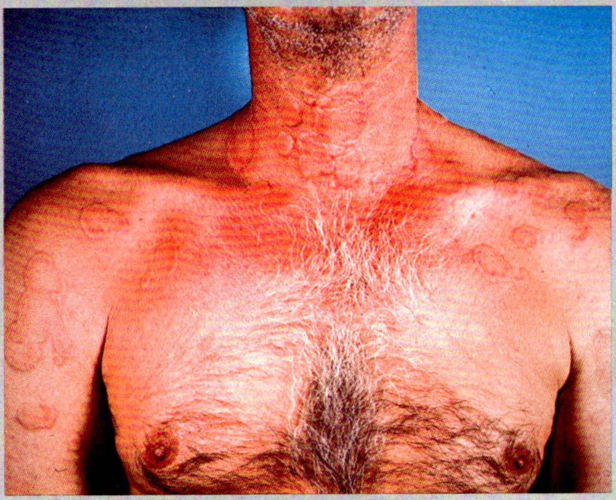

wedge-shaped, moderately dense, superficial and deep perivascular and interstitial infiltrate

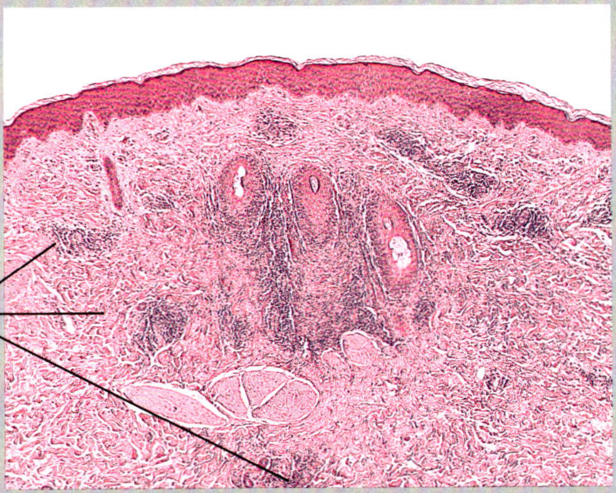

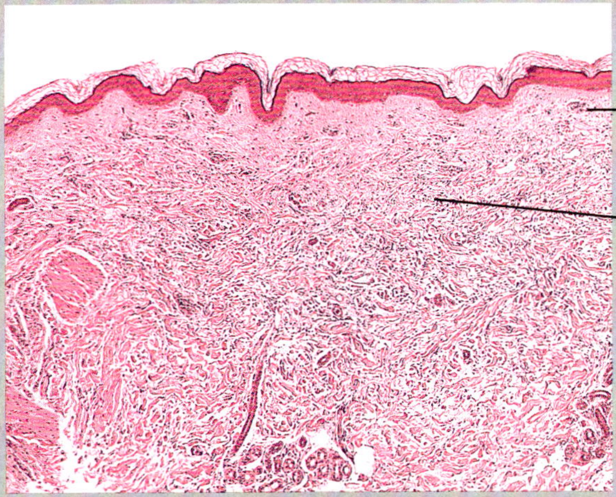

sparse perivascular infiltrate

sparse interstitial infiltrate

lymphocytes and eosinophils around a venule

eosinophil in the interstitium

lymphocytes and eosinophils around a venule

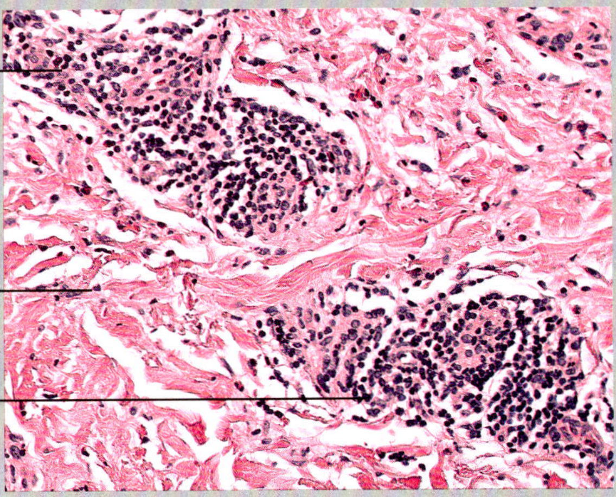

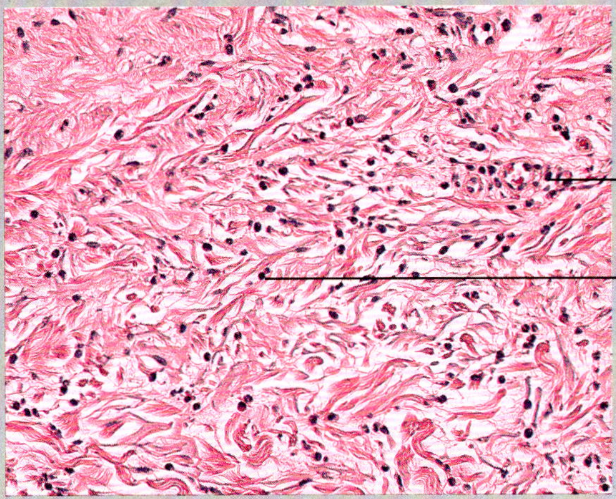

sparse perivascular infiltrate

sparse interstitial infiltrate

lymphocytes

eosinophils

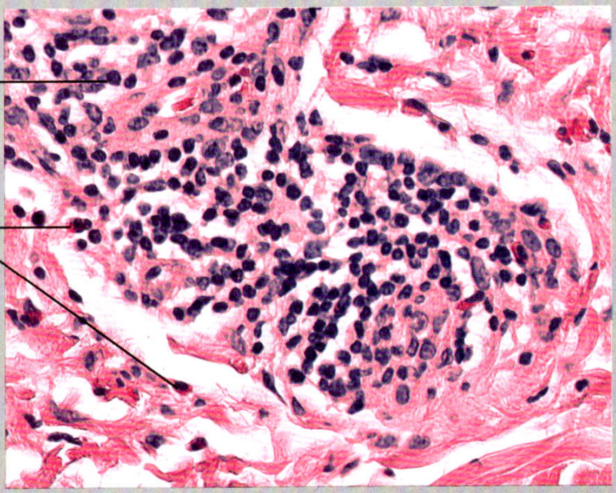

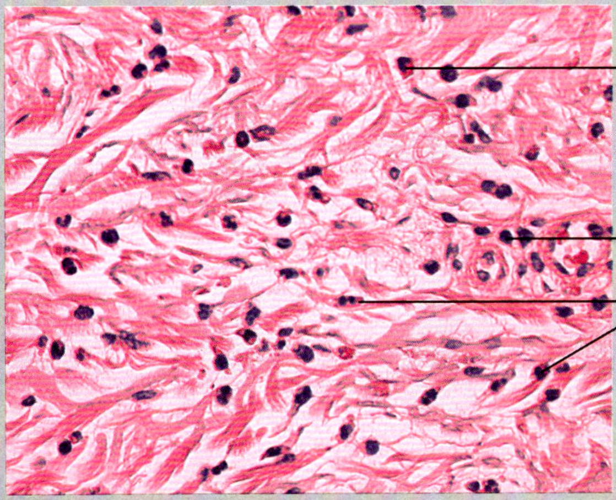

eosinophil

lymphocyte

neutrophils

In urticarial reactions to arthropod assaults and in lesions of urticaria, the infiltrate of inflammatory cells is mixed, contains at least lymphocytes and eosinophils, and is accompanied by extravasated erythrocytes and edema of the papillary dermis. Because of these features in common, the two conditions may need to be differentiated histopathologically by the criteria just listed, especially by the greater density and depth of the wedge-shaped infiltrate in arthropod reactions and the usual preponderance of neutrophils, rather than eosinophils, in the infiltrate of urticaria.

Reactions to arthropod assaults vary enormously in their histopathologic appearance depending upon the particular offending organism, the sensitivity of the host, the duration of the lesion at the time a biopsy is performed, and the part of the lesion sampled (e.g., the center, which may show both intra- and subepidermal vesiculation, or the periphery, which may demonstrate edema in the papillary dermis and no vesiculation). The usual histopathologic appearance of an entire lesion of a typical vesicular reaction to an arthropod assault is a superficial and deep perivascular and interstitial infiltrate of lymphocytes and eosinophils around blood vessels, eosinophils scattered interstitially, edema of the papillary dermis, and a central tense intra-epidermal vesicle. The changes in the dermis just described are seen in urticarial responses to arthropod assaults. There are few, if any, epidermal alterations in those lesions.

Subtle histopathologic differences exist, however, among responses to bites of various kinds. For example, mosquitoes seem to "bite" at the site of an ostium of a hair follicle, and that is reflected commonly in perifollicular infiltrates of inflammatory cells at the center of a lesion; "bites" of sand fleas are associated with neutrophils, rather than eosinophils; bee stings that leave a stinger behind in the dermis may be followed in weeks by a foreign body granulomatous reaction; mouth parts of a tick left in the dermis as the critter is pulled out may induce a pseudolymphomatous reaction replete with lymphoid follicles; and nodular lesions of scabies have denser and deeper infiltrates than the usual papular reactions to scabies in which mites and their products, such as fecal nuggets, are housed superficially in the cornified layer. Other metazoa may cause reactions in skin that are indistinguishable from those of arthropods, e.g., larvae of creeping eruption, cercariae of swimmer's itch, nematocysts of the Portuguese man-of-war, hairs of the puss caterpillar, and spines of sea anemones and coral. When the dermal changes common to those various inducing agents are spotted, careful search should be undertaken in the cornified layer for the mite of scabies, in the spinous layer for cercariae, and in and above the basal layer for hookworm larvae.

Lesions in response to arthropod assaults vary in number from one to innumerable, but appear mostly on uncovered parts, whereas the lesions of urticaria almost always are many and widespread. In most instances, no cause can be found for urticaria that is long-standing, in contrast to urticaria that is short-lived and for which the patient usually knows the cause, e.g., inhalants such as fumes, ingestants such as foods, and injections such as drugs. One cause of urticaria that persists for months or years is occult infestations, such as gastrointestinal parasites.

Clinically, individual lesions of long-standing urticaria may be indistinguishable morphologically from those of urticaria that is short-lived. All are edematous papules that may have pseudopods. Histopathologically, the lesions look different at different stages of their rather rapid evolution and devolution, i.e., a few hours to many hours. Very early lesions are associated with such sparse mostly perivascular infiltrates of a few neutrophils, eosinophils, and lymphocytes that, at first blush at scanning magnification, the section of skin seems to be normal. Fully developed lesions consist of slightly more dense perivascular and interstitial infiltrates of neutrophils and eosinophils, and resolving lesions may show only sparse perivascular infiltrates of lymphocytes and hardly any eosinophils.

It is artificial to designate lesions of urticaria that wax and wane for less than six weeks as "acute," and those that continue to come and go for more than six weeks as "chronic." Wheals, irrespective of cause, usually disappear entirely in a matter of hours. Hives, regardless of cause (e.g., allergen, pressure, sunlight), have the same clinical and histopathologic appearance. The differences among them mostly concern cause. When the condition is evanescent, the cause usually is obvious. When, however, the condition is of long duration, the cause of hives seldom is discovered.

12. Allergic (Leukocytoclastic) Vasculitis *vs.* Septic Vasculitis

Allergic (Leukocytoclastic) Vasculitis	*Septic Vasculitis*
1. Erosion and ulceration rare	1. Erosion and ulceration common
2. Epidermal damage (spongiosis and ballooning, intra-epidermal vesicles and pustules, and necrosis) sometimes	2. Epidermal damage (spongiosis and ballooning, intra-epidermal vesicles and pustules, and necrosis) nearly all the time
3. Neutrophils within the epidermis episodically	3. Neutrophils within the epidermis nearly consistently
4. Necrosis of epithelial structures of adnexa rare	4. Necrosis of epithelial structures of adnexa frequent
5. Vasculitis involves venules of the dermis and only occasionally those of the subcutaneous fat	5. Vasculitis involves arterioles as well as venules of both the dermis and the subcutaneous fat
6. Deep plexus usually, but not always, involved	6. Deep, as well as superficial, plexus involved virtually always
7. Thrombi rare	7. Thrombi common
8. Fibrin in and around walls of venules common	8. Fibrin in and around walls of small vessels rare
9. Leukocytoclasis, i.e., neutrophilic nuclear "dust," abundant	9. No nuclear "dust"
10. Eosinophils common	10. Eosinophils absent as a rule

Allergic (Leukocytoclastic) Vasculitis

Septic Vasculitis

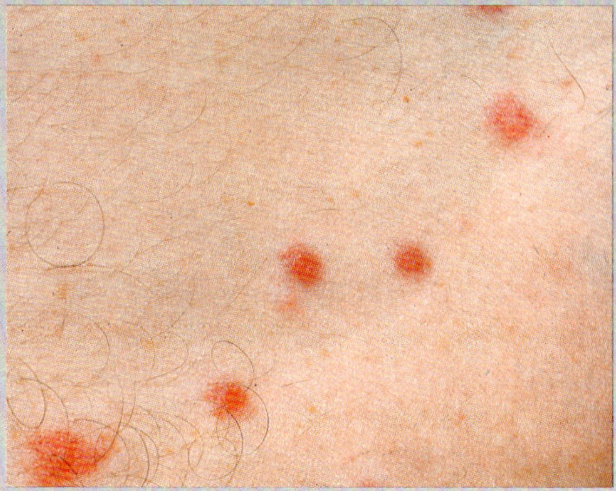

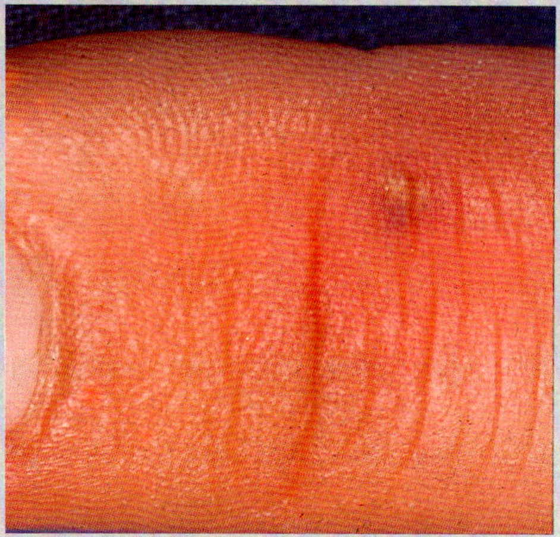

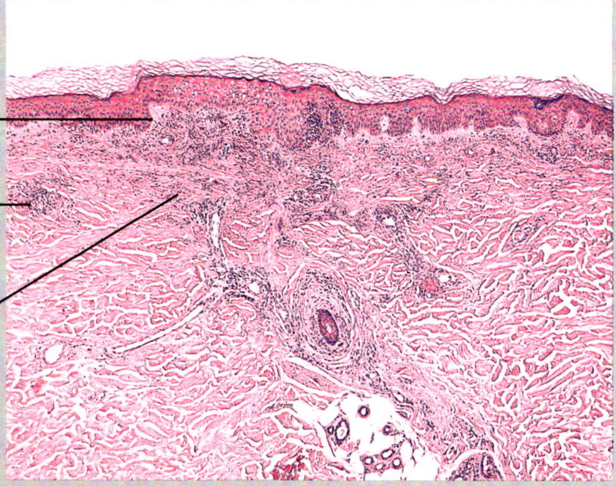

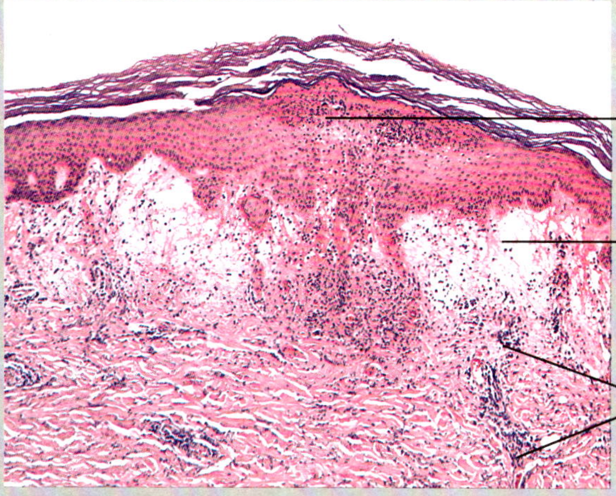

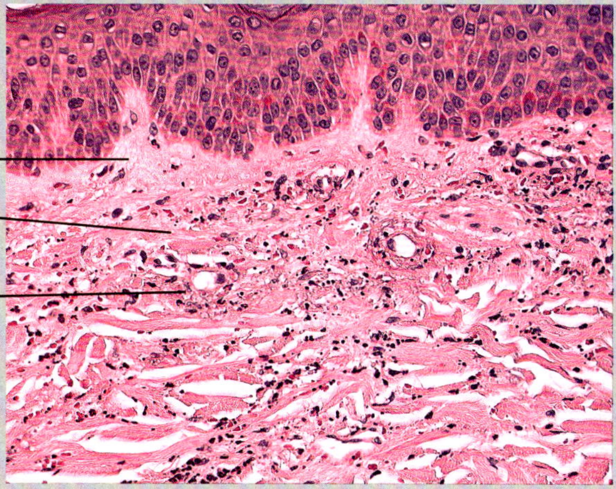

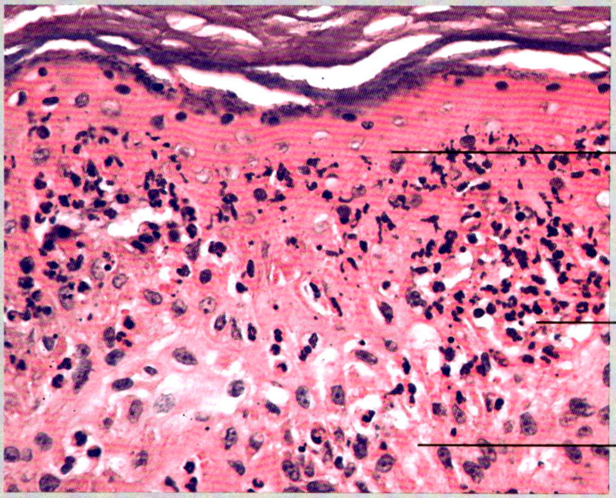

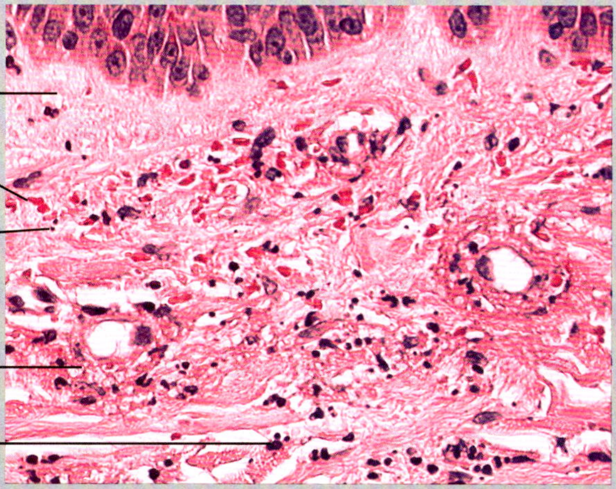

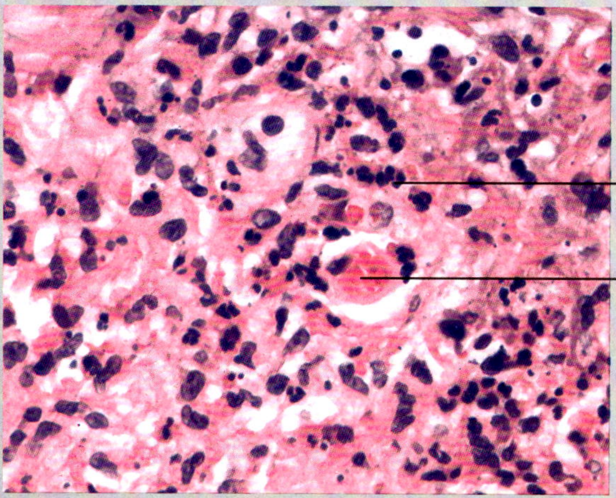

ALLERGIC (leukocytoclastic) vasculitis and septic vasculitis have several histopathologic features in common, namely neutrophils within and around the walls of small dermal blood vessels, neutrophils scattered interstitially, extravasated erythrocytes, and tendency to necrosis of the epidermis.

Small-vessel vasculitis is an inflammatory process that occurs partly within the walls of blood vessels and is attended by histopathologic evidences of fibrin within those walls, thrombi within lumina, or both. Extravasation of erythrocytes is concurrent nearly always. The presence of inflammatory cells within the walls of small blood vessels is not in itself sufficient for a diagnosis of vasculitis because those cells simply may be traversing the walls of blood vessels in their normal manner en route from lumina to surrounding tissue (diapedesis). For this reason, strict histopathologic criteria are requisite as guides to differentiation of vasculitis from the much more common perivascular infiltrates of inflammatory cells.

Vasculitis may be classified according to the type of inflammatory cells that predominate (e.g., neutrophils, lymphocytes, and histiocytes in granulomas) and the kind of blood vessels involved (e.g., arteries, veins, arterioles, venules, and capillaries). Allergic vasculitis and septic vasculitis are examples of neutrophilic vasculitis that affect small blood vessels of the dermis primarily. They may be distinguished from each other, however, by distinctive histopathologic differences. Neutrophilic nuclear "dust" and eosinophils usually are abundant in and around the walls of venules of allergic vasculitis, but are not present at all in septic vasculitis; thrombi develop more commonly in septic than in allergic vasculitis, and arterioles, as well as venules and capillaries, are involved in septic, but not allergic, vasculitis. There also are immunopathologic differences between these different types of small-vessel vasculitis: deposits of immunoglobulins and complement are found in early lesions of leukocytoclastic vasculitis, but not in septic vasculitis.

Allergic vasculitis occurs as an expression of many conditions, e.g., drug reactions, systemic lupus erythematosus, rheumatoid arthritis, Henoch-Schoenlein syndrome, cryoglobulinemia, and Lucio's phenomenon (erythema necroticans), and in association with internal malignant neoplasms, to mention but a few of many examples. A specific cause cannot be inferred of leukocytoclastic vasculitis from histopathologic changes alone, except in leprosy where foamy histiocytes (Virchow cells) are present and in lues maligna where there are typical features of secondary syphilis. Leukocytoclastic vasculitis, irrespective of cause (and often no cause is attributable), has the same appearance when viewed through a conventional microscope.

Clinical lesions of leukocytoclastic vasculitis, whatever the cause, also are similar in appearance. They usually begin as edematous papules ("urticarial vasculitis") that progress quickly to purpuric papules ("palpable purpura") and then may evolve into vesicles, bullae, pustules, or ulcers. The legs are sites of predilection, but no part of the skin is exempt. In some conditions, such as Henoch-Schoenlein syndrome, skin lesions do not evolve beyond the stage of purpuric papules or nodules. In lesions of granuloma faciale and of erythema elevatum diutinum, leukocytoclastic vasculitis may persist for years. These conditions are characterized by plaques and nodules rather than by edematous papules, vesicles, or ulcers.

Septic vasculitis may be caused by gonococci, meningococci, pseudomonads, and staphylococci, as well as by other microorganisms. Skin lesions caused by each of these agents have features in common, namely, purpura (petechial and ecchymotic), vesiculopustules (often with gray roofs that signify epidermal necrosis), hemorrhagic bullae and, occasionally, ulceration. Chronic gonococcemia and chronic meningococcemia characteristically have only a few lesions that are confined to the extremities, especially acral parts. Those lesions are petechiae surrounded by a broad rim of erythema, vesiculopustules associated with epidermal necrosis and, rarely, hemorrhagic bullae.

The histopathologic changes of septic vasculitis just described are seen typically in chronic gonococcemia and meningococcemia. The vasculitis associated with pseudomonad septicemia (echthyma gangrenosum) and staphylococcal septicemia have some features in common with gonococcemia and meningococcemia. There are significant differences between them, however, such as the density of the infiltrate of inflammatory cells (e.g., sparse in pseudomonad septicemia, usually moderately dense in gonococcal septicemia), the number of organisms that can be detected in tissue sections (e.g., many in pseudomonad septicemia, usually none in gonococcal), and the amount of tissue destruction (e.g., great in pseudomonad septicemia, slight in gonococcal).

In some instances, it may be impossible to distinguish histopathologically between incipient lesions of septic vasculitis and those of allergic vasculitis, especially in rare cases in which there are thrombi in allergic vasculitis, and leukocytoclasis and fibrin in septic vasculitis. Very early lesions of allergic vasculitis usually are devoid of fibrin. Such early lesions may show a predominance of intact neutrophils or, occasionally, a preponderance of neutrophilic nuclear "dust." When neutrophilic nuclear "dust" predominates in what seems to be a superficial or superficial and deep perivascular dermatitis, the diagnosis of leukocytoclastic vasculitis may be made with confidence.

13. Granuloma Annulare *vs.* Necrobiosis Lipoidica

Granuloma Annulare	*Necrobiosis Lipoidica*
1. Epidermis not thinned	1. Epidermis thinned with effacement of rete ridges
2. Upper part of the dermis usually more involved than the lower part; subcutaneous fat spared in papular lesions	2. Lower part of the dermis (and the subcutaneous fat) usually more involved than the upper part
3. Changes focal, i.e., intervening zones of normal dermis within a 4-mm punch biopsy specimen	3. Changes diffuse with no intervening zones of normal dermis within a 4-mm punch biopsy specimen
4. Discrete foci of histiocytes in palisaded and/or interstitial array within the dermis; dermis around those foci is normal	4. Diffuse involvement of the dermis by palisaded and interstitial infiltrates of histiocytes; no normal reticular dermis in the specimen usually
5. No linear arrangement of infiltrates of inflammatory cells in tiers within the dermis	5. Linear arrangement of inflammatory cells in two or three tiers within the dermis as a rule
6. Histiocytes form palisades around foci rich in acid mucosubstances that cause bundles of collagen to separate; slight degeneration of collagen bundles	6. Histiocytes form palisades around zones of marked degeneration of collagen bundles; no acid mucosubstances in these foci
7. Mast cells increased in mucinous foci within zones of granulomatous inflammation	7. Mast cells not increased in number in zones of degenerated collagen bundles
8. No plasma cells or only a few of them	8. Plasma cells usually numerous
9. No panniculitis except in the uncommon subcutaneous variant	9. Granulomatous septal panniculitis usual
10. Resolution with near restoration of normal structure; no sclerosis	10. Progression to sclerosis of the reticular dermis and widened sclerotic septa in the subcutaneous fat

Granuloma Annulare

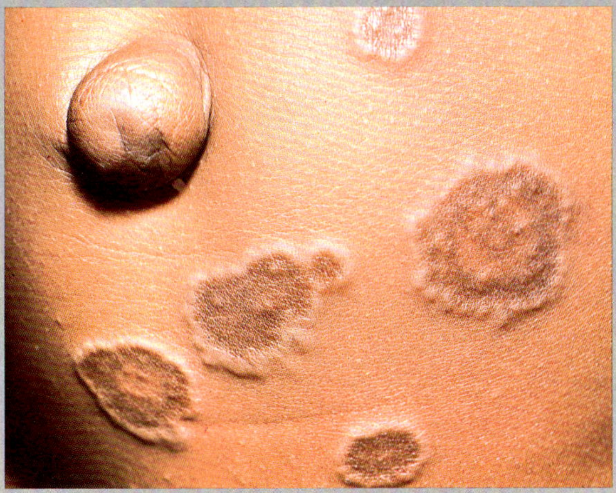

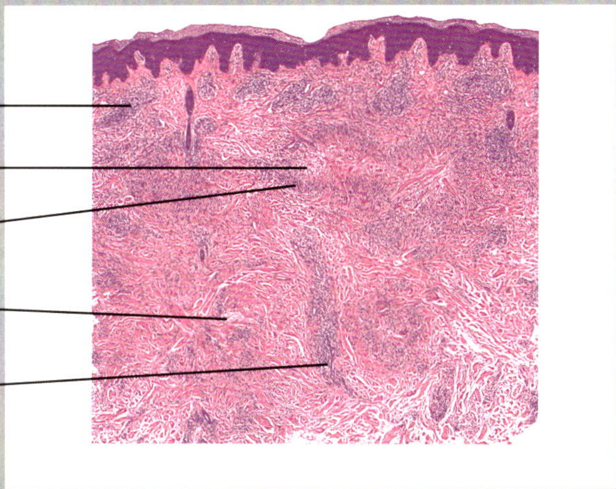

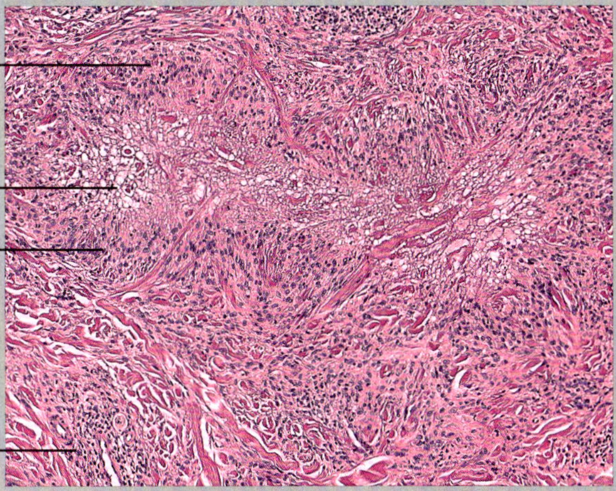

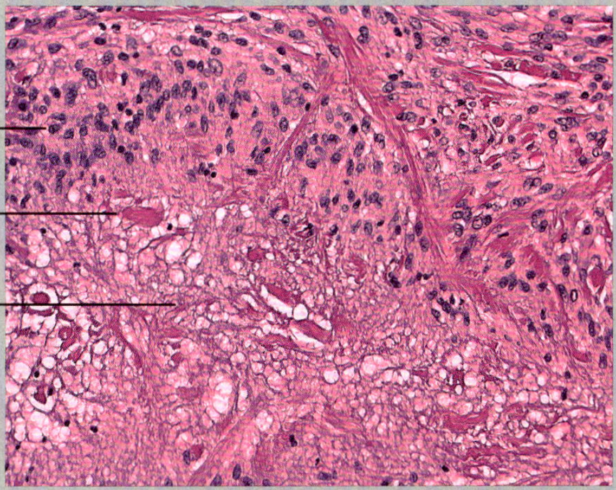

Necrobiosis Lipoidica

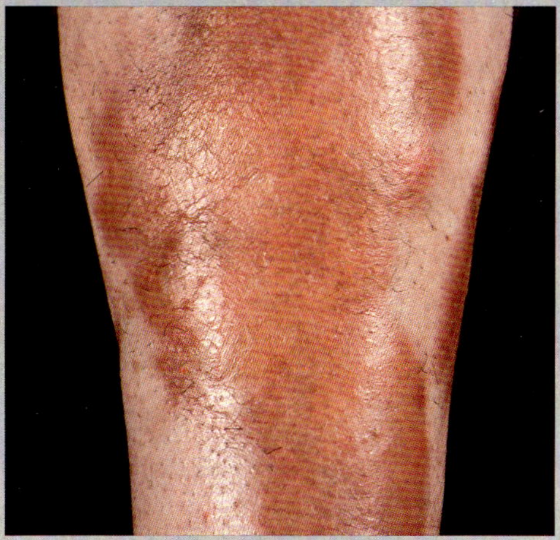

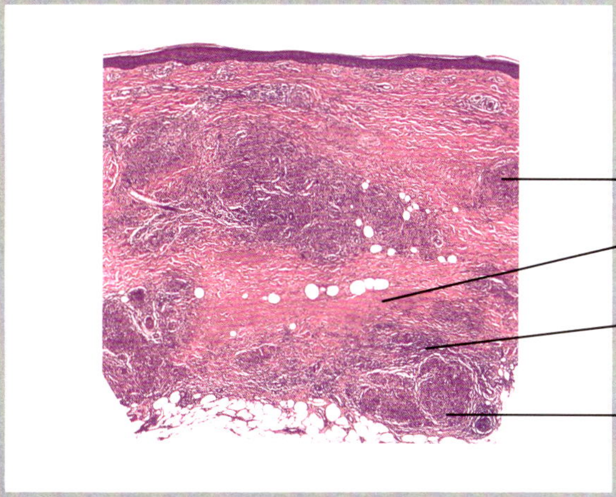

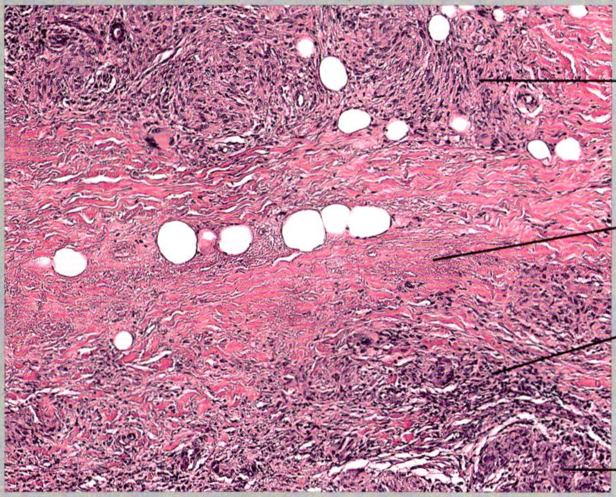

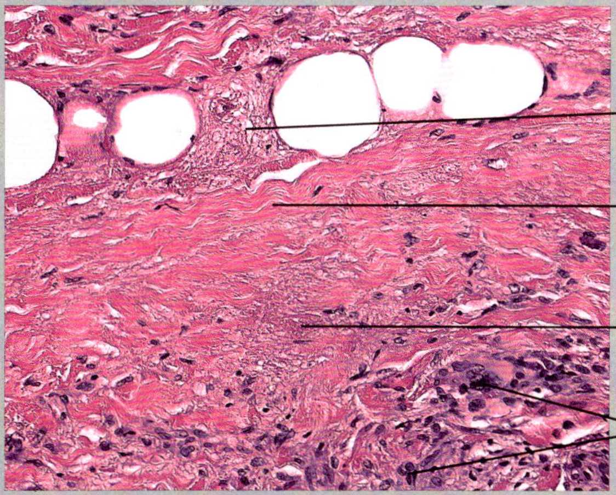

BOTH granuloma annulare and necrobiosis lipoidica are characterized by palisaded granulomatous dermatitis, superficial and deep perivascular predominantly lymphocytic infiltrates, and some degeneration of bundles of collagen, as well as deposits of fibrin in centers of palisades of histiocytes. Stains for elastic tissue reveal that elastic fibers are decreased or absent from foci of degenerated collagen bundles in both diseases.

The major histopathologic differences between granuloma annulare and necrobiosis lipoidica are the patchy quality of the granulomatous process in granuloma annulare (i.e., in several discrete foci amid otherwise normal dermis), abundant deposits of acid mucosubstances in foci of granulomatous inflammation, absence of tiers of granulomatous inflammation aligned parallel to the skin surface within the dermis, and sparing of subcutaneous tissue usually. In contrast, the pathologic process in necrobiosis lipoidica is diffuse, i.e., it involves the entire dermis with no intervening normal zones, degeneration of collagen bundles is prominent, no deposits of acid mucosubstances can be detected, two or three tiers of granulomatous inflammation tend to be present in the dermis and, almost always, the subcutaneous fat is involved by the process.

Of great value in differentiation of these two palisaded and interstitial granulomatous dermatitides is the fact that acid mucosubstances, recognizable readily in sections stained by hematoxylin and eosin as granular and feathery, slightly basophilic material, are near constant accompaniments of granuloma annulare, but practically never are discernible in necrobiosis lipoidica. When, episodically, it is exceedingly difficult to differentiate granuloma annulare from necrobiosis lipoidica in sections stained by hematoxylin and eosin, a stain for acid mucosubstances, such as colloidal iron or alcian blue, may enable definitive diagnosis. In granuloma annulare, abundant mucin usually is demonstrable in the center of palisaded granulomas and in zones of interstitial involvement by histiocytes, whereas in necrobiosis lipoidica none is visible.

In very early lesions of granuloma annulare and necrobiosis lipoidica, hints of neutrophilic vasculitis with formation of thrombi may be discerned. In granuloma annulare, a small degenerated venule associated with fragments of neutrophilic nuclei may be identified on occasion within the center of a palisade of histiocytes. In necrobiosis lipoidica, similarly affected dermal vessels are found in the midst of degenerated collagen bundles in the deep reticular dermis and within the subcutaneous fat. The neutrophilic vasculitis seen in early lesions of necrobiosis lipoidica often is followed by granulomatous vasculitis and eventual obliteration of the affected small blood vessels.

Several clinical presentations of granuloma annulare are recognizable. The most common is one or several rings of papules that surround seemingly normal or slightly hyperpigmented skin. Uncommon is a widespread (in a photodistribution sometimes) papular form of discrete, tiny, smooth-surfaced papules, many of which have an almost indiscernible central dell. One type is composed of patches of hyperpigmentation at the periphery of which subtle papules coalesce to form a gently elevated rim. A subcutaneous form occurs mainly on the extremities in children and, in times past, often was misinterpreted histopathologically as "pseudo-rheumatoid nodule." In actuality, all so-called pseudorheumatoid nodules are examples of subcutaneous granuloma annulare. Last, there is a perforating type of granuloma annulare in which mucin and bundles of degenerated collagen are extruded from the papillary dermis, through the epidermis onto the skin surface where they form tiny crusts atop discrete papules.

Necrobiosis lipoidica begins as a patch that becomes a reddish plaque which, in years, evolves into an atrophic, yellowish, telangiectatic patch. Trauma, including biopsy, often results in indolent ulcers. The long-standing process is most common on the anterior aspect of the legs below the knees of young diabetic women, but it may develop anywhere on the skin. Necrobiosis lipoidica sometimes may appear in individuals who do not manifest overt signs of diabetes, but all patients with necrobiosis lipoidica should be followed closely to ensure that diabetes is not concurrent or in the offing.

14. Tuberculoid Leprosy *vs.* Sarcoidosis

Tuberculoid Leprosy	*Sarcoidosis*
1. Oblong tubercles of epithelioid histiocytes	1. Roundish tubercles of epithelioid histiocytes
2. Granulomas predominantly in the lower part of the dermis, less often in the upper part alone	2. Granulomas predominantly in the upper part of the dermis, uncommonly in the lower part alone or in the subcutaneous fat
3. Moderately dense infiltrate of lymphocytes around the tubercles of histiocytes	3. Sparse infiltrate of lymphocytes around the tubercles ("naked tubercles") usually
4. Infiltrate of lymphocytes and histiocytes in and around cutaneous nerves and adnexal epithelium in the deep reticular dermis	4. No infiltrate of inflammatory cells within nerves or adnexal epithelium usually
5. Cutaneous nerves often destroyed by inflammatory cells and their products	5. Cutaneous nerves preserved
6. No fibrin within tubercles as a rule	6. Fibrin within tubercles sometimes
7. Little or no fibrosis	7. Fibrosis in late lesions sometimes
8. Acid-fast bacilli demonstrable rarely	8. No acid-fast bacilli
9. Asteroid bodies in histiocytes rare	9. Asteroid bodies in histiocytes common, especially multinucleated ones

Tuberculoid Leprosy

Sarcoidosis

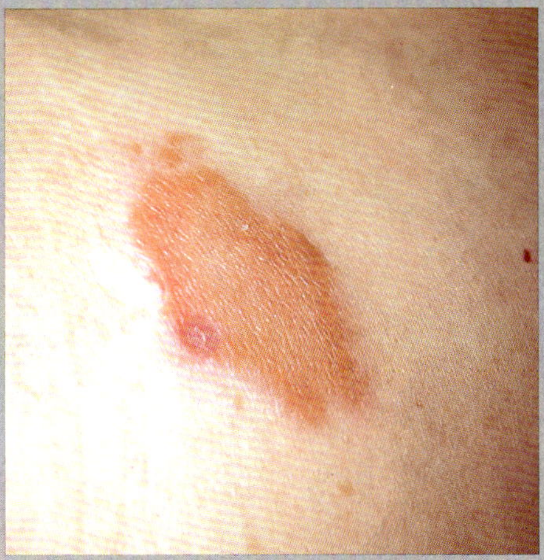

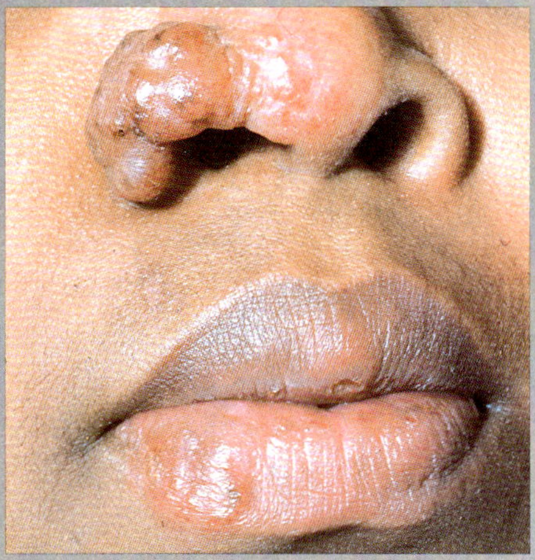

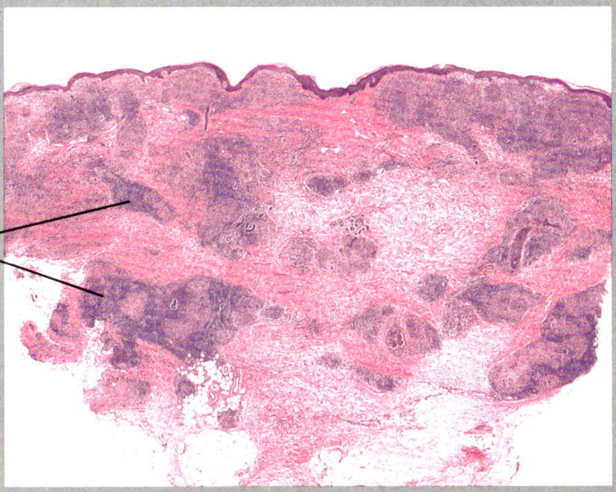

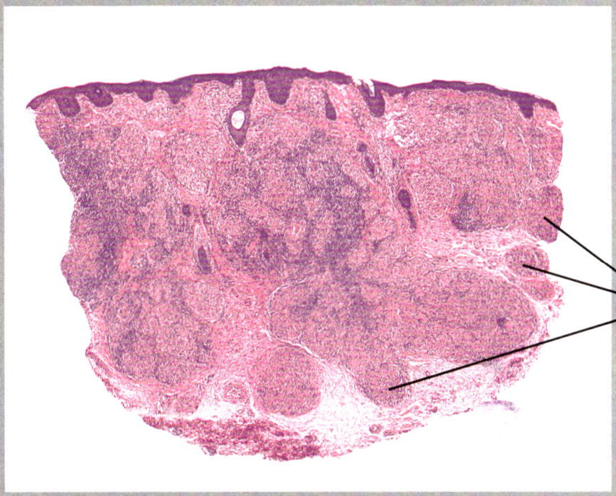

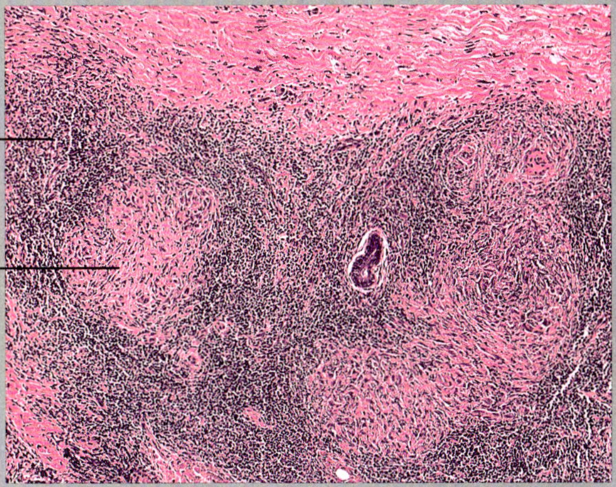

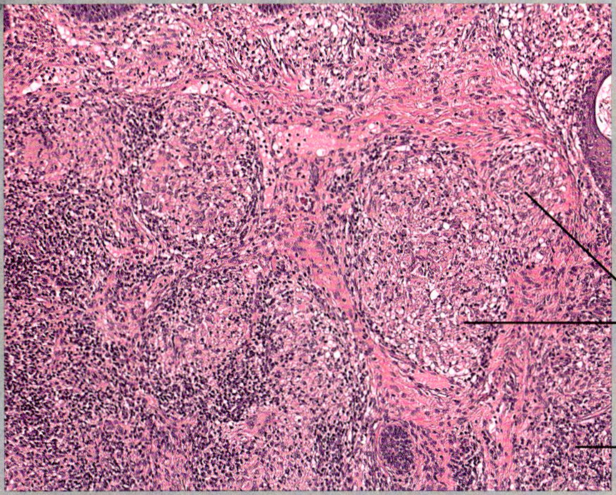

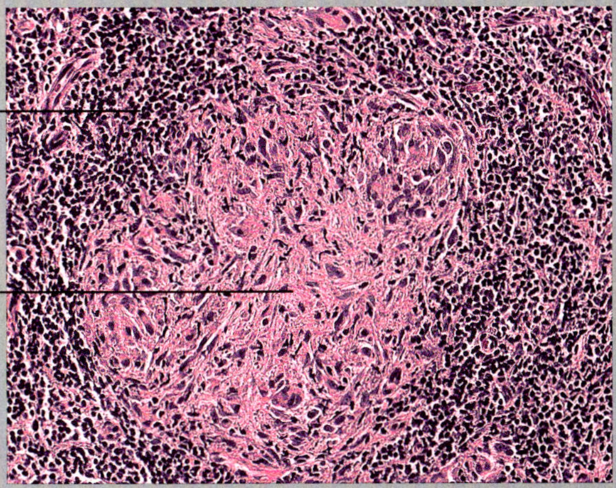

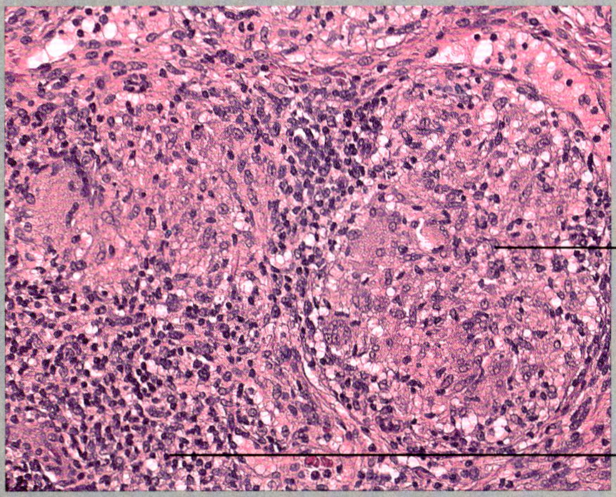

Tuberculoid leprosy and sarcoidosis are granulomatous dermatitides that resemble one another histopathologically because both consist of tubercles of epithelioid histiocytes in the dermis and sometimes in the subcutaneous fat. Despite these similarities, sarcoidosis may be differentiated from tuberculoid leprosy in most instances if the preceding criteria are sought and found.

Tuberculoid leprosy is one of the two major expressions of leprosy, a disease caused by acid-fast bacilli *(Mycobacterium leprae).* Clinically, tuberculoid leprosy is characterized stereotypically by one or several discrete, hypopigmented anesthetic patches. Peripheral nerves may be thickened palpably in patients with this form of the disease. Patients with tuberculoid leprosy are capable of expressing delayed hypersensitivity, whereas those with sarcoidosis often are not. Rarely are bacilli demonstrable with the Fite stain in the tuberculoid form of leprosy. With the assistance of the electron microscope, however, lepra bacilli may be detected, albeit with difficulty, within histiocytes in tuberculoid leprosy.

In contrast to tuberculoid leprosy, cutaneous sarcoidosis presents itself clinically as numerous firm orange-brown papules, nodules, and plaques that favor the face (especially the zones around the eyes, nose, and mouth), but may be widespread. The disease is much more common in blacks. A rare form of sarcoidosis (Darier-Roussy type) consists of granulomatous infiltrates in the subcutaneous fat. When lesions of sarcoidosis manifest themselves in the skin, the likelihood is that other organs are involved concurrently by the disease. The cause of sarcoidosis is not yet known.

Other granulomatous dermatitides that may be indistinguishable histopathologically from sarcoidosis are caused by silica, beryllium, and zirconium. Silica is readily apparent when tissue sections are examined by polarized light. Micro-incineration and x-ray diffraction techniques are required to detect beryllium. Zirconium may be identified by spectrographic analysis.

Papular lesions of rosacea may have granulomatous features that can be confused with those of sarcoidosis, especially because both diseases have a predilection for the face. In contrast to tuberculoid leprosy, granulomatous expressions of rosacea consist of poorly circumscribed epithelioid tubercles, marked edema and telangiectases in the upper part of the dermis, and a perivascular and perifollicular mixed-cell infiltrate. Suppurative folliculitis sometimes accompanies granulomas in rosacea.

The histopathologic differential diagnosis of tuberculoid leprosy includes lupus vulgaris and the relapsing form of leishmaniasis. Lupus vulgaris involves predominantly the upper portion of the dermis by well-circumscribed epithelioid tubercles within which necrosis may be found. The infiltrates of inflammatory cells in lupus vulgaris do not involve small nerves within the dermis. The recidivans form of leishmaniasis more closely resembles lupus vulgaris than it does tuberculoid leprosy.

Sometimes, lesions of sarcoidosis may be joined by dense lymphocytic infiltrates in concert with epithelioid tubercles. In such instances, it may not be possible to differentiate histopathologically among sarcoidosis, tuberculoid leprosy, lupus vulgaris, and the recidivans form of leishmaniasis. Rarely, numerous plasma cells may be seen in lesions of sarcoidosis, in concert with epithelioid tubercles, and such lesions must be distinguished from those of late secondary and tertiary syphilis. That is accomplished most reliably by serological studies.

15. Keloid *vs.* Hypertrophic Scar

Keloid	*Hypertrophic Scar*
1. Lesion elevated markedly above the skin surface usually; little tendency to regression without therapy	1. Lesion elevated slightly above the skin surface; later, even without treatment, becomes flush with the skin surface or depressed below it as an atrophic scar
2. No tendency to subepidermal clefts or vesicles	2. Subepidermal clefts or vesicles occasionally
3. Markedly thickened, homogeneous bundles of collagen with few fibrillary bundles of collagen in fully developed lesions	3. Fibrillary bundles of collagen only; no markedly thickened ones
4. Collagen bundles brightly eosinophilic	4. Collagen bundles slightly eosinophilic or amphophilic
5. Collagen bundles in haphazard array	5. Collagen bundles generally oriented parallel to the skin surface
6. Fibrocytes alongside thickened collagen bundles also in haphazard pattern	6. Fibrocytes alongside fibrillary bundles of collagen arranged mostly parallel to the skin surface
7. Widely dilated blood vessels oriented randomly	7. Widely dilated blood vessels oriented somewhat perpendicular to the skin surface
8. Abundant mucin between bundles of collagen often	8. Little mucin between bundles of collagen except in early lesions when it may be abundant
9. Infiltrates of lymphocytes around dilated blood vessels at the periphery of a lesion especially	9. Infiltrates of lymphocytes around dilated blood vessels throughout a lesion

Keloid | *Hypertrophic Scar*

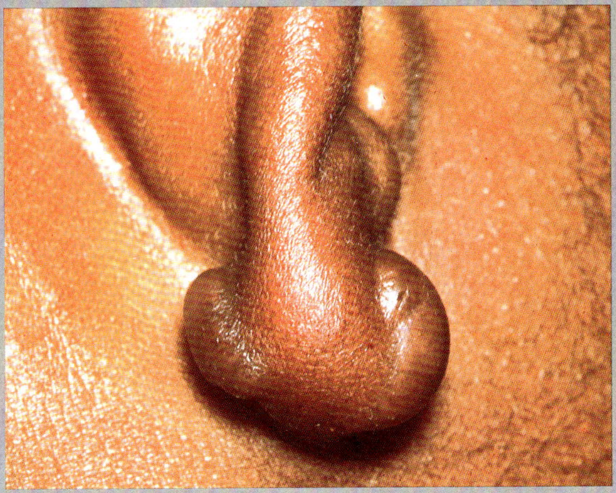

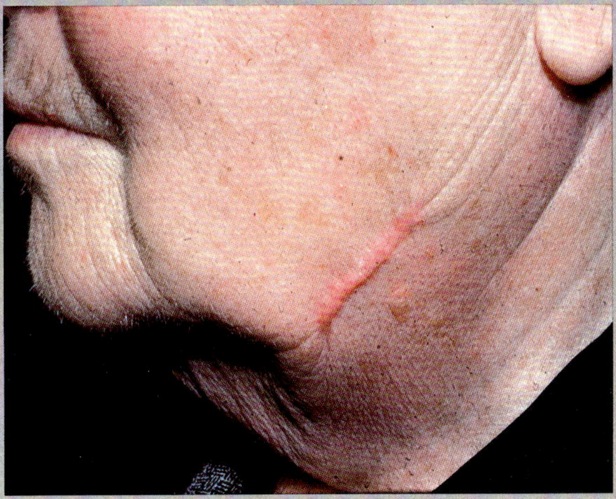

thick bundles of collagen in haphazard array

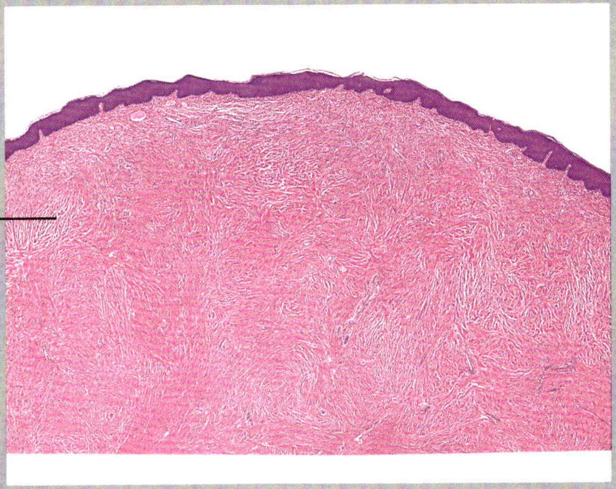

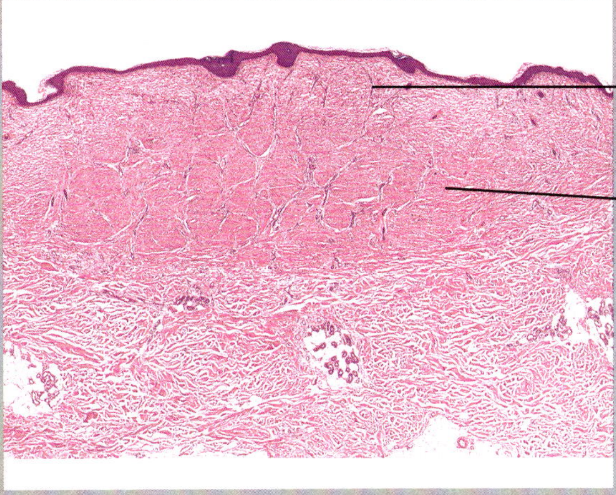

venule perpendicular to skin surface

thin bundles of collagen parallel to skin surface

thick collagen bundles arranged randomly

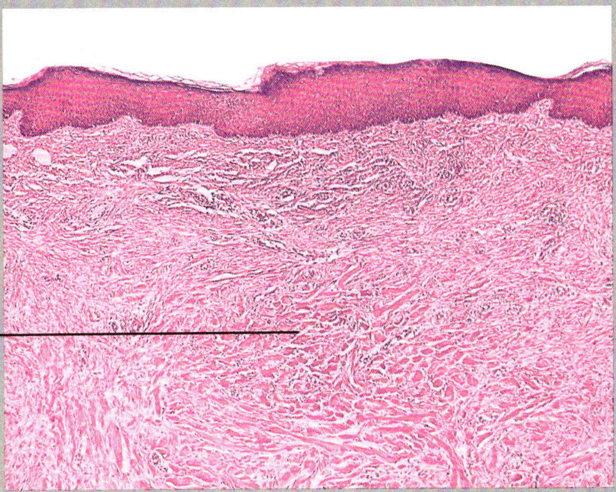

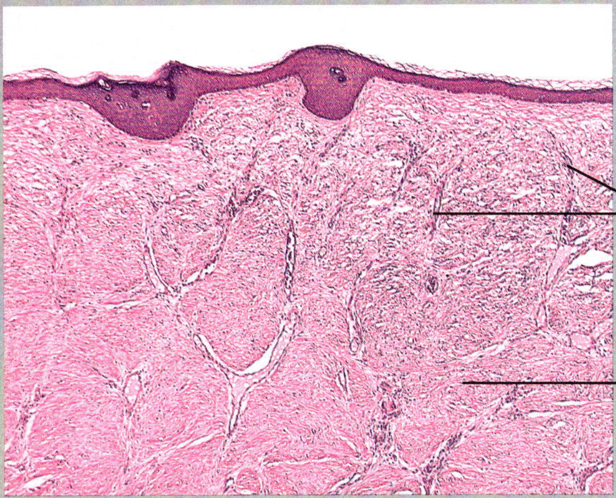

venules perpendicular

collagen bundles parallel

thick bundles of collagen

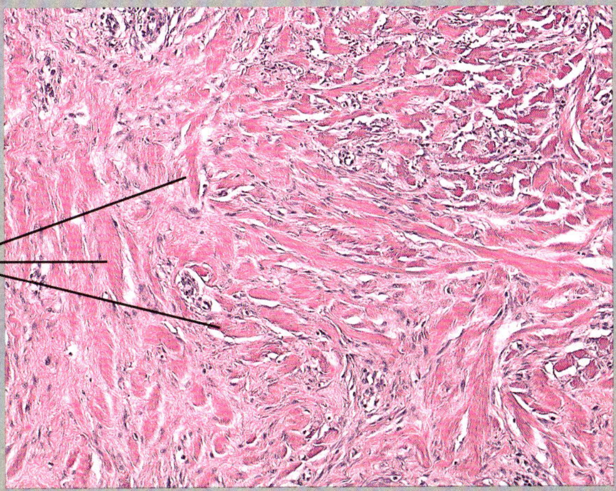

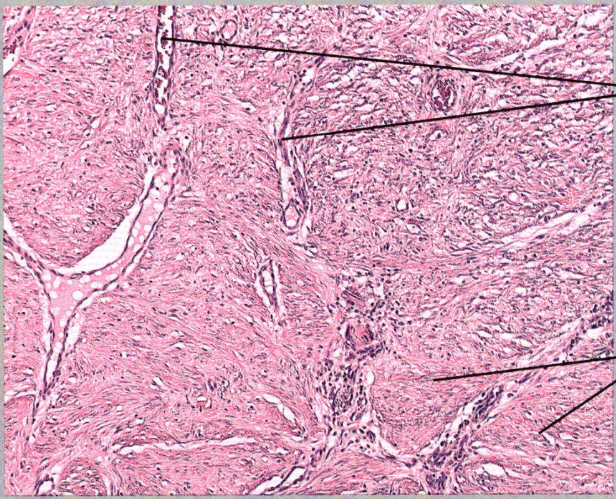

vertical orientation of venules

horizontal orientation of collagen bundles

KELOIDS and hypertrophic scars have many histopathologic features in common (e.g., fibroplasia, telangiectases, inflammatory-cell infiltrates, mucin) and, in some instances, features of what seem to be both keloid and hypertrophic scar may be found in sections from the same biopsy specimen. When distinct keloidal features are present in the form of brightly eosinophilic, thick bundles of collagen in haphazard array, the diagnosis, by convention, is keloid. On the other hand, when there are no such bundles of collagen, the diagnosis is hypertrophic scar.

Hypertrophic scars usually are linear lesions that follow traumas such as surgical incisions and accidental lacerations. These scars have no predilection for individuals of any particular intensity of pigmentation. As a rule, hypertrophic scars tend to flatten over time without treatment, whereas keloids do not shrink appreciably.

Both keloids and hypertrophic scars are types of fibrosing dermatitis, i.e., inflammatory processes that resolve with fibroplasia. The entire spectrum of inflammation from granulation tissue to sclerosis may be found in keloids and hypertrophic scars, depending upon when in their course a biopsy specimen is obtained.

In early lesions of keloids, only abundant fibrillary bundles of collagen are present in nodular aggregations that contain numerous plump fibrocytes in haphazard array. No thickened, homogeneous, brightly eosinophilic bundles of collagen are found in early keloids. The best clue to diagnosis of keloids, even at this early stage, is the presence of fibrillary bundles of collagen like those of a scar in a lesion whose configuration is distinctly nodular. In time, within such a lesion, foci of markedly thickened brightly eosinophilic collagen bundles arranged randomly appear within the mass of fibrillary collagen bundles. Those thickened bundles of collagen, in that particular setting, are signs of a keloid. The histopathologic diagnosis of keloid has important implications for a patient vis-à-vis prevention of future keloids and treatment of existing ones.

Thickened collagen bundles like those in keloids also are seen, episodically, in otherwise typical lesions of dermatofibromas (fibrosing inflammation with keloidal features), nodular fasciitis (fibrosing inflammation with keloidal features), and basal-cell carcinomas (malignant neoplasms associated with keloidal features). The factors that induce fibrocytes to manufacture collagen with various morphologic appearances are not understood, e.g., thick collagen bundles in haphazard array, as in a keloid; fibrillary collagen bundles, as in a scar; short, coarse collagen bundles in haphazard array, as in a dermatofibroma; thickened collagen bundles arranged compactly and in parallel, as in scleroderma; wiry bundles of collagen in random distribution associated with lichenoid infiltrates of lymphocytes as in mycosis fungoides; bundles of collagen in lamellae in the papillary dermis immediately beneath nests of melanocytes at bases of rete ridges and parallel to undulations of rete ridges as in melanocytic proliferations like simple lentigines, junctional nevi, and malignant melanoma in situ; sclerotic collagen in the upper part of the dermis, as in lichen sclerosus et atrophicus; and concentric whorls of collagen bundles around hair follicles, as in fibrous papules of the face (perifollicular fibroma).

Why fibrocytes produce bundles of collagen arranged in vertical streaks in a thickened papillary dermis is known well. Those coarse bundles that appear in lichen simplex chronicus, prurigo nodularis, and picker's nodule result from prolonged, persistent rubbing of the skin. The mechanisms whereby these characteristic changes occur have yet to be learned.

16. Lichen Sclerosus et Atrophicus *vs.* Scleroderma

Lichen Sclerosus et Atrophicus	*Scleroderma*
1. Marked laminated or compact orthokeratosis of the stratum corneum	1. Normal stratum corneum
2. Infundibula and acrosyringia plugged by orthokeratotic cells often	2. Adnexal ostia not plugged by corneocytes as a rule
3. Thinned epidermis with loss of the normal pattern between epidermal rete ridges and dermal papillae	3. Normal epidermis including the pattern between epidermal rete ridges and dermal papillae
4. Melanin decreased uniformly across the entire epidermis	4. Melanin decreased in epidermal foci and increased in others sometimes
5. Vacuolar alteration at the dermo-epidermal junction	5. Little or no vacuolar alteration at the junction
6. Papillary dermis thickened by sclerosis ("homogenized")	6. Papillary dermis relatively unaffected in most lesions; indistinguishable from lichen sclerosus in a minority of lesions
7. Reticular dermis practically unaffected	7. Reticular dermis thickened by thickened bundles of collagen arranged compactly and parallel to the skin surface
8. Moderately dense, perivascular, predominantly lymphocytic infiltrate with occasional plasma cells beneath a thickened papillary dermis	8. Moderately dense, superficial and deep, perivascular and sometimes interstitial infiltrate of lymphocytes, plasma cells and, sometimes, eosinophils
9. Epithelial structures of adnexa mostly preserved	9. Epithelial structures of adnexa mostly destroyed
10. No involvement of the subcutaneous fat	10. Septal panniculitis and subsequent thickening of septa by compactly arranged thickened bundles of collagen
11. No fasciitis	11. Fasciitis occasionally; process may extend into skeletal muscle rarely and into bone exceedingly rarely

Lichen Sclerosus et Atrophicus | *Scleroderma (Morphea)*

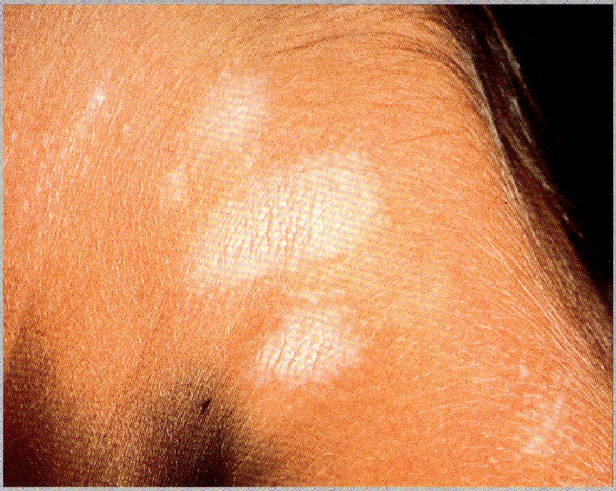

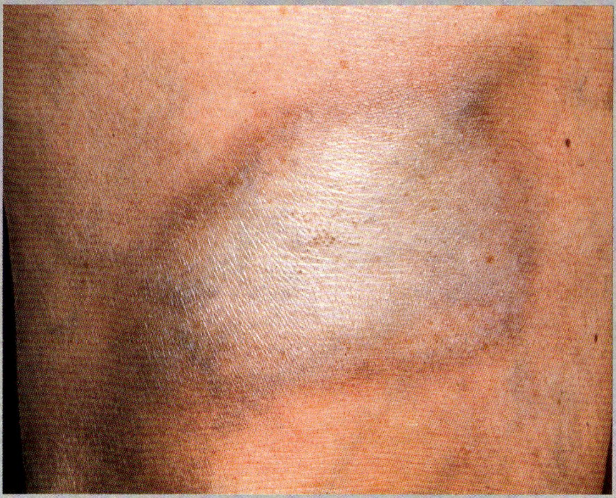

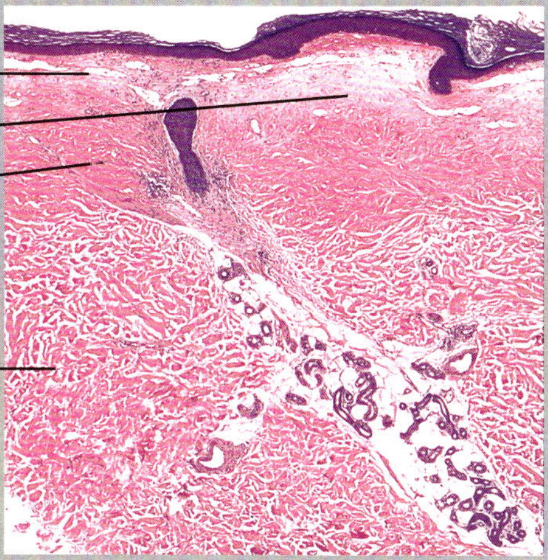

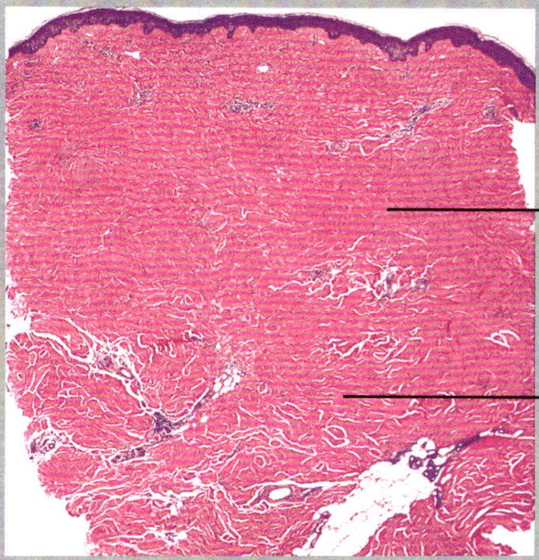

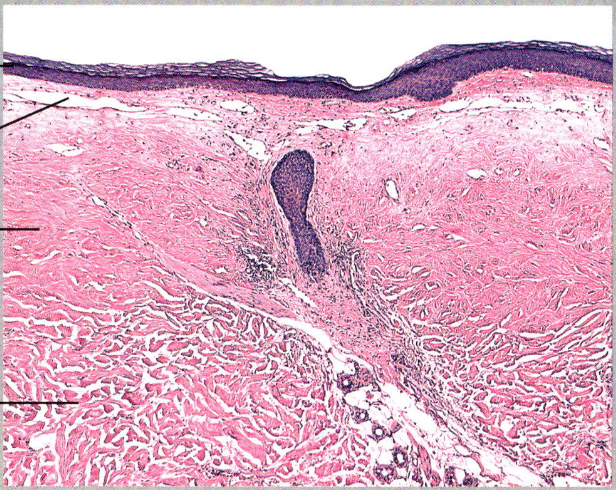

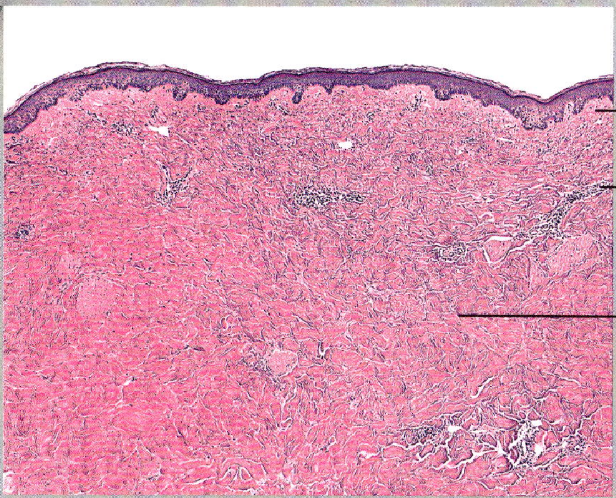

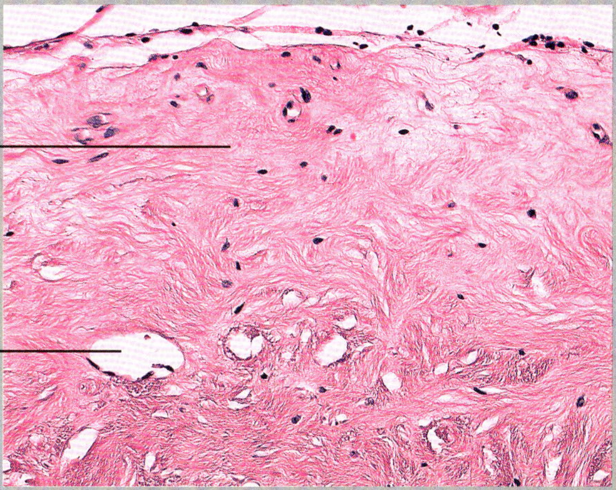

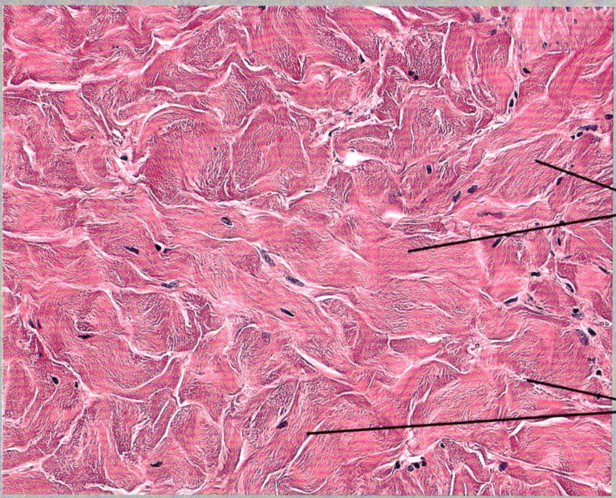

LICHEN sclerosus et atrophicus and scleroderma are inflammatory processes associated with marked alteration of collagen bundles, i.e., sclerosis in the papillary dermis of lichen sclerosus and thickened bundles in the reticular dermis and septa of the subcutaneous fat in scleroderma. Sclerosis is synonymous with "homogenization" of bundles of collagen and represents an end stage of fibrosis. Collagen bundles are thickened in scleroderma, but their integrity is preserved; there is no sclerosis except episodically in the papillary dermis. In lichen sclerosus et atrophicus, the inflammatory changes are confined to the upper portion of the dermis, whereas in scleroderma the entire dermis, especially the lower half, the subcutaneous fat and, episodically, the fascia are involved.

On occasion, histopathologic changes that resemble those of lichen sclerosus et atrophicus may be seen in the papillary dermis in lesions of indubitable morphea. Sometimes typical lesions of lichen sclerosus and of morphea, as judged both clinically and histopathologically, are seen independent of one another in the same patient. Some colleagues have suggested that these changes represent examples of two different diseases occurring together in the same specimen and the same patient, whereas others have proposed that lichen sclerosus et atrophicus and morphea are parts of a spectrum of a single pathologic process. We now interpret the histopathologic changes that resemble lichen sclerosus et atrophicus in otherwise typical lesions of morphea to be a manifestation of scleroderma and not lichen sclerosus. We have come to think of lichen sclerosus et atrophicus as morphea confined to the papillary dermis and superficial vascular plexus.

Clinically, the lichen sclerosus et atrophicus expression of morphea presents itself in sequence as rose-colored macules and patches, then as whitish papules and plaques, and last as atrophic patches, some of which are dotted by dilated follicular ostia filled with plugs of corneocytes. The typical patient is a middle-aged or older woman who complains of severe itching in the vulvar, perineal, and/or perianal areas. When such lesions have been rubbed persistently, the clinical and histopathologic features of lichen simplex chronicus may be found superimposed upon those of the underlying vulvar lichen sclerosus et atrophicus. The lichen simplex chronicus takes the form of extensive compact orthokeratosis and hypergranulosis that resembles the upper two layers of epidermis on a palm or sole. Lichen sclerosus et atrophicus may involve the glans penis, where it has been termed balanitis xerotica obliterans. It also may develop in children, where it is said to disappear "spontaneously" and completely on occasion.

The whiteness of the lesions of lichen sclerosus et atrophicus is caused by a combination of hyperkeratosis, loss of melanin from the epidermis, and sclerosis of the papillary dermis. The atrophy results from obliteration, by sclerosis, of the normal relationship between dermal papillae and epidermal rete ridges and, in particular, from loss of cutaneous volume as a consequence of effacement of dermal papillae.

Clinically, the skin changes of scleroderma, i.e., guttate, morphea (including the idiopathic atrophoderma of Pasini and Pierini), linear (including facial hemiatrophy), diffuse fasciitis with eosinophilia, acrosclerosis, and diffuse sclerosis, have features in common. It is obvious, however, that these names do not represent a single disease. Nonetheless, all the cutaneous expressions of so-called scleroderma are characterized by hardness that results from alterations in bundles of collagen within the dermis, the subcutaneous fat, and the fascia, and by pigmentary alterations that follow loss of melanin from the epidermis into dermal macrophages. The "salt and pepper" effect of intermingled spotty hypo- and hyperpigmentation results from contiguous foci of increased and decreased melanin within the epidermis. When subcutaneous fat and fascia are replaced subsequently by thickened bundles of collagen, the skin in scleroderma has a "hide-bound" quality. Fasciitis with eosinophilia seems merely to be a deep variant of scleroderma, as does the tryptophan-myalgia syndrome. Lichen sclerosus et atrophicus seems merely to be a superficial variant of one type of localized scleroderma, to wit, morphea.

17. Erythema Nodosum *vs.* Nodular Vasculitis

Erythema Nodosum	*Nodular Vasculitis*
1. No ulceration	1. Ulceration often
2. Sparse infiltrate of lymphocytes around blood vessels in the dermis	2. Dense, mixed-cell infiltrate throughout the lower part of the dermis
3. Involvement mostly of septa in the subcutaneous fat	3. Involvement mostly of lobules in the subcutaneous fat
4. Granulation tissue between septa and lobules in the subcutaneous fat	4. Granulation tissue in the subcutaneous fat randomly distributed within lobules
5. Granulomas in thickened fibrotic septa	5. Granulomas around foci of necrosis and suppuration in lobules
6. No vasculitis	6. Vasculitis of large vessels in the deep reticular dermis and the subcutaneous fat
7. Necrosis of adipocytes slight, usually reflected as foam cells	7. Necrosis of adipocytes extensive, usually in the form of necrosis en masse, fat "microcysts," and membranous fat necrosis, as well as of foam cells
8. No suppuration in the subcutaneous fat	8. Suppuration in the subcutaneous fat
9. Eosinophils often; frequently numerous	9. Eosinophils seldom; usually few

Erythema Nodosum | *Nodular Vasculitis*

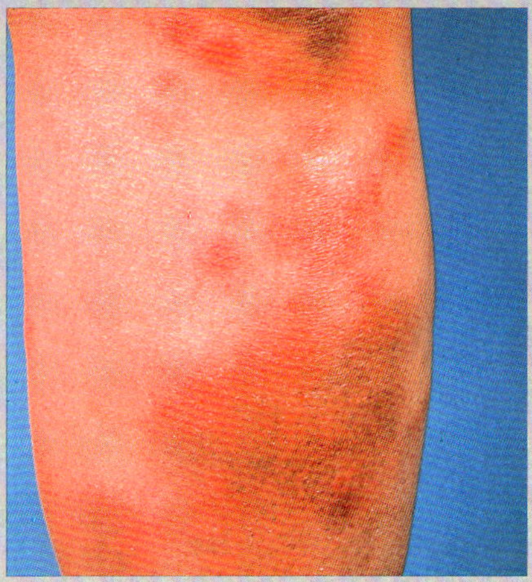

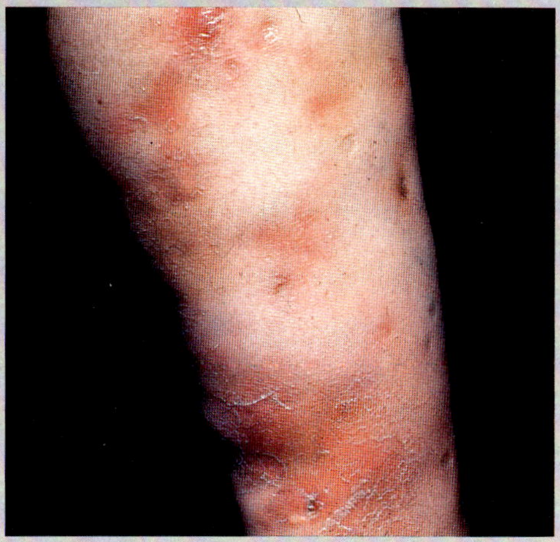

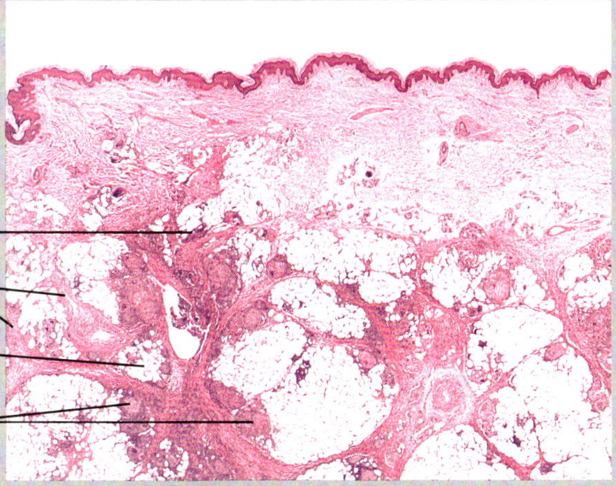

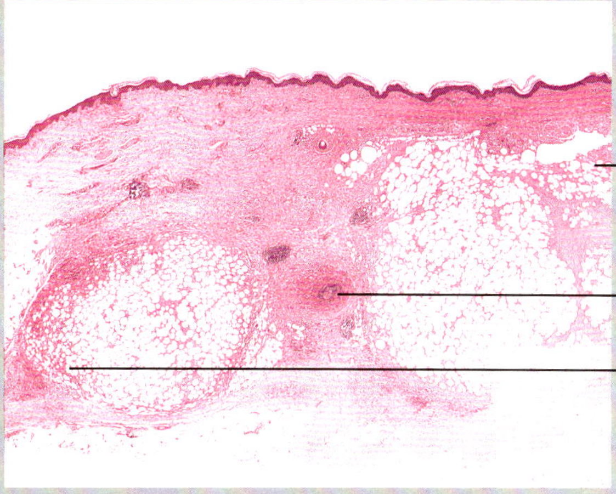

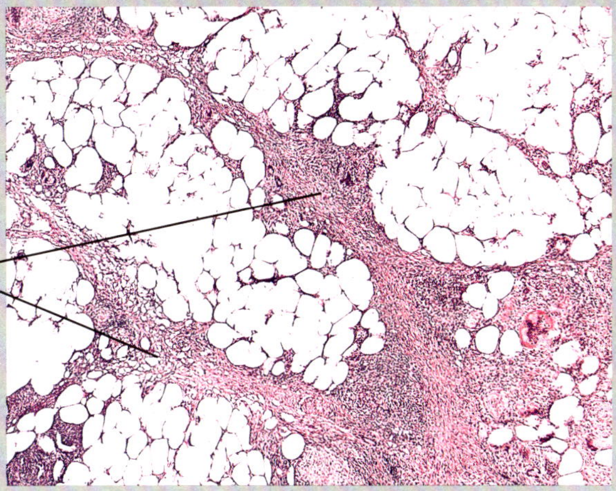

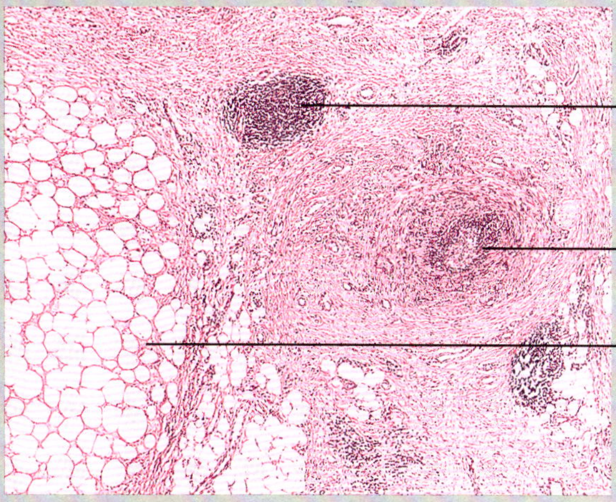

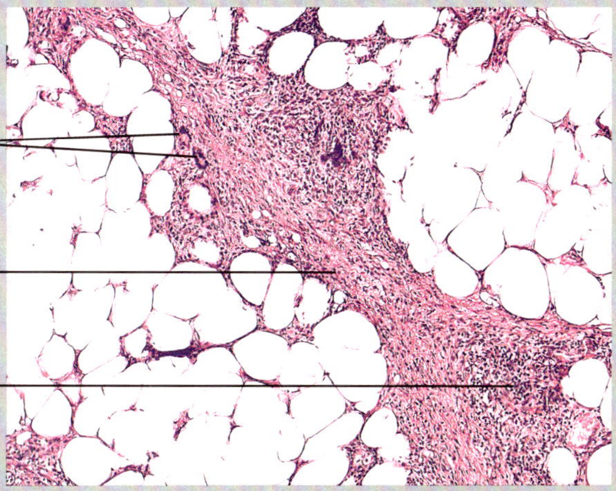

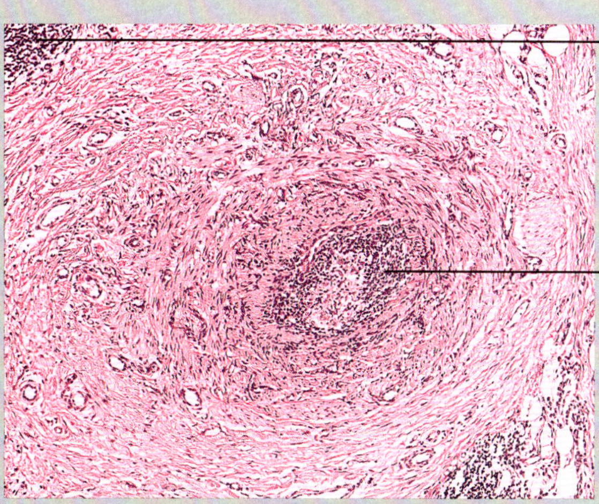

ERYTHEMA nodosum and nodular vasculitis are stereotypes of septal and lobular panniculitis, respectively. When fully developed, erythema nodosum is a granulomatous septal panniculitis and nodular vasculitis is a necrotizing, suppurative, and granulomatous lobular panniculitis secondary to severe arteritis. Because the damaged artery courses within a septum in the subcutaneous fat, nodular vasculitis must involve septa as well as lobules. The most prominent histopathologic changes in nodular vasculitis, however, as viewed with the scanning objective of a conventional microscope, are in the fat lobules. In erythema nodosum, when inflammatory cells in septa spill over into the peripheries of fat lobules, they induce granulation tissue and eventually fibrosis in the zones between septa and lobules. Thus, although erythema nodosum is fundamentally a septal process as observed with the scanning objective, the peripheries of fat lobules are involved inevitably in the pathologic process. In some instances, granulomatous changes are present in the centers of fat lobules in erythema nodosum, as well as at the peripheries of them. In these circumstances, it is easy to misinterpret erythema nodosum as subcutaneous sarcoidosis.

Erythema nodosum and nodular vasculitis, like most panniculitides, are not of short duration, but tend to last for weeks and usually months. Individual lesions of nodular vasculitis may be especially long-standing. Depending upon when biopsy specimens are taken, different histopathologic features are found in the undisturbed progression of lesions.

Clinically, erythema nodosum and its more chronic variant, the subacute nodular migratory panniculitis (Vilanova and Pinol), begin as bright, red, shiny, warm, exquisitely tender patches or plaques that usually are distributed symmetrically on the extensor surfaces of the lower extremities of young women. Histopathologically, a typical early lesion shows:

1. Edema in fibrous septa of the subcutaneous fat
2. Neutrophils and occasional lymphocytes, histiocytes, and eosinophils within septa and at the junction of fat lobules
3. Few necrotic adipocytes.

Later lesions of erythema nodosum are violet to brown, nontender nodules. Sections cut from biopsy specimens of such lesions reveal:

1. Granulomas within widened septa; numerous multinucleated histiocytic giant cells usually
2. Fibrosis that may predominate over granulation tissue in the zones between septa and lobules
3. Variable numbers of histiocytes, including foam cells, within lobules.

Uncommonly, granulomas in erythema nodosum may pepper lobules throughout the subcutaneous fat and, in those instances, the condition may be difficult to differentiate from subcutaneous sarcoidosis. A helpful clue to resolution of that conundrum is concurrent extensive septal involvement in erythema nodosum.

Clinically, early lesions of nodular vasculitis are dull red, faintly tender, slightly elevated nodules distributed asymmetrically on the calves of thick-legged young and middle-aged women. Histopathologically, such lesions show:

1. Mixed-cell infiltrates in the wall and in the lumen of an artery situated within a septum in the subcutaneous fat
2. Coagulation necrosis of fat and suppuration in lobules.

Later lesions of nodular vasculitis are characterized clinically by dusky nodules that ulcerate and heal with hyperpigmented scars that may be topped by scales. The histopathologic findings in such lesions are:

1. Ulceration
2. Focal necrosis, suppuration, granulation tissue, and granulomatous inflammation within lobules
3. Extensive fibrosis that distorts completely the normal architecture of the subcutaneous fat.

Because of the combination of severe fat necrosis and granulomatous inflammation, nodular vasculitis was thought, in former times, to be a manifestation of tuberculosis, i.e., a "tuberculid," and was named erythema induratum. Nowadays, tuberculous cause is rare, and therefore we use the term nodular vasculitis as a general designation of the condition under discussion here, no matter what its cause.

The histopathologic distinctions between erythema nodosum and nodular vasculitis are apparent readily when sections from a deep, generous biopsy specimen delivered by scalpel is presented to a histopathologist. In sections from such a specimen, erythema nodosum can be recognized as a panniculitis fundamentally and not a vasculitis; nodular vasculitis can be identified as a vasculitis basically and a panniculitis only secondarily.

18. Alopecia of Discoid Lupus Erythematosus *vs.* Alopecia of Lichen Planus

Alopecia of Discoid Lupus Erythematosus	*Alopecia of Lichen Planus*
1. Epidermis thinned usually	1. Epidermis normal usually, but typical changes of lichen planus may be present focally
2. No wedge-shaped hypergranulosis of follicular infundibula	2. Wedge-shaped hypergranulosis of follicular infundibula
3. Vacuolar alteration at the junction between epidermis and dermis, and between follicular epithelium and dermis	3. Vacuolar alteration mostly at the junction of follicular epithelium and dermis
4. Thickened basement membrane beneath epidermal and infundibular epithelium	4. No thickened basement membrane
5. Abundant deposits of acid mucosubstances in the reticular dermis	5. No increase of acid mucosubstances in the dermis
6. Patchy, predominantly lymphocytic infiltrates along the length of hair follicles	6. Band-like, predominantly lymphocytic infiltrates along the length of hair follicles
7. No peri-infundibular fibroplasia and no clefts between follicles and dermis	7. Peri-infundibular fibroplasia with clefts between thinned infundibula and altered dermis
8. Fibrotic tracts at sites of extinct hair follicles, as well as sclerosis in the upper part of the dermis	8. Fibrotic tracts at sites of extinct hair follicles, but no sclerosis in the interfollicular dermis

Alopecia of Discoid Lupus Erythematosus

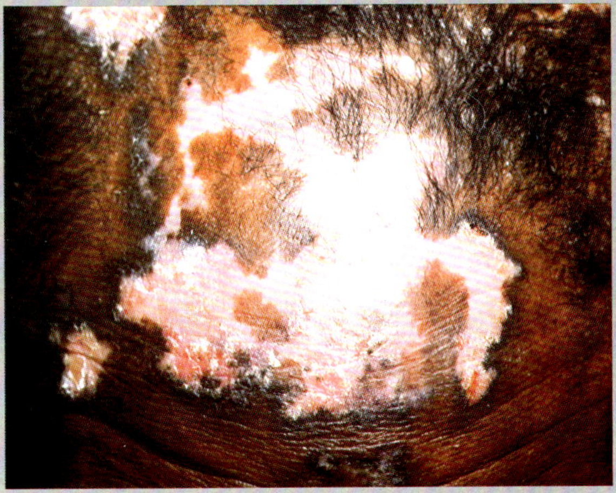

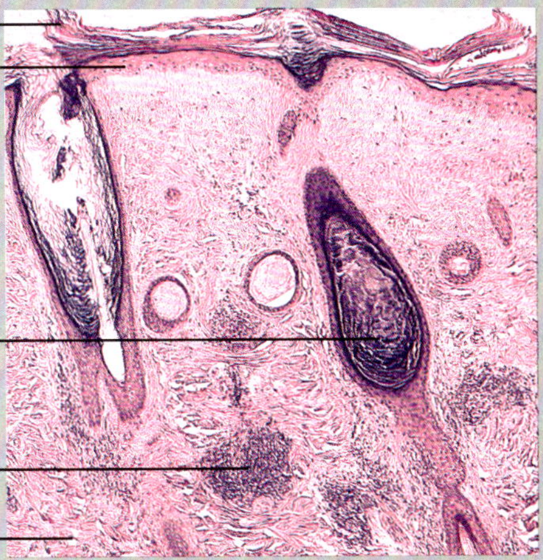

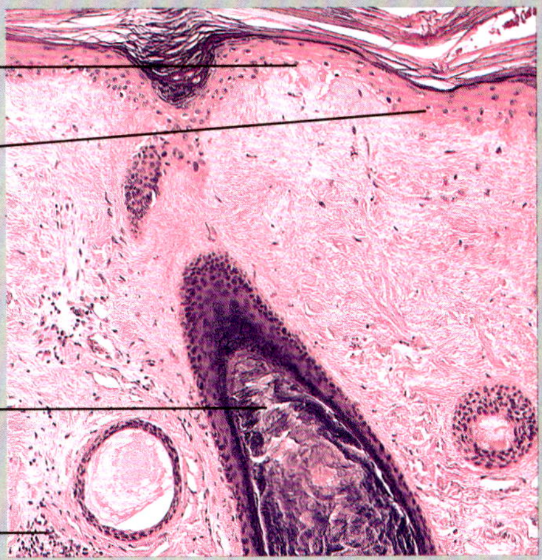

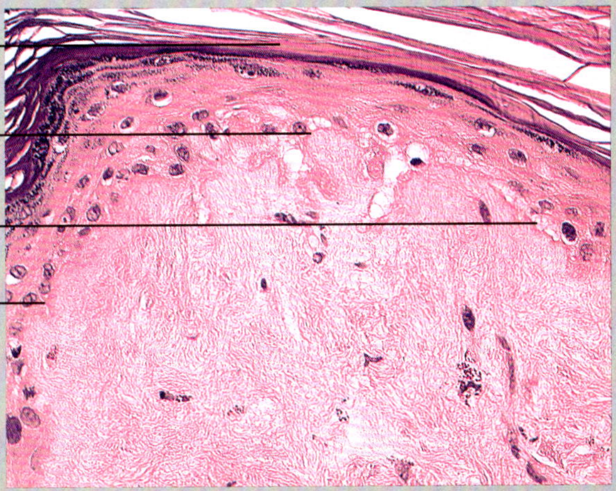

Alopecia of Lichen Planus (Lichen Planopilaris)

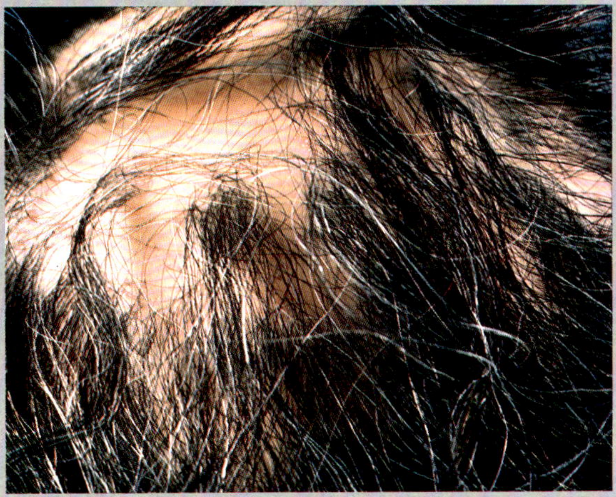

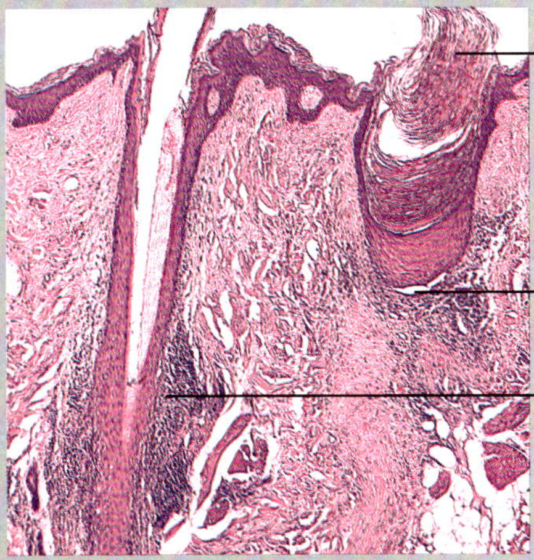

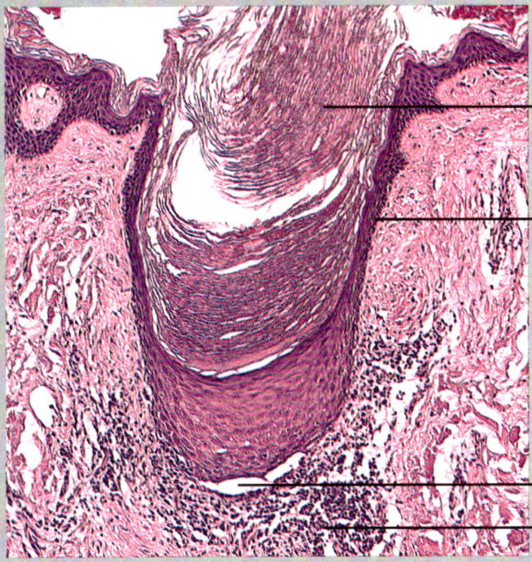

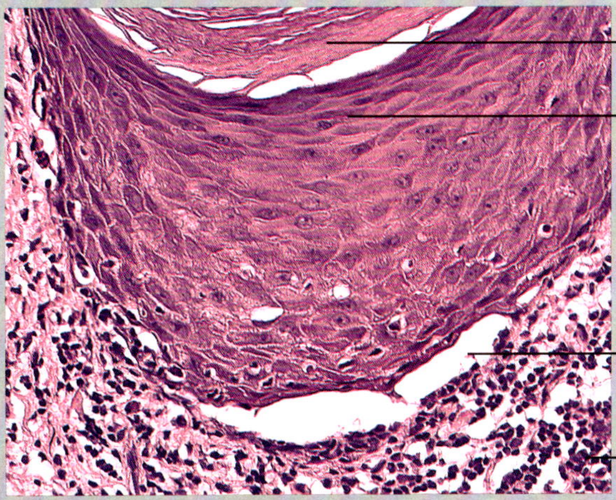

THE alopecias of discoid lupus erythematosus and of lichen planus share these histopathologic features: predominantly lymphocytic perivascular and perifollicular infiltrates, vacuolar alteration at the junction between follicular epithelium and the dermis, infundibula plugged by orthokeratotic corneocytes, and fibrotic tracts along the paths of extinct hair follicles.

The crucial features for differentiation histopathologically of the alopecia of discoid lupus erythematosus from that of lichen planus are found at the dermo-epidermal interface. In long-standing lesions of discoid lupus erythematosus, vacuolar alteration and a thickened basement membrane are present beneath a thinned epidermis, whereas in lesions of lichen planopilaris, the junction between epidermis and dermis often is normal. Occasionally, however, typical changes of lichen planus may be seen in the vicinity of the dermo-epidermal junction as irregular epidermal hyperplasia, focal hypergranulosis, a lichenoid infiltrate of lymphocytes, and vacuolar alteration. In short, the alopecia of chronic discoid lupus erythematosus is associated with involvement of both epidermal and follicular epithelia, whereas that of lichen planus tends to spare the epidermis and involve follicular epithelium only.

In discoid lupus erythematosus, studies by direct immunofluorescence show granular deposits of immunoglobulins and complement at the dermo-epidermal junction; that is not the case in lichen planus.

Clinically, lesions of discoid lupus erythematosus may progress through stages of red macules, papules, and plaques associated with scales and keratotic plugs of follicles, and may regress as atrophic scars. During the process, alopecia may supervene in zones of scars, the centers of which usually are hypopigmented and telangiectatic, the peripheries strikingly hyperpigmented, especially in dark-skinned people. Keratotic plugs also may be apparent in ostia of the hairless follicles. Alopecic lesions of discoid lupus erythematosus favor the face and scalp, but they may occur in discoid lesions elsewhere on the skin.

In contrast, follicular lesions of lichen planus, known as lichen planopilaris, begin as violaceous papules that soon become keratotic. With time, they evolve into atrophic scars that are devoid of hairs. The scarring alopecia of lichen planopilaris may be accompanied by typical lesions of lichen planus elsewhere on the skin, in nail units, and on mucous membranes.

Pseudopelade (i.e., psuedo-alopecia areata) refers to the end stage of scarring alopecias in general. The most common inflammatory disease to result in these lesions, which have been likened clinically to "footprints in the snow," is the alopecia of lichen planus. Similar alopecic lesions, however, may be seen as a consequence of chronic discoid lupus erythematosus.

Alopecias may be permanent and nonscarring histopathologically. For example, common (androgenic) alopecia is noninflammatory, nonscarring, and permanent, and alopecia areata is inflammatory, nonscarring, and may be permanent. The alopecias of discoid lupus erythematosus and lichen planus are inflammatory, scarring, and permanent alopecias in which fibrosis is mostly localized to sites where follicles once resided. In contrast, alopecias consequent to physical and chemical burns are inflammatory, scarring, and permanent as a result of diffuse fibrosis throughout the dermis. A variation on that theme occurs in the inflammatory disease scleroderma, in which thickened bundles of collagen distributed throughout the dermis obliterate hair follicles.

19. Alopecia Areata vs. Trichotillomania

Alopecia Areata	*Trichotillomania*
1. Sparse lymphocytic infiltrate around the blood vessels of the superficial and deep plexuses	1. Practically no infiltrate of inflammatory cells
2. In early lesions, infiltrate of lymphocytes in follicular papillae and in fibrous sheaths that surround follicular bulbs	2. Little or no infiltrate of inflammatory cells around hair follicles
3. Increased number of mast cells and melanophages in association with dilated capillaries in linear arrangement in fibrous tracts and at sites where follicular papillae once were	3. No increased number of mast cells, melanophages, or blood vessels in follicular papillae or in fibrous tracts
4. More follicles in catagen and telogen than in anagen usually	4. More follicles in anagen than in catagen or telogen usually
5. Few intervening follicles in anagen	5. At least several intervening follicles in anagen
6. No everted outer sheaths	6. Everted outer sheaths occasionally
7. No trichomalacia	7. Trichomalacia (pleated hair shafts that contain clumps of melanin) within infundibula of follicles invariable, but not necessarily in every section of a specimen
8. In long-standing lesions, at sites of follicular papillae in the deep reticular dermis, whorls of wiry collagen bundles house degenerated glassy membranes and melanophages	8. No whorls of wiry collagen bundles
9. No superimposition of lichen complex chronicus or of erosion and crusts	9. Lichen simplex chronicus, in the form of compact orthokeratosis, superimposed sometimes; erosions and crusts are uncommon findings

Alopecia Areata

Trichotillomania

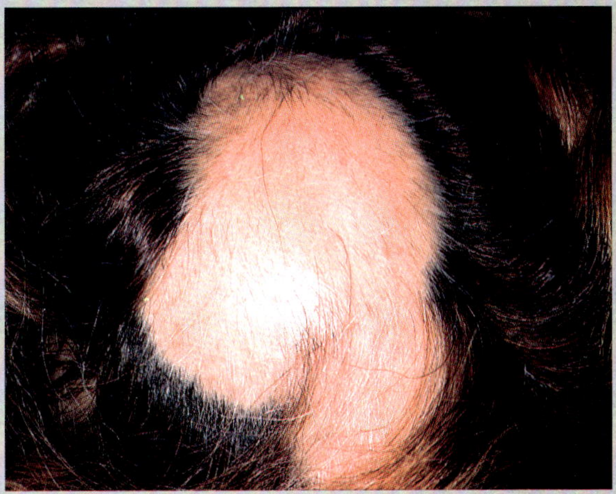

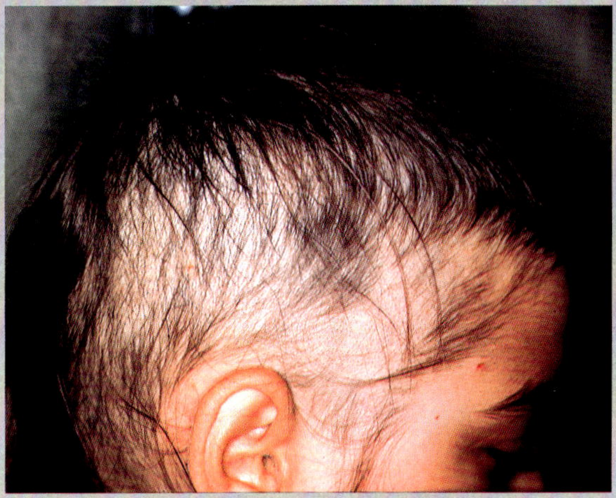

follicles in catagen

lymphocytes at base of follicle

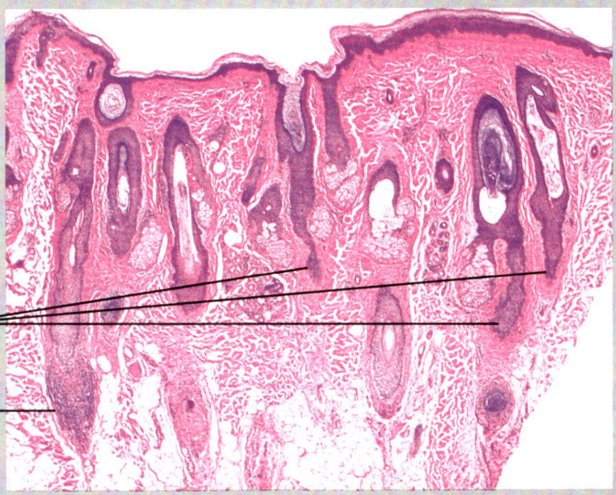

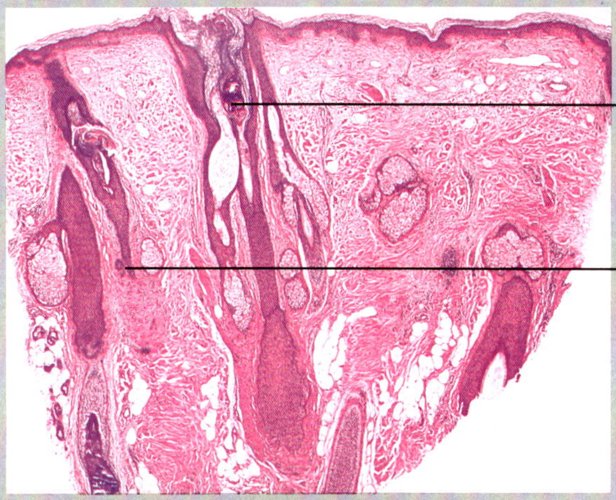

trichomalacia

follicle in catagen

follicle in anagen

lymphocytes around lower segment of the follicle

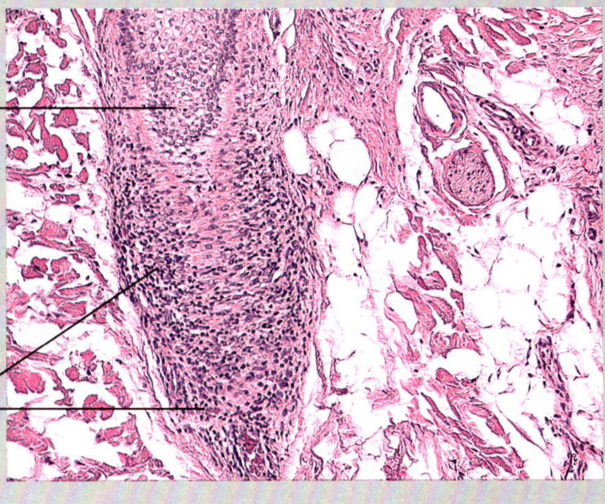

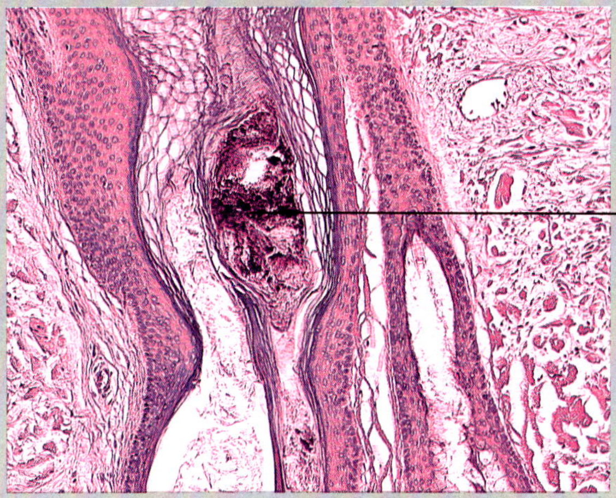

trichomalacia

lymphocytes scattered in follicular epithelium

dilated capillary

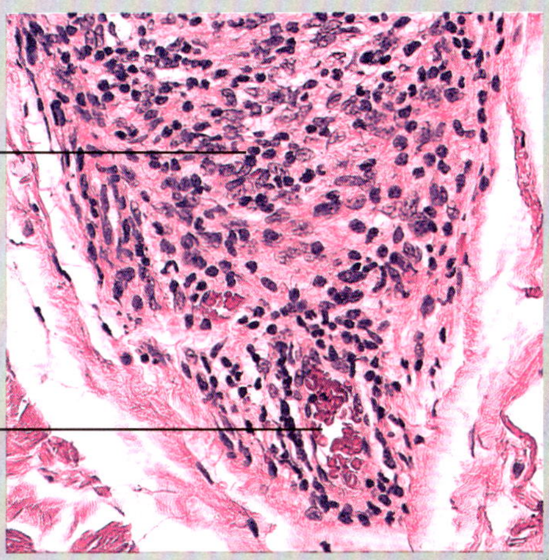

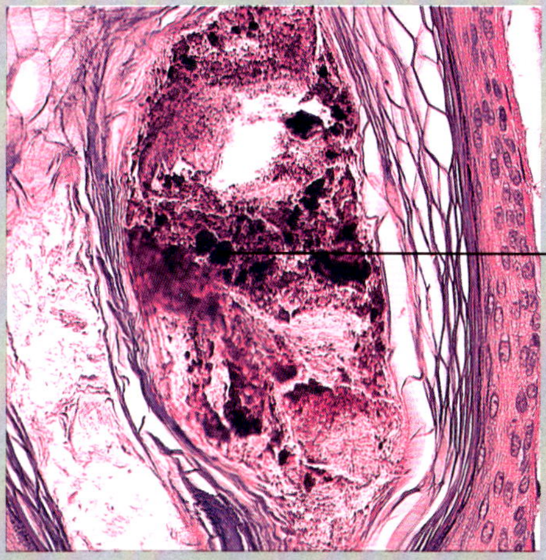

clumps of melanin in a pleated hair shaft

ALOPECIA areata and trichotillomania have several histopathologic features in common, namely, some follicles in catagen and often in telogen, long fibrous tracts behind shortened follicles and, in some specimens, hardly any perivascular infiltrates of inflammatory cells in the dermis. Granulomatous inflammation is a rare common denominator of alopecia areata and trichotillomania, occurring at the base of every involved follicle in exceptional examples of the former and as a focus of foreign-body reaction to a hair in the latter.

Alopecia areata is an inflammatory disease in which the perifollicular connective tissue at the base of follicles is affected mostly, whereas trichotillomania is a factitious condition that results from persistent twisting of hairs, as well as plucking and pulling of them.

Clinically, alopecia areata consists of sharply circumscribed, smooth, round to oval patches of skin devoid of hairs. It is especially frequent on the scalp and face. When the process involves the entire scalp, rather than discrete patches of it, the condition is termed alopecia totalis, and when the malady affects the entire hair-bearing integument, it is called alopecia universalis. The more widespread the condition and the longer its duration, the worse the prognosis for return of hair. Vitiligo and pitting of nails may be concurrent with alopecia areata and its more extensive variants.

Histopathologically, fibrous, rather than fibrotic, tracts form in the wake of catagen and telogen follicles in alopecia areata. Absence of whorls of wiry bundles of collagen in the deep reticular dermis at bases of follicles now withered is thought to presage regrowth of hairs. In some cases of long-standing alopecia areata and its variants, whorls of wiry bundles of collagen that contain remnants of thickened, degenerated "glassy" membranes and melanophages appear in the deep reticular dermis. These whorls are signs that units of follicular matrix cells and papillae are no longer extant and, as a consequence of the inhospitable collagenous environment, hairs cannot grow at those sites again.

Trichotillomania consists clinically of irregularly shaped, partially alopecic, "rat-eaten" patches of hairs that have broken off at different distances from the surface of the scalp. The patches have a ragged appearance as a result of persistent manipulation, i.e., twisting of the hairs especially. If a patient can forego twisting of and tugging at hairs, the pelage is likely to return to normal.

Trichomalacia, a cardinal histopathologic sign of trichotillomania, results from persistent twisting back and forth of hair with consequent fraying and breakage, and dispersal of melanin in variously sized clumps within bits of broken hair shafts. The number of follicles in catagen or telogen in trichotillomania depends upon how soon after hairs are uprooted the biopsy specimen is obtained (i.e., the nearer to the time that hairs are pulled out, the greater the number of follicles in catagen). Catagen follicles are identified histologically by necrotic keratinocytes in the outer sheath and by markedly thickened corrugated glassy membranes that envelop their lower portions.

The foregoing statements about the interpretation of histopathologic characteristics of alopecia areata and trichotillomania depend upon various factors, among them duration of the disease, the site of biopsy, and the breadth and depth of the biopsy specimen.

A not uncommon accompaniment of trichotillomania is one or more signs of lichen simplex chronicus, particularly of the hyperkeratotic variant. Unlike conventional lichen simplex chronicus consequent to prolonged and persistent rubbing of the skin on the trunk and extremities typified not only by epidermal hyperplasia but by coarse bundles of collagen arranged in vertical streaks in the thickened papillary dermis, the hyperkeratotic variant of lichen simplex chronicus on a scalp (and elsewhere, such as the vulva, scrotum, and perianal region) is characterized by marked compact orthokeratosis that resembles the normal cornified layer on palms and soles. Features of hyperkeratotic lichen simplex chronicus appear sometimes on the scalp of patients with trichotillomania, in addition to the stereotypical features of trichotillomania already enumerated, a result of the same anxiety that prompts twisting and plucking out of hairs. Just as the hairs are twisted as a consequence of unresolved emotional conflicts, so, too, may the scalp be exposed to "neurotic excoriations" which result in production of erosions, ulcerations, and crusts.

20. Follicular Cyst, Infundibular Type *vs.* Follicular Cyst, Isthmus-Catagen Type

Follicular Cyst, Infundibular Type	*Follicular Cyst, Isthmus-Catagen Type*
1. Cyst lining consists of stratified squamous epithelium that resembles normal infundibulum if a follicle (and normal epidermis), i.e., the cells flatten as they mature; the granular zone persists	1. Cyst lining consists of stratified squamous epithelium that resembles normal outer sheath of a follicle at the isthmus and early in catagen, i.e., the cells become paler as they mature; no granular zone is present
2. Cyst opens to skin surface through an infundibular ostium (demonstrable if serial sections are cut)	2. Cyst does not open to skin surface as a rule
3. Normal pattern of rete ridges and dermal papillae preserved along circumference of the cyst often	3. No pattern of rete ridges and dermal papillae along circumference of the cyst
4. Lining epithelium does not project into the cyst cavity	4. Lining epithelium projects as scallops into the cyst cavity
5. Cornified cells within a cyst arranged in basket-weave and laminated pattern	5. Cornified cells within a cyst arranged compactly
6. No calcification of cornified contents of cyst	6. Calcification of cornified contents of cyst common
7. Melanin and melanocytes present in the lining epithelium, and melanin alone within the cornified cells of contents	7. Neither melanin nor melanocytes are present in the lining epithelium
8. Sebaceous (bluish granular) material among the cyst contents	8. No sebaceous material among the cyst contents
9. No cholesterol clefts within a cyst	9. Cholesterol clefts within a cyst often
10. Bacteria and yeasts within a cyst often	10. No bacteria or yeasts within a cyst usually

Follicular Cyst, Infundibular Type

Follicular Cyst, Isthmus-Catagen Type

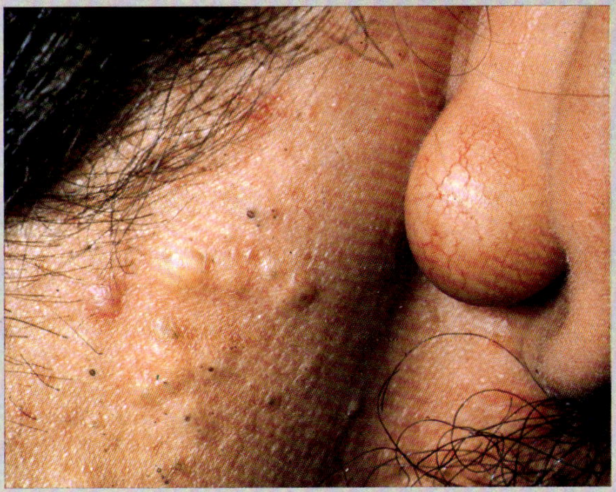

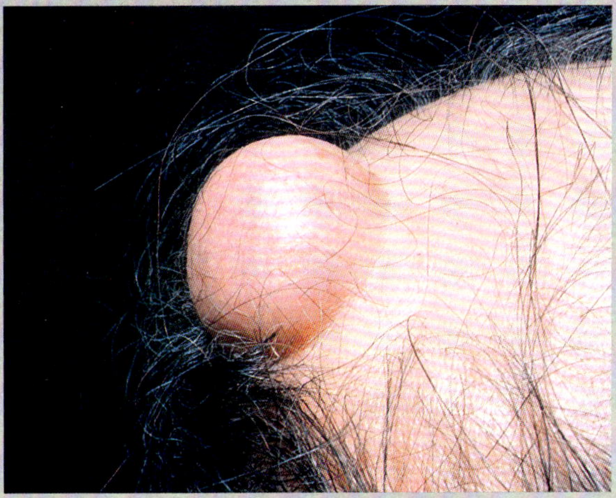

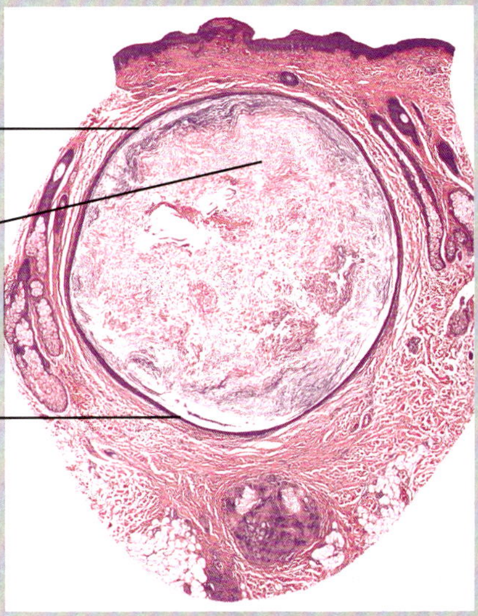

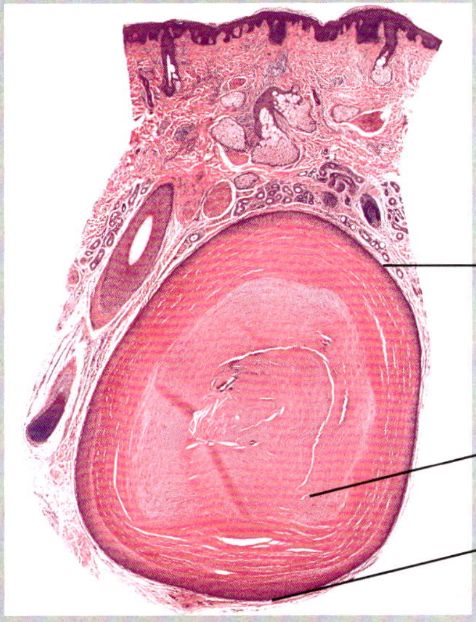

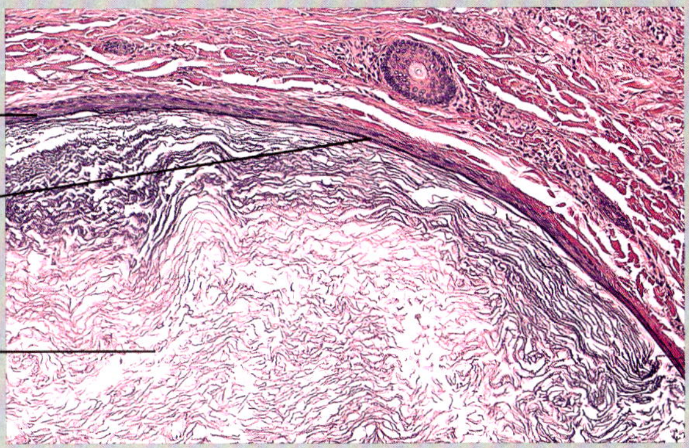

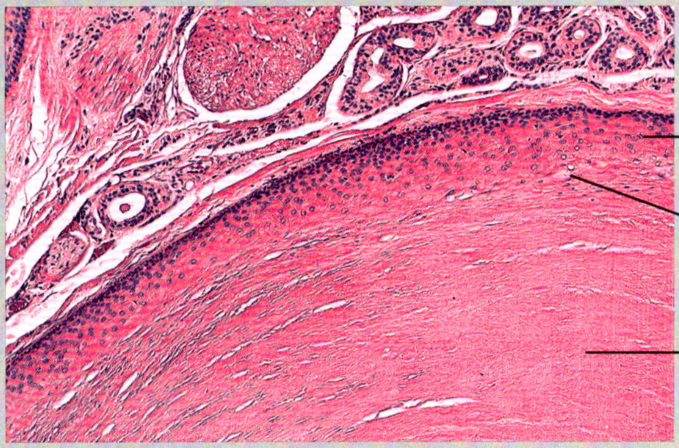

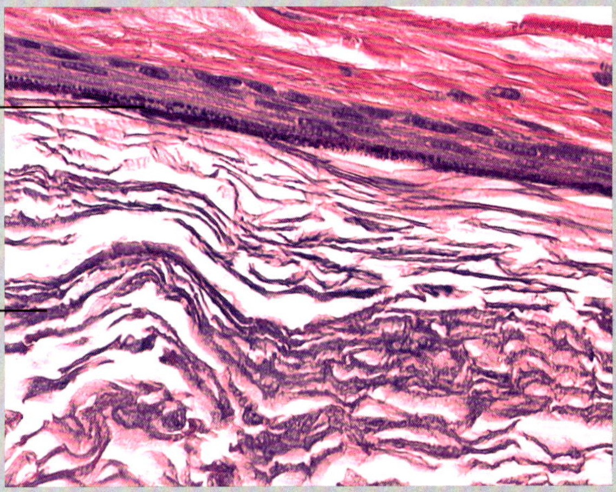

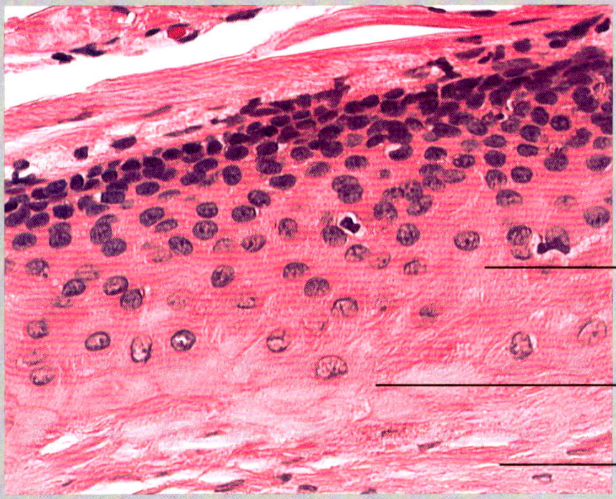

THESE two common cutaneous cysts have several features in common, namely, follicular nature, lining of stratified squamous epithelium, and cornified cells within their cavities.

We name cysts according to the normal epithelial structure of adnexa that the lining of the cyst resembles most closely, e.g., infundibular and isthmus-catagen cysts. Conventionally, hair follicle cysts of the infundibular type have been termed epidermoid or epidermal cysts, epidermal inclusion cysts, and retention cysts. Because the lining of these cysts resembles the epithelium of the infundibular portion of hair follicles, we call them infundibular cysts. The epithelial lining of an infundibulum closely resembles the epidermis histologically, as would be expected from its origin embryologically. Therefore, the term epidermoid cyst also is accurate from a morphologic vantage. Milia are simply small infundibular cysts (and rarely eccrine duct cysts).

Infundibular cysts develop especially on the face and upper part of the trunk. Frequently, a comedo marks their center. They are slow-growing, round, and moderately firm orbs. Upon gross sectioning, a rancid odor is emitted as a consequence of the effects of bacteria upon the sebaceous material within them. Sebaceous secretion enters infundibular cysts from lobules of sebaceous glands via sebaceous ducts that are continuous with bases of them.

When infundibular cysts rupture, a foreign body reaction ensues in response to contents of the cysts that are spewed into the dermis. At first there is suppuration, then granulomatous inflammation, and finally fibrosis.

Historically, hair follicle cysts of the isthmus-catagen type have been called tricholemmal cysts, pilar cysts, sebaceous cysts, and wens. The lining of isthmus-catagen cysts is the same as that of the outer sheath at the isthmus (the uppermost part of the inferior segment of a follicle) and of a follicle early in catagen (the involutional stage in a normal follicular cycle). "Tricholemmal" is a synonym for the entire outer sheath, and the lining of the cyst under discussion is like that of the upper part of the tricholemmal sheath only, namely, the isthmic portion. "Pilar" means hair and, therefore, neither infundibular nor "isthmic-catagen" cysts are truly pilar sheaths. Neither contains discernible hairs as a rule, although rarely a hair shaft may be spied in an infundibular cyst. Paradoxically, some cystic hamartomas, such as steatocystomas and folliculo-sebaceous cystic hamartomas, nearly always contain hairs, but they are not designated pilar cysts.

Isthmus-catagen cysts, in contrast to infundibular cysts, usually develop on the scalp, are hard as a result of the compact arrangement of corneocytes and of calcification of those corneocytes, and rupture infrequently.

A variant of isthmus-catagen cyst is proliferating isthmus-catagen cyst, known also as proliferating tricholemmal cyst, proliferating pilar cyst, proliferating epidermoid cyst, pilar tumor of the scalp, and subepidermal acanthoma. Histopathologically, "proliferating isthmus-catagen cyst" actually is a cystic neoplasm lined by epithelium just like that of an isthmus-catagen cyst. Proliferations of similar epithelium in aggregations of different sizes and shapes extend from the lining far into the cyst cavity. Because these neoplastic cells may exhibit nuclear atypia, mitotic figures, and signs of dyskeratosis, a proliferating isthmus-catagen cyst may be misinterpreted as a squamous-cell carcinoma. The continuous epithelial lining at the periphery of the cystic neoplasm enables it to be distinguished from a squamous-cell carcinoma. In former times, proliferating isthmus-catagen cystic neoplasms (which, for ease of communication, we term "proliferating follicular cystic neoplasm") were considered to be squamous-cell carcinomas that arose in pre-existing cysts.

Rarely, a hair follicle cyst may have a lining that in one part resembles infundibular epithelium and in another part isthmic epithelium. That combination has been referred to as a "hybrid cyst."

Last, epidermoid cysts that occur on the palms and soles are identical histopathologically to infundibular cysts, but, of course, in those locations cannot arise in pre-existing hair follicles. Whether epidermoid cysts on palms and soles are dilations of eccrine ducts or true inclusions of epidermis into the dermis secondary to puncture wounds, or both, is not yet known.

21. Syringocystadenoma Papilliferum *vs.* Hidradenoma Papilliferum

Syringocystadenoma Papilliferum	*Hidradenoma Papilliferum*
1. Not truly cystic (not a sac encircled by epithelium)	1. Truly cystic (a sac enclosed completely or almost completely by epithelium)
2. Surface of skin papillated and hyperkeratotic	2. Surface of skin domed; cornified layer normal
3. Surface of specimen covered by three types of epithelium: epidermal, follicular, and apocrine	3. Surface of specimen covered by epidermis only
4. Papillations lined by apocrine epithelium extend along the length of a cup-shaped cavity that connects at several foci with infundibular structures that lead to the skin surface	4. Numerous thin trabeculae lined by apocrine epithelium intersect a large cyst lined by apocrine epithelium within the dermis
5. Numerous sites of connection between apocrine glandular lining epithelium and epidermis; infundibular epithelium serves as conduits between those two epithelia	5. No connection between apocrine glandular epithelium and epidermis as a rule; rarely a connection exists at a single site
6. Numerous discrete apocrine glands deep in the dermis often, and sometimes in the subcutaneous fat	6. No increased number of apocrine glands in the dermis or subcutaneous fat
7. Dense infiltrate mainly of plasma cells	7. Sparse infiltrate of lymphocytes mainly, but also of plasma cells and mast cells
8. Marked edema and telangiectases	8. Little edema and no telangiectases
9. Concurrent adnexal neoplasms and other abnormalities (e.g., nevous sebaceus, hidrocystoma, hidradenoma, milia) present in sections from the same specimen	9. No association with other neoplasms or abnormalities

Syringocystadenoma Papilliferum

Hidradenoma Papilliferum

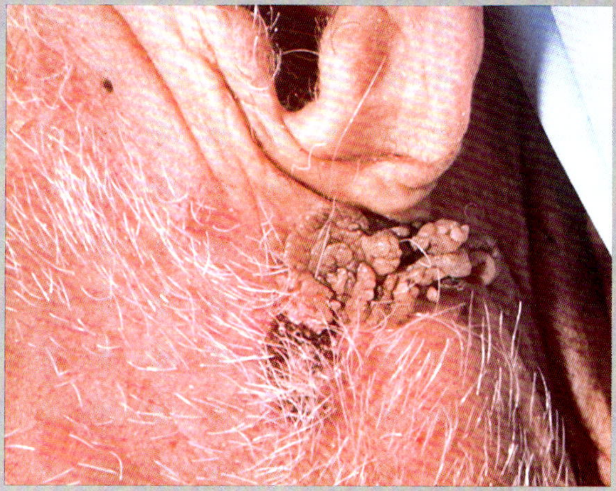

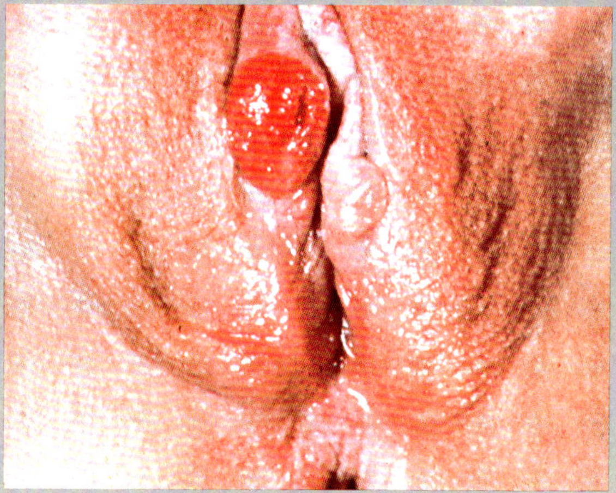

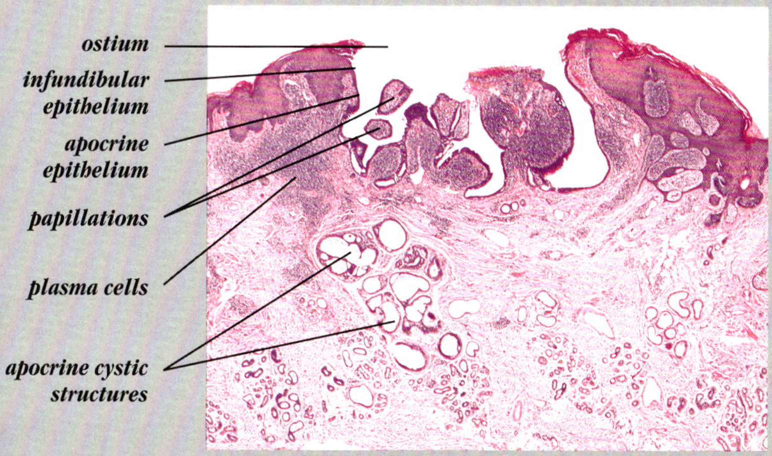

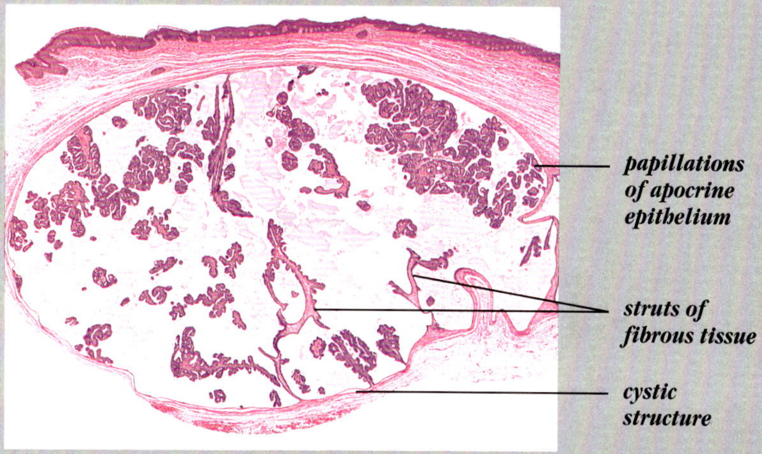

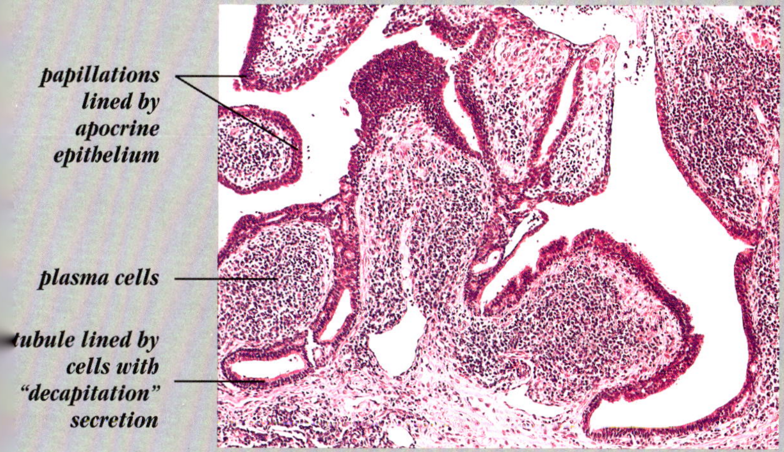

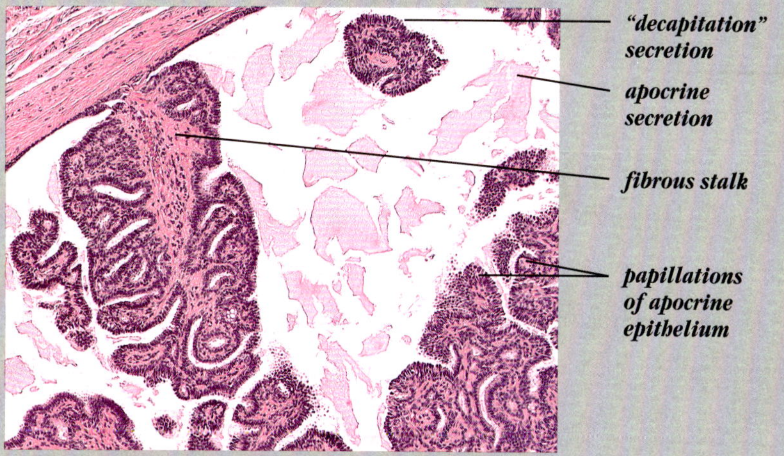

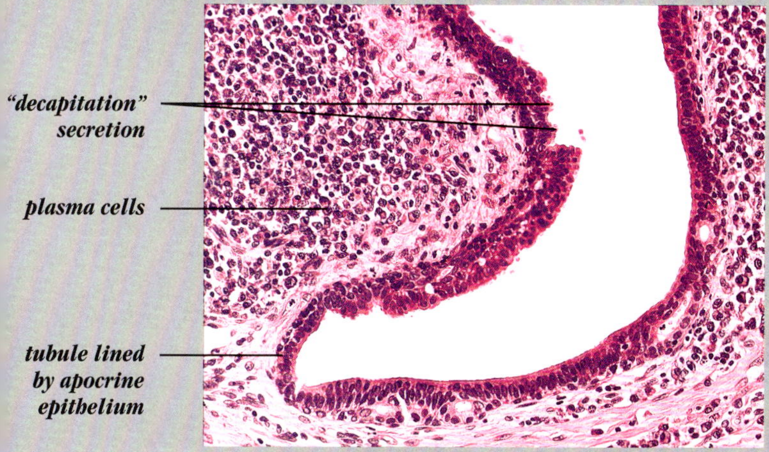

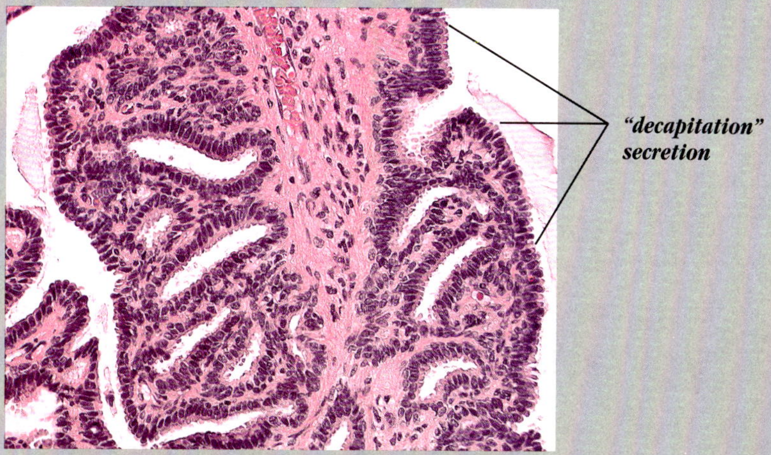

SYRINGOCYSTADENOMA papilliferum and hidradenoma papilliferum are apocrine papillated cystadenomas. The former is a hamartoma and the latter is a benign neoplasm. As a consequence of these differences, they have different clinical and histopathologic patterns.

Clinically, syringocystadenoma papilliferum appears at birth or in early childhood as a crusted, often weeping, verrucous plaque, predominantly on the scalp. Occasionally, the hamartoma occurs on the face and less frequently on the trunk or the extremities. In contrast, hidradenoma papilliferum almost always develops in adult women in the perineal or perianal areas, especially on the vulva, where it is seen to be a smooth-surfaced cystic nodule.

Histopathologically, the patterns of these two conditions are unlike, despite the fact that both are lined by apocrine glandular epithelium arranged in two rows, an outer columnar layer that shows "decapitation secretion" typical of cells of apocrine glands and an inner cuboidal one. Syringocystadenoma papilliferum is characterized by bulbous projections above the skin surface and papillations into a cup-shaped cavity that connects to the skin surface, whereas hidradenoma papilliferum consists of delicate trabecula within a cystic structure that is confined to the dermis.

Often in syringocystadenoma papilliferum, the papillated cystadenomatous endophytic component is continuous with widely dilated follicular infundibula that are filled with corneocytes. When one considers that apocrine epithelium takes origin embryologically from follicular infundibula, it is not surprising that a relationship exists between apocrine epithelium and infundibular epithelium in the hamartomatous syringocystadenoma papilliferum. Those infundibula connect directly to the epidermis.

The association, episodically, between syringocystadenoma papilliferum and nevus sebaceus of Jadassohn is well established. Many authors contend that this phenomenon occurs often, but the incidence is low in our experience. Syringocystadenoma papilliferum is but one of many hamartomas and benign and malignant neoplasms that may arise within nevus sebaceus, a hamartoma marked by alterations of the dermis, the epidermis, and the epithelial structures of adnexa.

Clinically, it is relatively easy to suspect the presence of a syringocystadenoma papilliferum in association with a nevus sebaceus. The former lesion is often verrucous and reddish-brown, and its surface is moist as a consequence of secretions from apocrine glandular cells. In contrast, the latter lesion is yellowish, and its surface is like cobblestones and dry.

Syringocystadenoma papilliferum, hidradenoma papilliferum, and the apocrine type of mixed tumor are the three most common cutaneous cystadenomatous conditions with apocrine differentiation. "Decapitation secretion" is the sine qua non for establishing the apocrine nature of cysts, hamartomas, and neoplasms. Only exceedingly rarely do syringocystadenoma papilliferum and hidradenoma papilliferum eventuate in apocrine carcinoma.

A few words should be written about an important cystadenomatous analogue of hidradenoma papilliferum that may be situated on a nipple. This cystic adenoma is known by a variety of names, among them nipple adenoma, subareolar papillomatosis, and erosive adenomatosis. It is considered to be a pseudo-malignancy because at times it has been misinterpreted histopathologically as a primary carcinoma of the breast. Such confusion has resulted in unnecessary mastectomy. Nipple adenoma, like many benign neoplasms, is symmetrical, well-circumscribed, and wedge-shaped.

22. Ichthyosis Vulgaris *vs.* X-linked Ichthyosis

Ichthyosis Vulgaris	*X-linked Ichthyosis*
1. Cornified layer thickened, but less than half the thickness of the remainder of the epidermis	1. Cornified layer thickened and often at least half the thickness of the remainder of the epidermis
2. Compact laminated orthokeratosis associated often with plugs of infundibula by corneocytes (keratosis pilaris)	2. Compact laminated orthokeratosis, but no plugs of infundibula by corneocytes usually
3. Granular zone thinned (to about one row of cells) or nearly absent	3. Granular zone normal (two or three rows of cells) or even slightly thickened to as many as five rows of cells
4. Thinned suprapapillary plates	4. Normal suprapapillary plates
5. Thinned epidermis with muted rete ridges	5. Normal or slightly thickened epidermis with preserved rete ridges
6. Undulations between epidermal rete ridges and dermal papillae shallow or flat	6. Normal undulations between epidermal rete ridges and dermal papillae
7. Mitotic figures in the basal layer rare	7. Mitotic figures in the basal layer occasionally

Ichthyosis Vulgaris | *X-linked Ichthyosis*

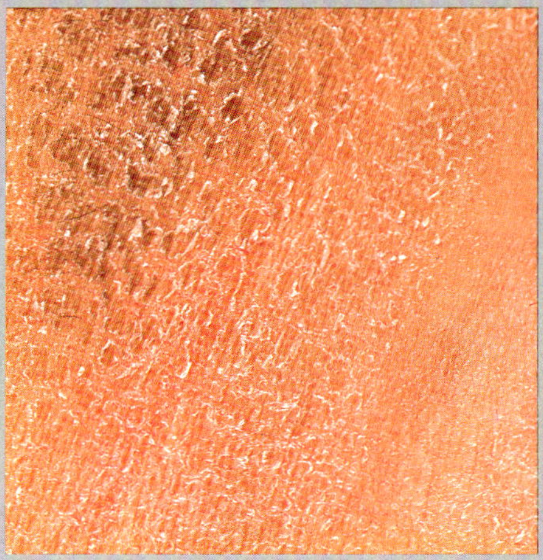

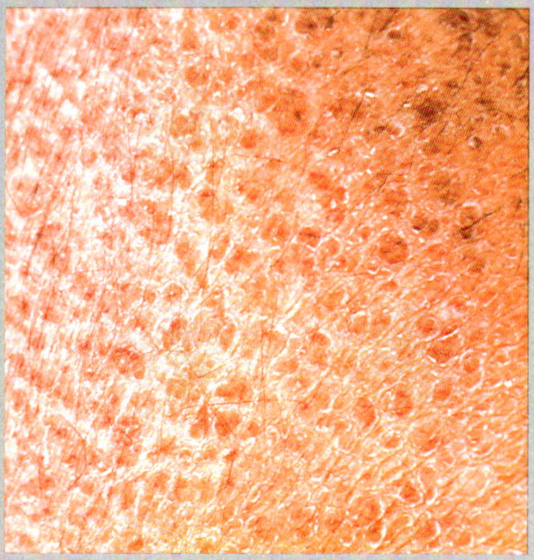

cornified cells in basket-weave and laminated patterns

rete ridges not prominent

dilated infundibulum plugged by cornified cells

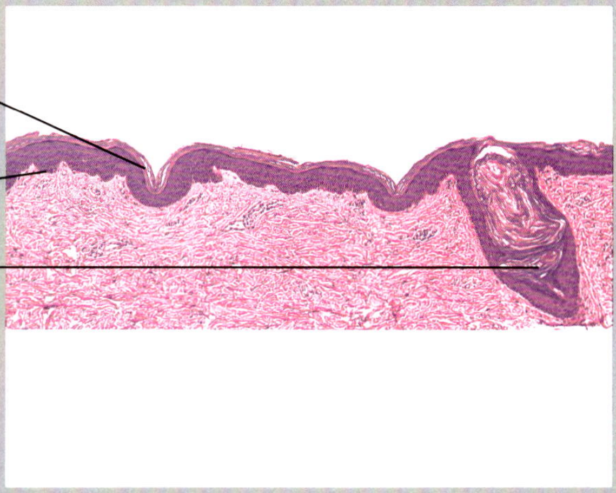

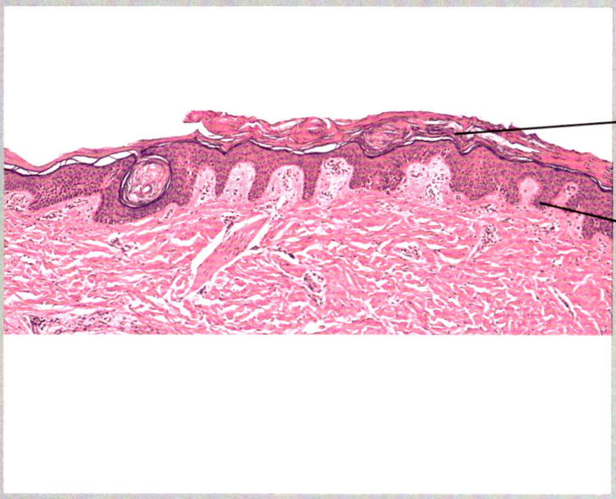

cornified cells in laminated array

rete ridges prominent

cornified cells in laminated and basket-weave patterns

infundibulum plugged by cornified cells

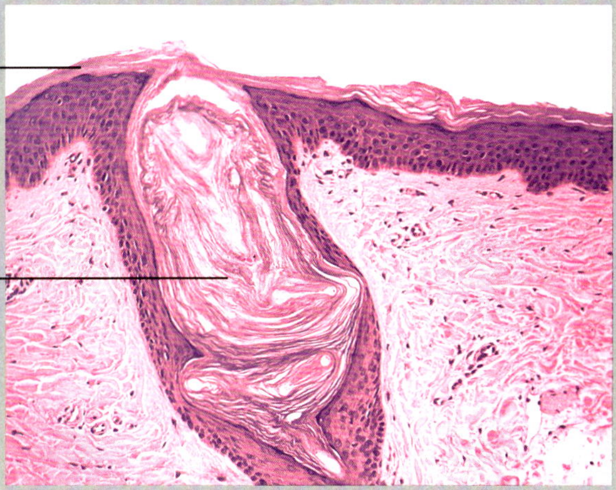

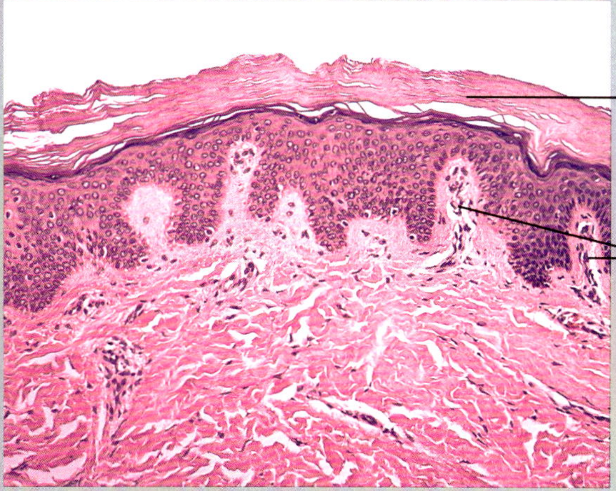

laminated arrangement of cornified cells

undulations between rete ridges and dermal papillae

laminated orthokeratosis

granular layer but one cell thick

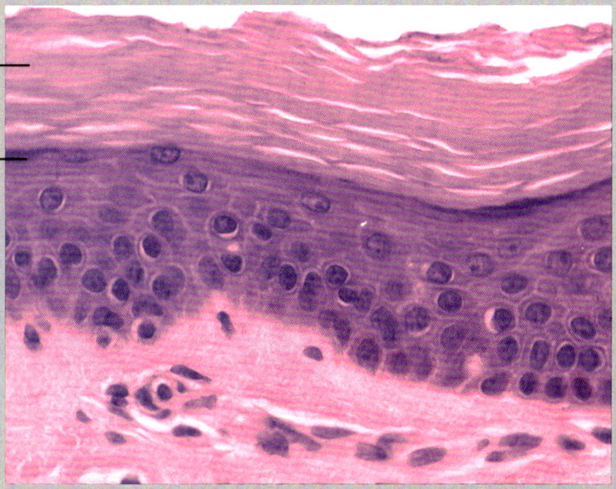

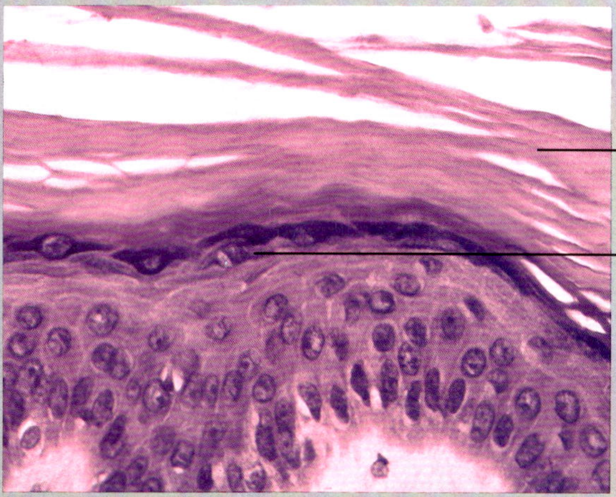

compact and laminated orthokeratosis

granular layer several cells thick

ICHTHYOSIS vulgaris and X-linked ichthyosis are true ichthyoses because the clinical appearance of their scales resembles those of fish (In Greek, *ichthos* means fish, and *-osis* means a condition of). As in all ichthyoses, the scales are thickest on the legs. Histopathologically, the scales of both ichthyosis vulgaris and X-linked ichthyosis consist mostly of compactly arranged laminated orthokeratosis. The epidermal turnover time in both conditions is about normal.

Ichthyosis vulgaris is an autosomal dominant condition that develops early in childhood. Affected individuals usually show widespread fine scaling of the skin, most apparent on the trunk and extremities, but with a tendency to spare the flexures. Common concurrents of ichthyosis vulgaris are atopic diathesis and propensity to keratosis pilaris. Youngsters with ichthyosis vulgaris have such severe accentuation of the normal skin markings on the palms and soles that the volar surfaces of their hands and feet often resemble those of elderly persons.

Ichthyosis vulgaris, as the name suggests, is more common than X-linked ichthyosis. The latter condition, in its fullest expression, affects males only; female heterozygotes, however, may be affected slightly. Present at birth or shortly thereafter, X-linked ichthyosis tends to involve much of the body surface including the sides of the face, neck, and flexural areas. Unlike ichthyosis vulgaris, there are no abnormalities of skin markings on the palms and soles of persons with X-linked ichthyosis. Corneal opacities may be found in patients with X-linked ichthyosis and in female carriers of the disease.

A third true ichthyosis is lamellar ichthyosis. Lamellar ichthyosis is characterized histopathologically by markedly thickened, compactly organized, laminated orthokeratosis (much thicker than that of either ichthyosis vulgaris or X-linked ichthyosis), hypergranulosis (sometimes more than seven cells thick), psoriasiform hyperplasia (the long rete ridges usually are also broad), increased numbers of mitotic figures within the basal layer of the epidermis (epidermopoiesis is increased markedly), and a sparse, superficial, perivascular infiltrate of lymphocytes. Lamellar ichthyosis is uncommon compared to X-linked ichthyosis and rare in comparison to ichthyosis vulgaris. It is transmitted in autosomal recessive fashion, and infants who have the condition often are born with skin that appears to be covered by a tight shiny envelope that resembles collodion or a baked apple. When this shiny membrane is shed, erythroderma and large, plate-like scales are revealed. The scales are widespread.

Non-bullous congenital ichthyosiform erythroderma is a fourth example of true ichthyosis and the only one characterized by evidence of an inflammatory process. The histopathologic pattern is slight spongiotic psoriasiform dermatitis with parakeratosis. Clinically, those afflicted exhibit an erythroderma covered by fish-like scales. Ectropion is a common complication and may invite injuries to the cornea.

Another type of ichthyosis emerges in adulthood as an acquired condition, apparently as a consequence of an underlying disease like Hodgkin's disease, carcinoma of the breast, and lepromatous leprosy. Individual scales of acquired ichthyosis have the clinical and histopathologic features of ichthyosis vulgaris.

Bullous congenital ichthyosiform erythroderma, listed invariably in classifications of the ichthyoses, is not truly an ichthyosis for several reasons, the most important of which is its total lack of resemblance clinically to scales of fish. Clinically, bullous congenital ichthyosiform erythroderma is characterized by widespread verrucous keratoses and histopathologically by epidermolytic hyperkeratosis. Intra-epidermal blisters may develop in children with the disorder, sometimes as a result of superimposed bacterial infection of the skin. Bullous congenital ichthyosiform erythroderma is inherited as an autosomal dominant trait, is evident at birth, and is one type of widespread epidermal nevus. A circumscribed form of the disorder is known as ichthyosis hystrix, and it, too, is an epidermal nevus, rather than an expression of ichthyosis. A localized form of this particular epidermal nevus with distinctive histopathologic features of epidermolytic hyperkeratosis is confined to palms and soles.

The term ichthyosis also has been applied incorrectly to conditions like ichthyosis linearis circumflexa.

23. Epidermolytic Hyperkeratosis *vs.* Plane Wart

Epidermolytic Hyperkeratosis	*Plane Wart*
1. Laminated and/or compact orthokeratosis; basket-weave orthokeratosis in foci uncommon	1. Basket-weave orthokeratosis and/or parakeratosis
2. Prominent papillated (sometimes digitated) thickened epidermis	2. Slightly papillated epidermal hyperplasia
3. Epidermis may be thickened markedly	3. Epidermis thickened slightly
4. Ill-defined, pale zones of various sizes around nuclei of keratinocytes throughout the viable epidermis	4. Well-defined, clear spaces of various sizes around nuclei of keratinocytes in the upper half of the epidermis
5. Keratinocytes lack distinct boundaries, which gives the epidermis a reticulated appearance	5. Keratinocytes have distinct boundaries; no reticulated appearance to the epidermis
6. Numerous large and small, irregularly shaped, basophilic keratohyaline-like bodies and often eosinophilic trichohyalin-like bodies throughout the epidermis, except for the basal layer	6. Large and small, irregularly shaped, basophilic keratohyaline-like bodies in cells of the upper spinous and granular zones; no trichohyalin-like bodies
7. No blue-gray bubbly cytoplasm of keratinocytes	7. Blue-gray bubbly cytoplasm of keratinocytes in early lesions
8. Increased number of mitotic figures in the lower portion of the epidermis	8. No increased number of mitotic figures in the epidermis
9. No arborization of rete ridges or adnexal epithelium at the periphery of a lesion	9. Slight arborization, i.e., inward turning of outermost elongated rete ridges or epithelial structures of adnexa at the periphery of a lesion common
10. Blood vessels in the papillary dermis not dilated prominently	10. Blood vessels in the papillary dermis markedly dilated and tortuous

Epidermolytic Hyperkeratosis

Plane Wart (Verruca Plana)

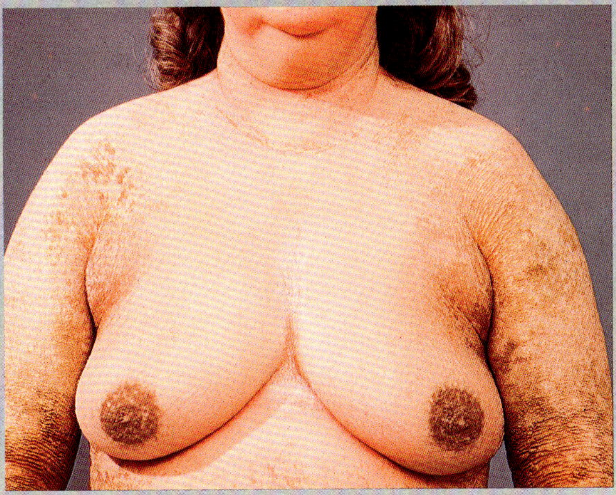

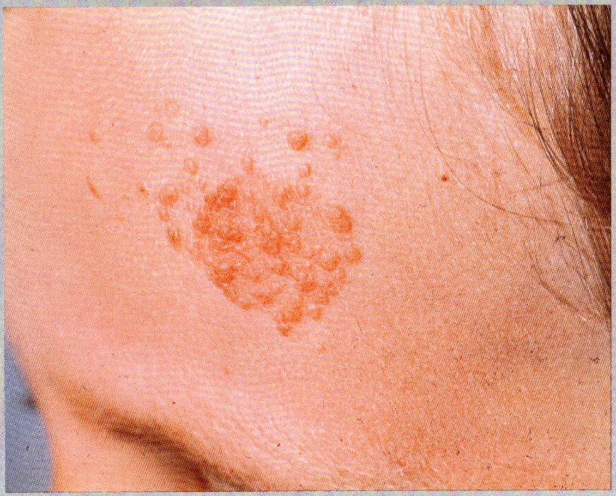

hyperkeratosis

papillated surface

pale keratinocytes

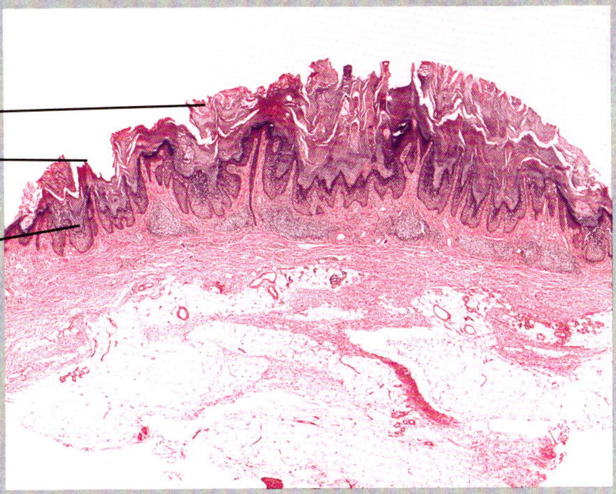

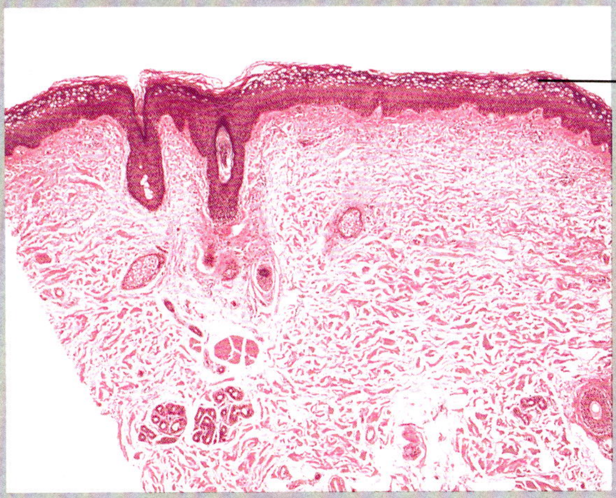

clear cells across a broad zone

compact and laminated orthokeratosis

papillation

ypergranulosis

"epidermolytic" changes in spinous and granular zone

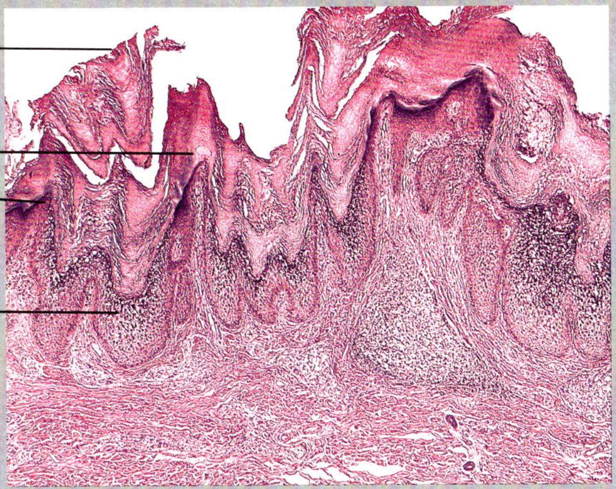

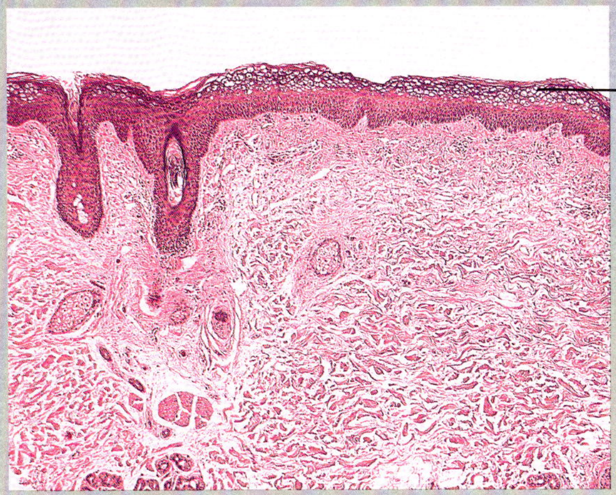

clear cells in the upper half of the epidermis

compact orthokeratosis

pergranulosis

poor cohesion etween keratinocytes ("epidermolysis")

pallor of keratinocytes

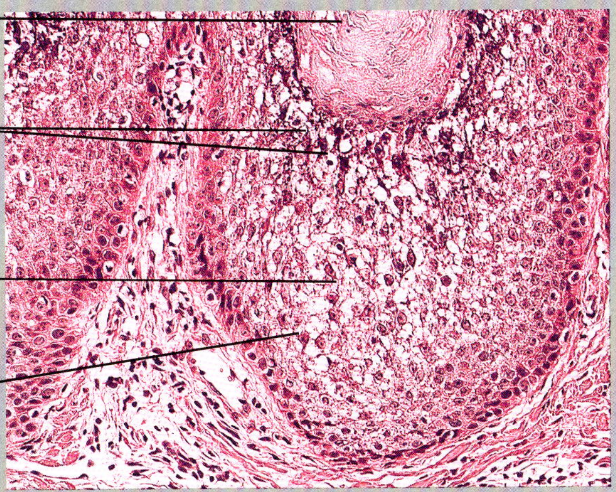

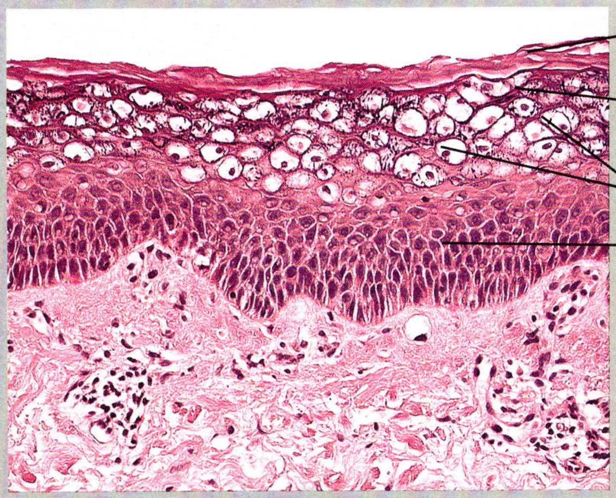

compact orthokeratosis

hypergranulosis

clear cells

normal appearing spinous cells

EPIDERMOLYTIC hyperkeratosis and a plane wart share several histopathologic features, namely, papillated and thickened epidermis, hypergranulosis, and cells with pale cytoplasm within the epidermis. The terms "epidermolytic hyperkeratosis" and "plane wart" are not in parallel with one another, however. Epidermolytic hyperkeratosis is a description of histopathologic findings that occur in several skin diseases, and plane wart is a designation for a specific disease. Because of their numerous similarities histopathologically, epidermolytic hyperkeratosis and plane wart form the basis for an authentic differential diagnosis.

Epidermolytic hyperkeratosis is a descriptive term for distinctive histopathologic changes that appear in several acquired and congenital conditions. As the term denotes, the epidermis appears to have lysed and is hyperkeratotic. In actuality, there is no lysis at all, only ill-defined boundaries between enlarged, pale keratinocytes in a thickened epidermis. This epidermis is characterized further by innumerable keratohyaline granules throughout the upper two thirds of it especially, and sometimes by a sprinkling of trichohyalin granules, too. These changes are topped by compact orthokeratosis.

When the term "epidermolytic hyperkeratosis" was introduced, it was meant to be specific for, diagnostic of, and synonymous with bullous congenital ichthyosiform erythroderma, a widespread epidermal nevus. Subsequently, the histopathologic features of epidermolytic hyperkeratosis were noted in other nevoid conditions of the epidermis, particularly ichthyosis hystrix and some hereditary keratodermas of the palms and soles. In addition, the phenomenon of epidermolytic hyperkeratosis has been reported in widespread follicular eruptions (nevoid follicular epidermolytic hyperkeratosis), follicular cysts, benign solitary keratoses (epidermolytic acanthomas), and solar keratoses, and as an incidental finding in tiny foci within the epidermis of various inflammatory diseases and benign and malignant neoplasms, especially malignant melanomas. As a histopathologic phenomenon, epidermolytic hyperkeratosis has been compared to other distinctive patterns of epithelial abnormalities in skin, namely, focal acantholytic dyskeratosis, cornoid lamellation, pale-cell acanthosis, and follicular mucinosis. Epidermolytic hyperkeratosis and focal acantholytic dyskeratosis may occur in the epidermis of the same specimen, either in separate discrete foci or side by side.

Plane warts are slightly elevated, mostly flat-topped, relatively smooth-surfaced, discrete papules that vary in color from that of normal skin to tan. They occur most commonly on the face and dorsal aspect of the distal parts of the upper extremities. The cause of verruca plana is papillomavirus.

Fully developed warts of different types on the skin, mucocutaneous surfaces, and mucous membranes have different architectural patterns. For example, plane warts are characterized by slightly mamillated epidermal hyperplasia, whereas condylomata acuminata show more markedly papillomatous epidermal hyperplasia, and fully developed lesions of verrucae vulgares exhibit digitated epidermal hyperplasia. In contrast, plantar warts are mostly endophytic, as a result of pressure exerted upon them by walking.

The papillomavirus responsible for warts also seems to be capable of causing squamous-cell carcinomas. Epidermodysplasia verruciformis, a condition that consists of numerous plane warts, is associated sometimes with the development of squamous-cell carcinomas at the sites of the plane warts. Giant condyloma acuminatum of Buschke-Löwenstein is a euphemism for verrucous squamous-cell carcinoma on the genitalia and, as the name suggests, is thought to arise in a pre-existing condyloma acuminatum. Carcinoma cuniculatum conceivably could arise in pre-existing mosaic warts, and florid oral papillomatosis may be squamous-cell carcinoma secondary to infection of that epithelium by papillomavirus.

Bowenoid papulosis consists of many small, innocuous-looking papules particularly on the genitalia of young adults. The papules, when viewed by conventional microscopy, have the silhouette of condylomata acuminata but the cytologic features of squamous-cell carcinoma in situ. Bowenoid papulosis represents condylomata acuminata that have eventuated in squamous-cell carcinomas in situ. We also have seen squamous-cell carcinomas that seem to have arisen within verrucae vulgares.

24. Nevus Verrucosus *vs.* Acanthosis Nigricans

Nevus Verrucosus	*Acanthosis Nigricans*
1. Orthokeratosis compact	1. Orthokeratosis in basket-weave and laminated patterns
2. Thick epidermis, either papillated or digitated	2. Thin epidermis
3. Hypergranulosis usually	3. Granular zone normal or slightly decreased
4. Epidermis sometimes hyperpigmented	4. Epidermis consistently hyperpigmented
5. Projections of elongated dermal papillae above the skin surface, but papillomatosis not prominent	5. Papillomatosis prominent

Nevus Verrucosus	Acanthosis Nigricans

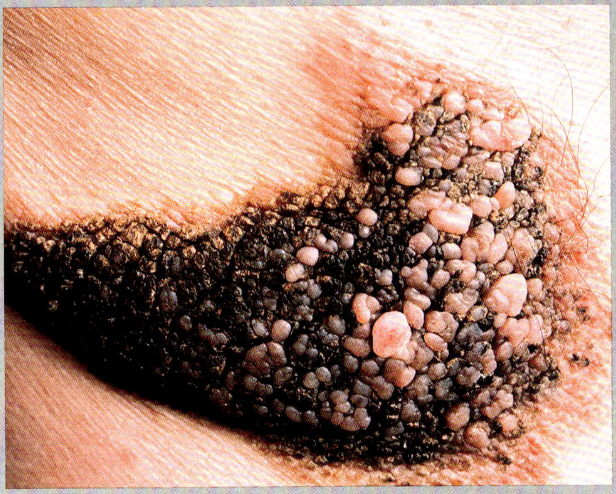

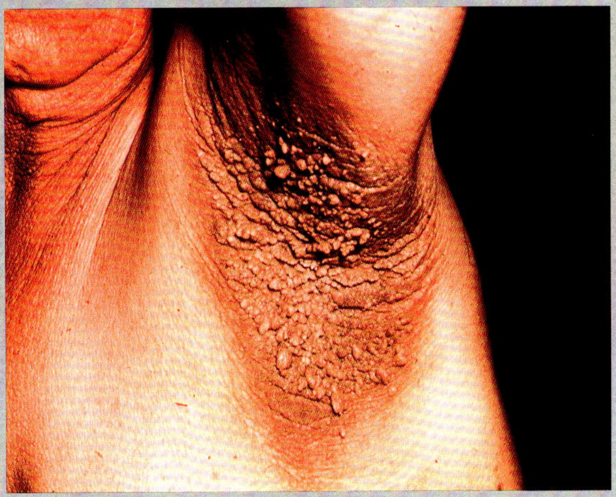

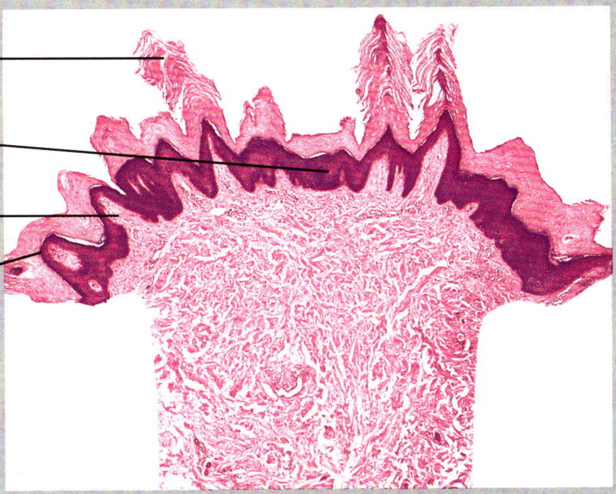

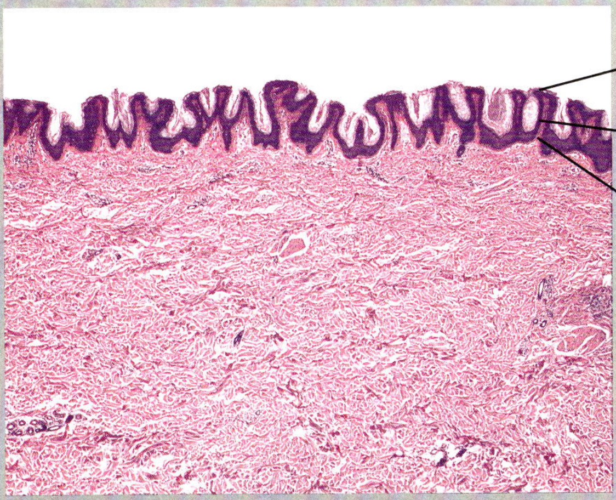

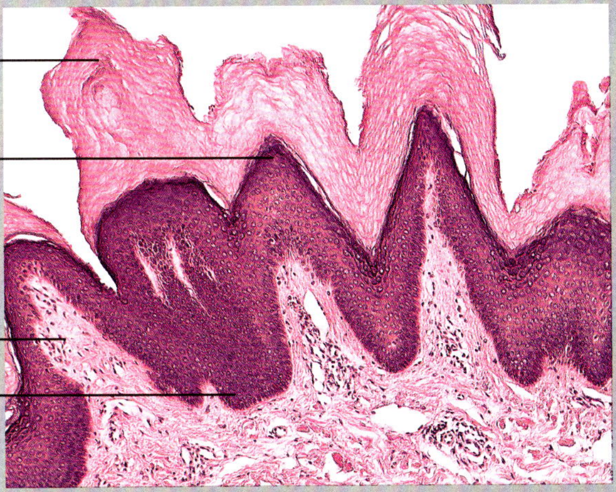

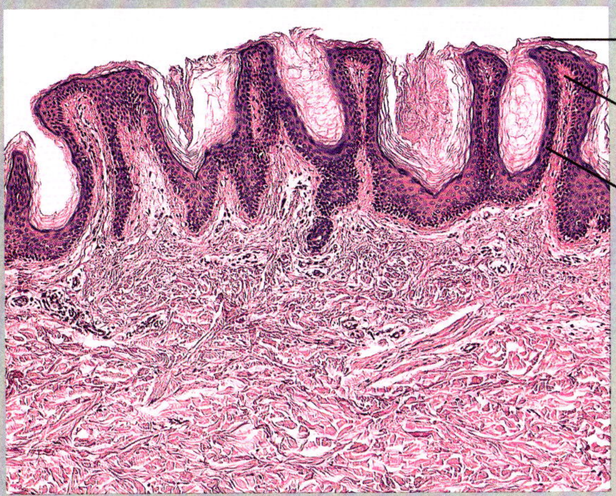

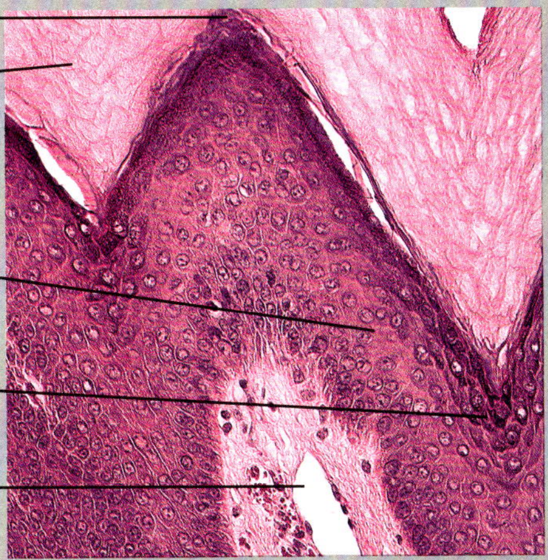

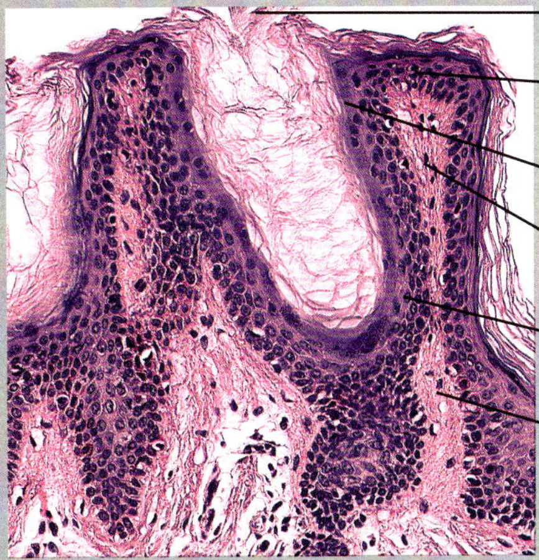

NEVUS verrucosus and acanthosis nigricans are processes that affect the papillary dermis and the epidermis. Both conditions may show hyperkeratosis, epidermal hyperpigmentation, papillomatosis, melanophages, and an increased number of fibrocytes in a thickened pale-staining papillary dermis.

Nevus verrucosus is an epidermal nevus, one among many. It usually starts to develop at birth or shortly afterward in the form of tan to brown, rough-surfaced, warty lesions. Like most other epidermal nevi of this type, nevus verrucosus usually is distributed in a circumscribed or systematized fashion, e.g., in linear or zosteriform pattern, and occasionally is widespread, e.g., on one half of the body. All unilateral epidermal nevi are termed nevus unius lateris. Rarely, nevus verrucosus may be universal, i.e., the entire integument is covered by it. The attributes of nevus verrucosus in general also apply to other types of epidermal nevi, such as those characterized histopathologically by epidermolytic hyperkeratosis (traditionally known as bullous congenital ichthyosiform erythroderma when widespread and as ichthyosis hystrix when more limited), focal acantholytic dyskeratosis (which is like Darier's disease histopathologically, but not clinically or biologically), cornoid lamellation (which usually is taken to be a histopathologic sign of porokeratosis), and seborrheic keratosis-like (which resembles a seborrheic keratosis histopathologically).

In contrast, acanthosis nigricans may be congenital or acquired. Clinically, irrespective of onset, the lesions are smooth rather than rough-surfaced, and histopathologically they are mostly papillomatoses, i.e., exaggerations of dermal papillae, rather than essentially keratoses. The velvety, tan to gray-brown excrescences of acanthosis nigricans tend to develop especially in intertriginous regions, such as the axillae and groin; the neck, umbilicus, and nipples are other favored sites. Conventionally, acanthosis nigricans has been classified into three types as follows: an autosomal dominant anomaly that appears in childhood ("benign" acanthosis nigricans); an aspect of an underlying endocrinologic abnormality, such as acromegaly, gigantism, diabetes insipidus, and Cushing's disease, or from obesity and ingestion of medications, such as corticosteroids and nicotinic acid ("pseudo"-acanthosis nigricans), and a portentous manifestation of an occult malignant neoplasm, usually an adenocarcinoma of the gastrointestinal or genital tract, breast, or lung ("malignant" acanthosis nigricans). Each of these forms of acanthosis nigricans, irrespective of the underlying cause, has the same fundamental clinical and histopathologic features.

The terms "benign," "pseudo," and "malignant" in the context of acanthosis nigricans are flawed. Morphologically (clinically and histopathologically) and biologically, acanthosis nigricans is a single pathologic process in the skin. It is neither benign nor malignant, and it is authentic, not pseudo. The factors responsible for it, however, are various. Obesity, in itself, is probably not one of them; the endocrinologic factors responsible for obesity probably are. In short, the accurate histopathologic diagnosis is "acanthosis nigricans," unmodified, and that diagnosis should prompt a clinician to consider and seek causes for it.

Other systematized congenital anomalies have clinical and histopathologic features reminiscent of acanthosis nigricans, some with such marked papillomatosis that they resemble innumerable fibro-epithelial polyps or papillomas (skin-"tags," acrochordons). They are malformations of the papillary dermis, i.e., connective tissue nevi. The confluent and reticulated papillomatosis of Gougerot and Carteaud resembles acanthosis nigricans closely histopathologically, although some authors continue to claim that it is an expression of amyloidosis.

In conclusion, the rough surface of nevus verrucosus signifies that it is basically an epidermal process, whereas the smooth surface of acanthosis nigricans indicates that it is primarily a dermal one.

25. Porokeratosis vs. Inflammatory Linear Verrucous Epidermal Nevus

Porokeratosis	*Inflammatory Linear Verrucous Epidermal Nevus*
1. Tall, thin, sharply circumscribed columns of parakeratosis (cornoid lamellae)	1. Short, broad, moderately well-circumscribed columns of parakeratosis
2. Columns of parakeratosis not perpendicular to the skin surface	2. Columns of parakeratosis perpendicular to the skin surface
3. Parakeratotic columns may be continuous with epidermal, acrosyringial, or infundibular epithelium	3. Parakeratotic columns are continuous with epidermis
4. Columns of parakeratosis are situated usually in valleys between papillations of thickened epidermis	4. Columns of parakeratosis are present usually at summits of papillations
5. Between foci of parakeratosis, the stratum corneum is hyperkeratotic, with alternations of basket-weave and compact patterns	5. Between zones of parakeratosis, the stratum corneum is hyperkeratotic in compact pattern
6. Beneath parakeratotic foci, no granular cells; dyskeratotic and vacuolated cells in the spinous zone are nearly invariable	6. Beneath parakeratotic foci, no granular, dyskeratotic, or vacuolated cells in the spinous zone
7. Beneath zones of orthokeratosis, the granular zone is normal or thickened	7. Beneath zones of orthokeratosis, the granular zone is thickened
8. Epidermis papillated, psoriasiform, or atrophic depending upon the type of porokeratosis and the stage of the disease	8. Epidermis thickened, usually papillated, and psoriasiform
9. Lichenoid infiltrate of lymphocytes in early lesions of the disseminated superficial type	9. Superficial perivascular lymphocytic infiltrate

Porokeratosis

Inflammatory Linear Verrucous Epidermal Nevus

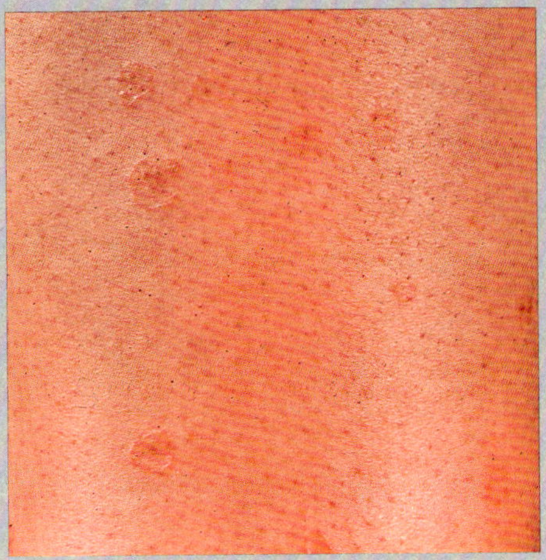

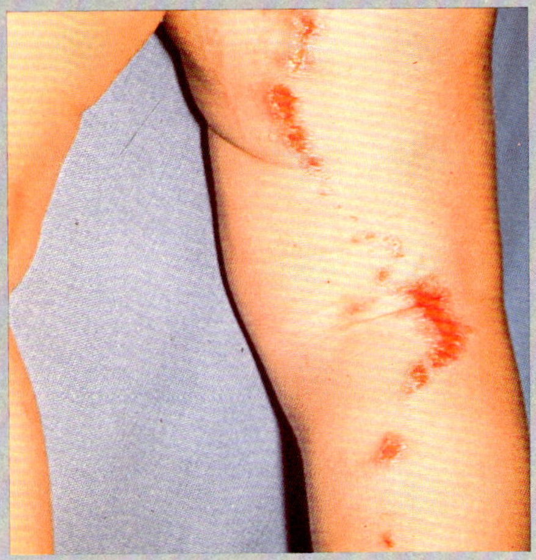

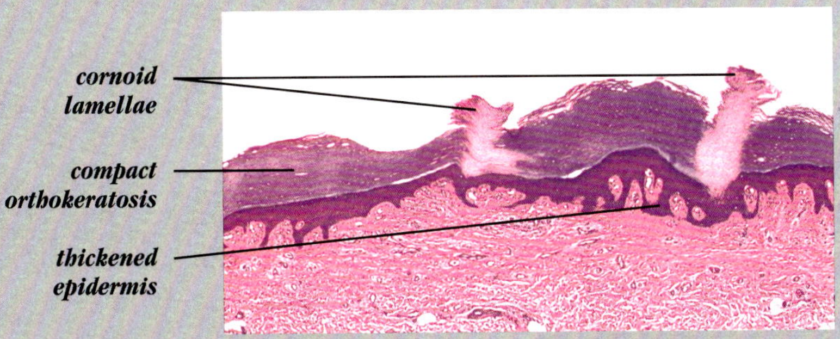

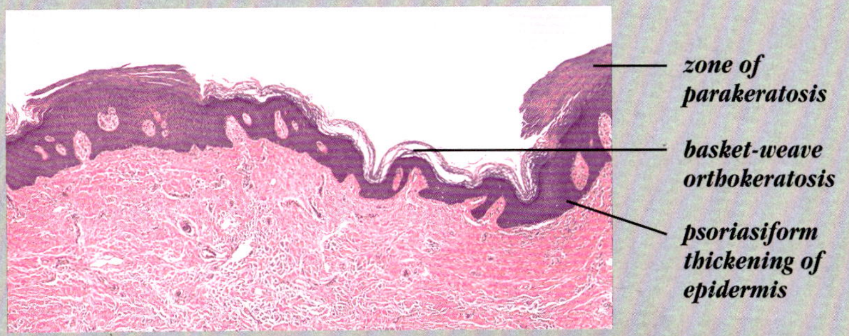

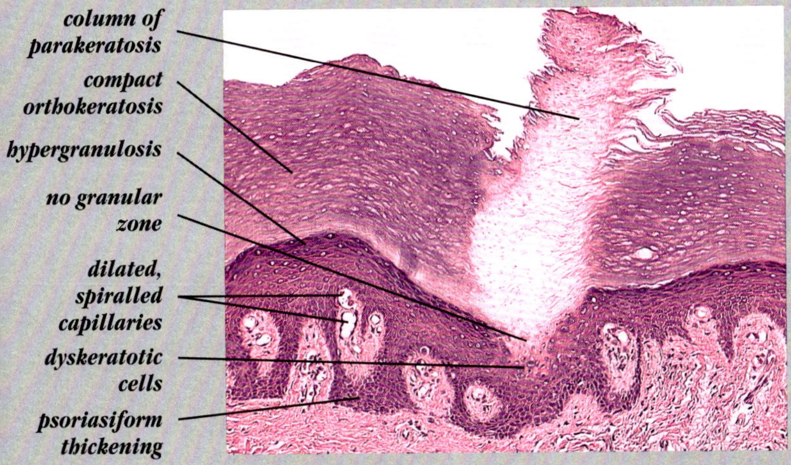

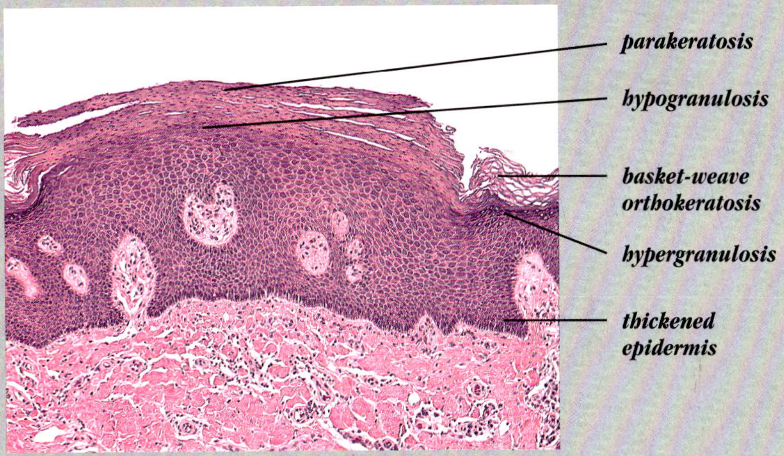

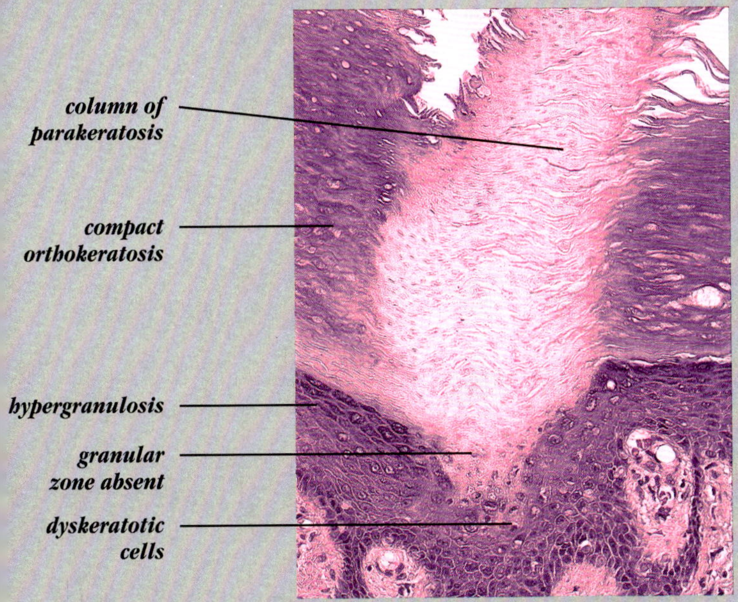

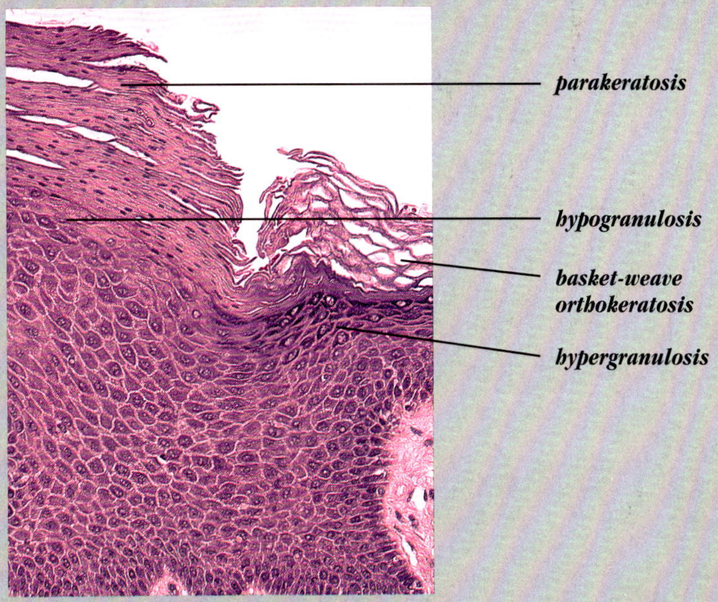

POROKERATOSIS in its various forms and the inflammatory linear verrucous epidermal nevus have in common well-circumscribed foci of parakeratosis beneath which the granular layer is absent, alternation of zones of ortho- and parakeratosis, and a lymphocytic infiltrate around dilated blood vessels in the upper part of the dermis. The several porokeratoses and inflammatory linear verrucous epidermal nevus are diseases that involve the epidermis predominantly and overtly, but the papillary dermis must be affected, too, if only covertly.

There are several varieties of porokeratosis, namely, porokeratosis of Mibelli, nevoid linear porokeratosis, punctate porokeratosis of the palms and soles, widespread punctate porokeratosis, and disseminated superficial porokeratosis (actinic and non-actinic types). The first to be recognized was porokeratosis of Mibelli, a genodermatosis that is inherited as an autosomal dominant trait. It may appear at any age, but usually is manifest early in childhood. The clinical lesions are papules and plaques delineated sharply from surrounding normal skin by a keratotic ridge marked by a slight central depression. Eventually, the centers of the lesions become atrophic. Lesions of porokeratosis of Mibelli may appear on any part of the skin and even may involve mucous membranes. They are asymptomatic and, in time, tend to increase in number and size; some may resolve without treatment.

A disseminated superficial type of porokeratosis, which is the most common expression of porokeratosis, was described in the 1970s by Chernosky. Prior to their recognition as distinctive phenomena, lesions of disseminated superficial actinic porokeratosis usually were deemed to be nothing more than solar keratoses. The condition presents itself as few or many, round or oval lesions rimmed by a thread-like keratotic border. Early in their evolution the centers are erythematous, but eventually they become gray or white and atrophic. Lesions of disseminated superficial porokeratosis have a predilection for sites that ordinarily are exposed to sunlight. Lesions indistinguishable from those of disseminated superficial actinic porokeratosis may appear on cutaneous parts that are not in the path of rays of the sun, such as the palms, soles, and genitals. This variant is termed "disseminated superficial porokeratosis."

Thin cornoid lamellae make up the thread-like rims of lesions in all forms of porokeratosis, and dense lichenoid lymphocytic infiltrates associated with dilated blood-filled venules are responsible for the erythematous appearance of centers of early lesions of the disseminated superficial actinic and non-actinic types. Clinical signs of atrophy in the centers of lesions result both from replacement of the normal papillary dermis by coarse bundles of collagen and from effacement of the normal undulating pattern formed by rete ridges and dermal papillae. Rarely, a squamous-cell carcinoma may develop in the atrophic center of a lesion of porokeratosis.

The inflammatory linear verrucous epidermal nevus appears at birth or shortly thereafter as a linear or patchy aggregation of reddish scaly papules most often, for inexplicable reasons, on a right leg of a girl. An arm also may be the extremity involved. Clinically, the condition must be differentiated from other examples of nevus unius lateris and from linear psoriasis, linear lichen planus, and lichen striatus.

26. Amputation Neuroma Secondary to Supernumerary Digit *vs.* Acquired Digital Fibrokeratoma

Amputation Neuroma Secondary to Supernumerary Digit

1. Increased number of large nerve trunks throughout the specimen
2. Nerve trunks and collagen bundles oriented perpendicular to the skin surface (i.e., parallel to the long axis of the elongated anomaly)
3. Fibrocytes not usually increased in number and are normal cytologically
4. Collagen bundles thick and coarse

Acquired Digital Fibrokeratoma

1. No nerve structures within the lesion itself
2. Collagen bundles arranged haphazardly
3. Fibrocytes markedly increased in number and often are large, stellate, or multinucleated
4. Collagen bundles mostly fibrillar; some are coarse

Amputation Neuroma Secondary to Supernumerary Digit

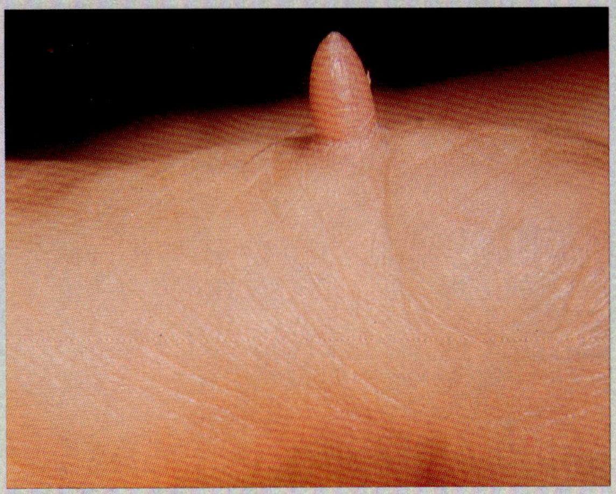

Acquired Digital Fibrokeratoma

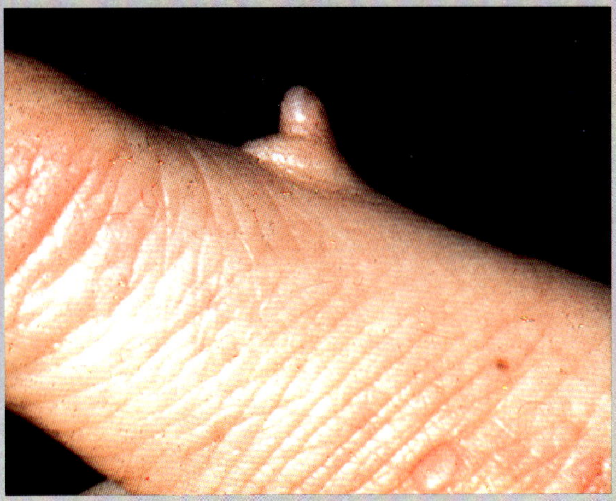

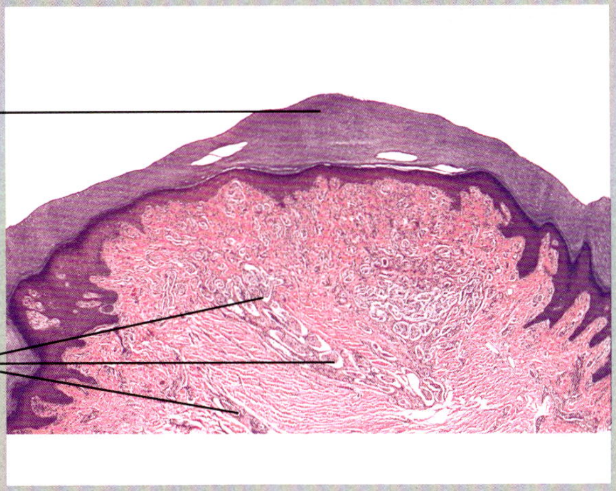

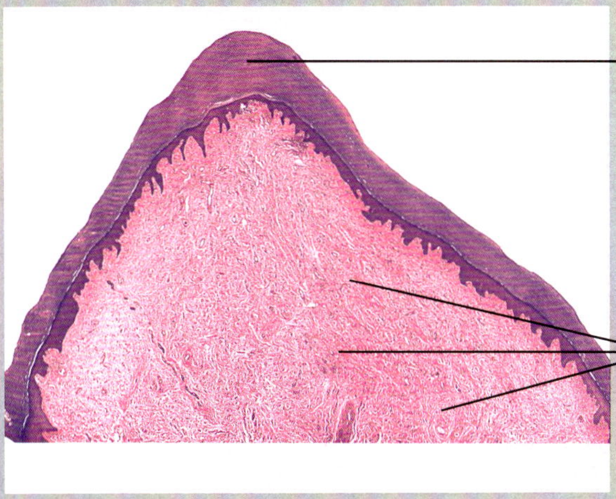

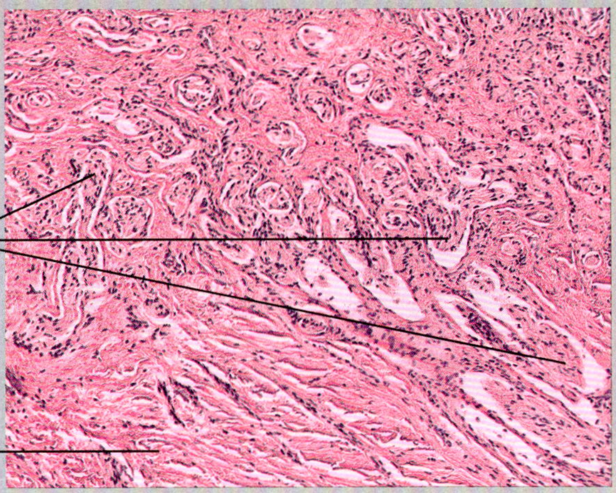

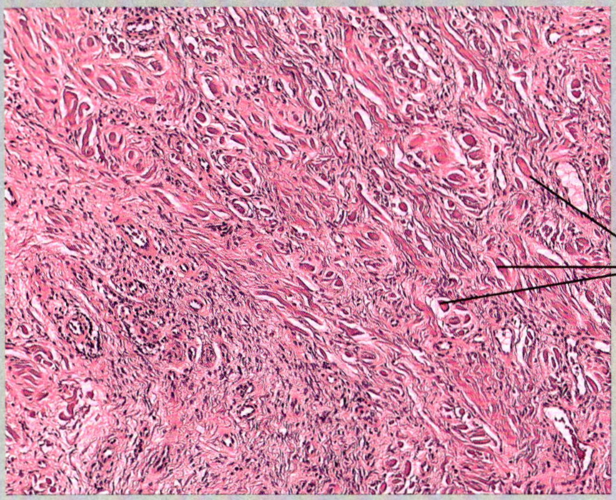

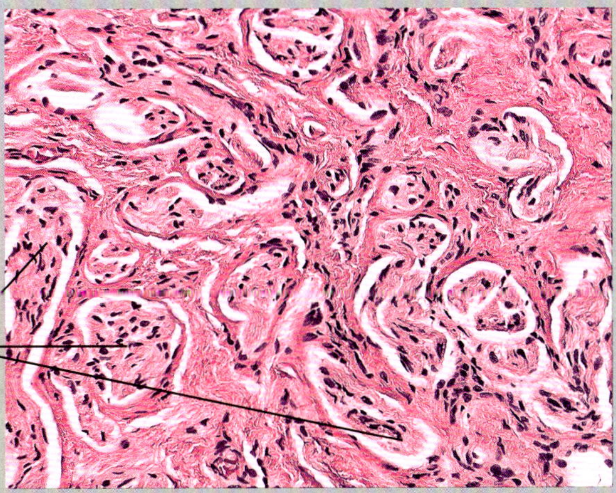

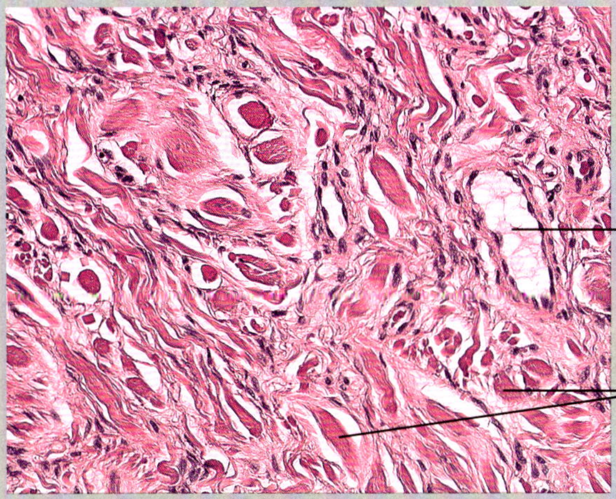

CLINICAL features common to amputation neuroma secondary to rudimentary supernumerary digit and acquired digital fibrokeratoma are location, shape, and consistency. Both conditions occur on or near fingers and both are firm, keratotic polypoid projections. Amputation neuromas are composed mostly of neural tissue; acquired digital fibrokeratomas are formed predominantly of fibrous tissue. In both abnormalities, widely dilated blood vessels tend to be present in the uppermost portion of the dermis, as are extravasated erythrocytes, which sometimes are found in the epidermis, too.

Amputation neuromas secondary to supernumerary digits are stubs present at birth that represent neural remnants in skin of supernumerary digits lost, presumably, in utero. Amputation neuromas frequently occur in pairs at lateral aspects of fifth fingers. They are comparable to those neuromas that develop later in life at sites of surgical amputations, but can be differentiated from them histopathologically by polypoid shape and a cornified layer characteristic of volar skin.

A supernumerary digit, by contrast, is not a neuroma but a miniature digit constituted of bone, cartilage, muscle, and other components, such as nail plate, of a normal finger.

Unlike amputation neuroma and supernumerary digit, acquired digital fibrokeratoma is a solitary excrescence that arises from the skin of an adult near interphalangeal joints of a finger. The projection may be elongated (polypoid) or domed (sessile), but is always keratotic. Other angiofibromas that have histopathologic features reminiscent of those in acquired digital fibrokeratomas are the papules of adenoma sebaceum, fibrous papules of the face, and pearly penile papules. The common denominators of these angiofibromas are marked vascularity and fibroplasia, the latter consisting mostly of fibrillar bundles of collagen and an increased number of large, stellate, and often multinucleated fibrocytes. Such fibrocytes tend to be found at sites of active, sustained manufacture of collagen bundles. Dark-staining inclusions are present sometimes in the cytoplasm of the distinctive fibrocytes, especially those in fibrous papules of the face. Although the aforementioned conditions have angiofibromatous features in common, they are not expressions of a single pathologic process. For example, fibrous papule is a hamartoma with prominent follicular and perifollicular components, whereas acquired digital fibroma is fundamentally a fibroma.

An interesting parallel exists between fibrous papules of the face and acquired digital fibrokeratomas on the one hand, and the cutaneous fibromas of tuberous sclerosis on the other. Fibrous papules of the face are identical histopathologically to papules of adenoma sebaceum in tuberous sclerosis, and acquired digital fibrokeratomas are indistinguishable, when viewed by conventional microscopy, from subungual and periungual fibromas that develop in children with tuberous sclerosis. Also noteworthy is the observation that the striking fibrocytes in cutaneous angiofibromas of tuberous sclerosis resemble closely glial cells in intracranial tubers of that phakomatosis. Perifollicular fibroma is a synonym for fibrous papule.

In sum, amputation neuroma secondary to loss in utero of a supernumerary digit and acquired digital fibrokeratoma look alike clinically and have similar silhouettes histopathologically. The former, however, is basically a neuroma, whereas the latter is a fibroma.

27. Verruca Vulgaris *vs.* Verrucous Solar Keratosis

Verruca Vulgaris	*Verrucous Solar Keratosis*
1. Compact orthokeratosis with focal parakeratosis mostly at the tips of digitations; orthokeratosis predominates	1. Parakeratosis in well-circumscribed broad columns that alternate with thin columns of orthokeratosis; parakeratosis predominates
2. Red blood cells in parakeratotic foci at tips of epidermal projections	2. No red blood cells at tips of epidermal projections usually
3. Granular zone intact or thickened	3. Granular zone decreased or absent beneath zones of parakeratosis
4. Clear spaces of various sizes around nuclei in the spinous and granular zones	4. No cells with clear spaces around nuclei
5. Few atypical keratinocytes, dyskeratotic cells, and mitotic figures, but when present they are in the basal region	5. Many atypical keratinocytes, some dyskeratotic cells, and occasional mitotic figures in at least the lower half of the epidermis
6. No buds of atypical keratinocytes	6. Buds of atypical keratinocytes extend into the papillary dermis
7. No suprabasal clefts	7. Suprabasal clefts episodically; often contain acantholytic dyskeratotic cells
8. Collarettes of adnexal epithelium	8. No epithelial collarettes as a rule
9. Intra-epidermal structures of adnexa (acrosyringia and acrotrichia) affected by the pathologic process	9. Intra-epidermal structures of adnexa (acrosyringia and acrotrichia) mostly spared by the process
10. "Squamous eddies" present sometimes	10. No "squamous eddies"
11. Marked tortuosity of capillaries in elongated dermal papillae	11. Slight tortuosity of capillaries in elongated dermal papillae
12. Slight to moderately dense infiltrate of lymphocytes in the upper part of the dermis	12. Moderately to markedly dense infiltrate of lymphocytes in the upper part of the dermis
13. Solar elastosis uncommon and incidental	13. Solar elastosis invariable and essential

Verruca Vulgaris

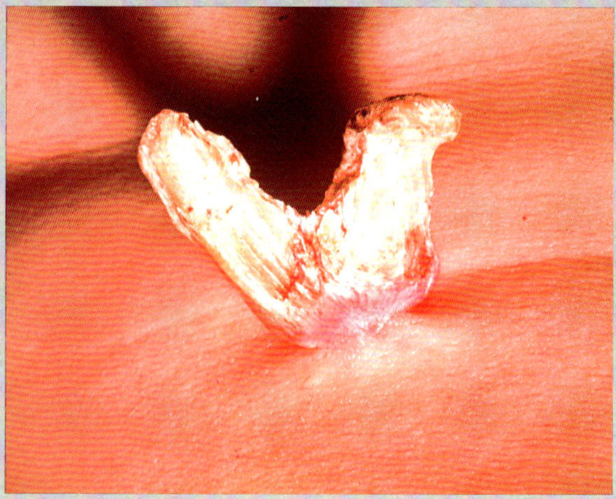

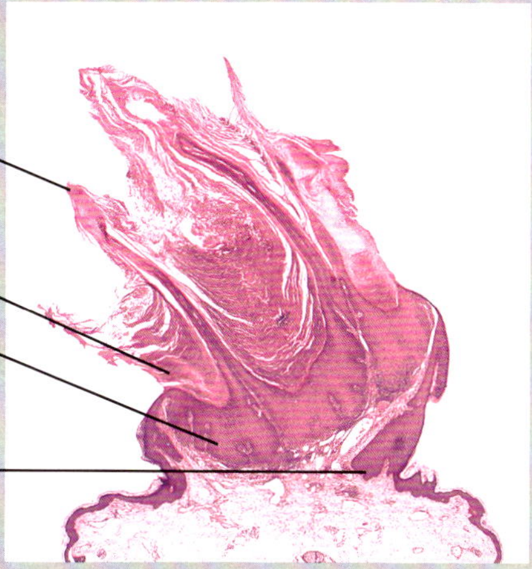

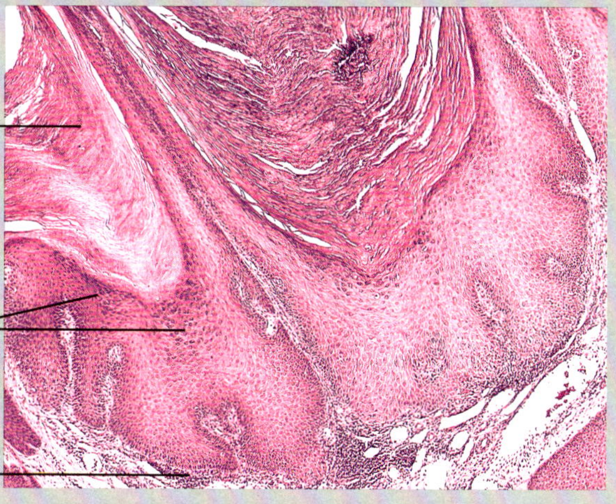

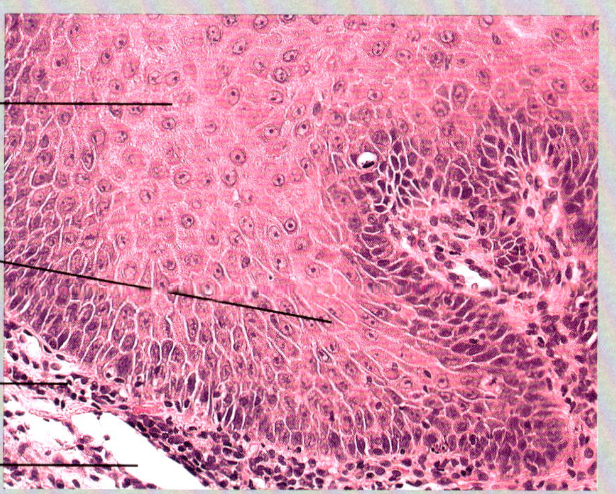

Digitated Solar Keratosis

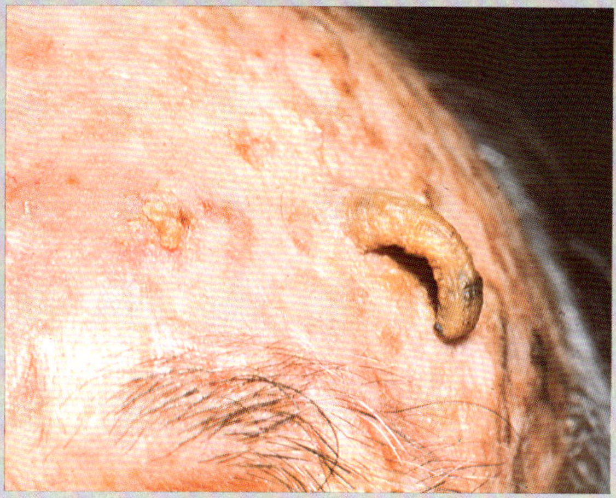

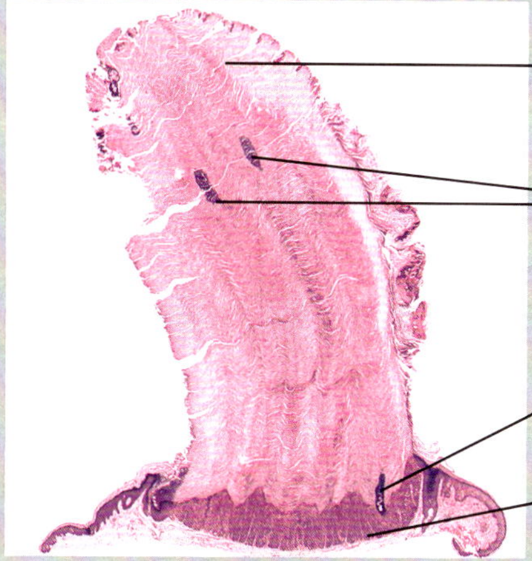

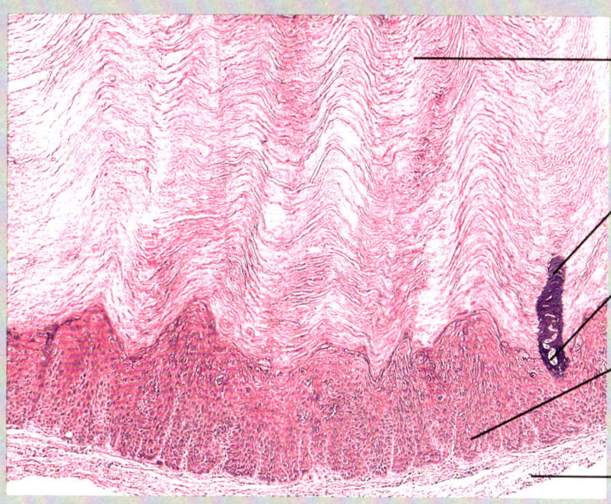

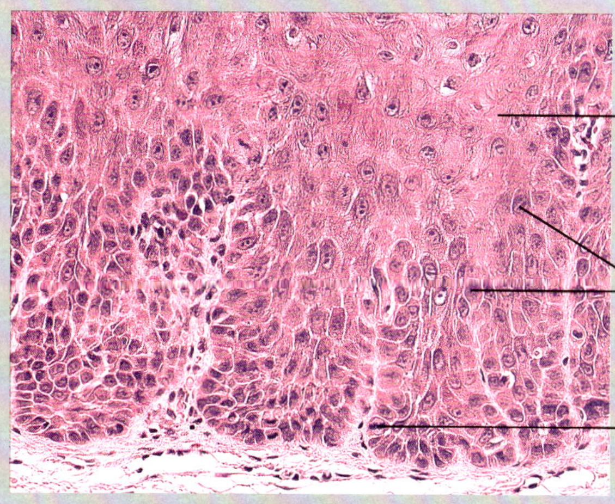

BOTH fully developed verrucae vulgares and digitated solar keratoses are examples of hyperkeratotic, verrucous, epidermal proliferations, but telling differences exist between them. Solar keratoses are atypical keratinocytic neoplasias of epidermal keratinocytes that spare intra-epidermal epithelial structures of adnexa, the eccrine ducts (acrosyringia), and the hair follicles (acrotrichia). The cytologically atypical epidermal keratinocytes of solar keratoses mature to become parakeratotic corneocytes. In contrast, verrucae vulgares are keratinocytic hyperplasias that involve intra-epidermal adnexal structures as well as epidermis, and the keratinocytes that constitute them mature into mostly orthokeratotic corneocytes. Epithelial structures of adnexa arborize in warts to form collarettes, but they do not do so in solar keratoses.

Histopathologic differentiation of warts from solar keratoses is of more than academic interest because verrucae behave in a wholly benign fashion, whereas solar keratoses are embryonic squamous-cell carcinomas that, if untreated, may enlarge to become destructive locally or, very rarely, to metastasize.

Although the histopathologic differentiation of warts and solar keratoses may be difficult sometimes, clinical differentiation between them may be even more so. Both conditions may present themselves as "cutaneous horns", i.e., hyperkeratotic projections well above the skin surface. The term "cutaneous horn" is a purely clinical one. A clinician can only speculate about what lies beneath a "cutaneous horn", e.g., a verruca, solar keratosis, and so on. Histopathologic examination alone of such a lesion can resolve the uncertainty.

Verrucae vulgares occur in both children and adults and on any area of the body, but they are more common on the fingers and hands. Warts are caused by a virus of the papilloma group.

Solar keratoses occur only on sites exposed to sunlight, and usually in older individuals with fair complexions. They are caused by the effects of sunlight on the epidermis and the dermis.

A subject of some debate among pathologists is the question of when a lesion marked by a proliferation of atypical keratinocytes should be diagnosed as "solar keratosis" and when it should be considered "squamous-cell carcinoma." The old shibboleth that a neoplasm is a squamous-cell carcinoma when it has "broken through the basement membrane" seems to have been abandoned by most pathologists. The concept of "invasion" is equally vague, because through a microscope everything is static, there is no movement of cells like that implied by the term "invasion," and wholly benign pseudocarcinomatous hyperplasia may extend deeper into the dermis than many authentic squamous-cell carcinomas. Histopathologic differentiation between them is accomplished by vigorous application of morphologic criteria based mostly upon silhouette, and not at all on the specious concept of "invasion."

What then is the boundary that enables a histopathologist to separate solar keratosis (or any squamous-cell carcinoma in situ, for that matter) from squamous-cell carcinoma? There is no clear-cut boundary, like a goal line in football, because these two conditions are a continuum. For purposes of communication and as guides to management of patients, we diagnose as solar keratoses those lesions whose atypical keratinocytes are confined to the papillary dermis. If a similar lesion, at a later stage, is present in the reticular dermis, we designate it a squamous-cell carcinoma. These distinctions are completely arbitrary because a solar keratosis *is* a squamous-cell carcinoma.

In brief, we consider solar keratoses to be early, evolving squamous-cell carcinomas that may remain embryonic for the lifetime of a patient or may grow to become fetal, neonatal, and eventually mature squamous-cell carcinomas. The same principle applies to Bowen's disease. It is a squamous-cell carcinoma confined to epithelium and, in this sense, is analogous to solar keratosis.

Last, verrucae may eventuate in squamous-cell carcinoma rarely, to wit, those that begin as epidermodysplasia verruciformis, condylomata that become bowenoid papulosis and "giant condylomata," and possibly mosaic warts that develop into carcinoma cuniculatum. These are but a few examples of the effects of papillomavirus on cutaneous epithelium, at first as hyperplasias (warts) and later as malignant neoplasias (squamous-cell carcinomas).

28. Leukokeratosis *vs.* Leukoplakia

Leukokeratosis	*Leukoplakia*
1. Orthokeratosis with few parakeratotic cells	1. Parakeratosis with few orthokeratotic cells
2. Hypergranulosis	2. Few, if any, granular cells if the lesion has not been rubbed
3. Epithelium thickened slightly	3. Epithelium thickened considerably
4. No atypical keratinocytes	4. Atypical keratinocytes
5. No mitotic figures	5. Mitotic figures usually
6. No dyskeratotic cells	6. Many dyskeratotic cells
7. Slight perivascular infiltrate of mononuclear cells	7. Moderately dense perivascular infiltrate of mononuclear cells

Leukokeratosis | *Leukoplakia*

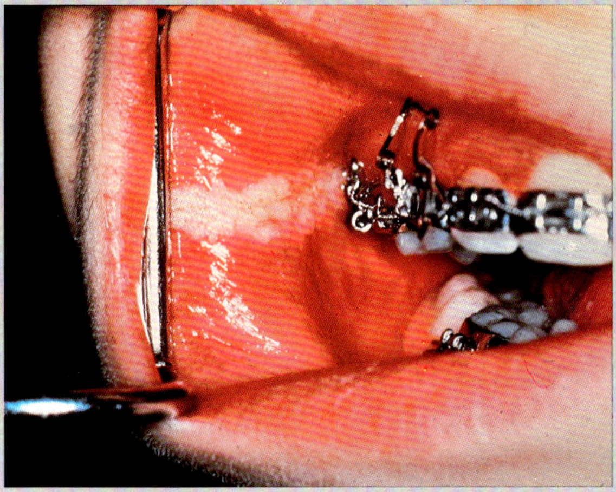

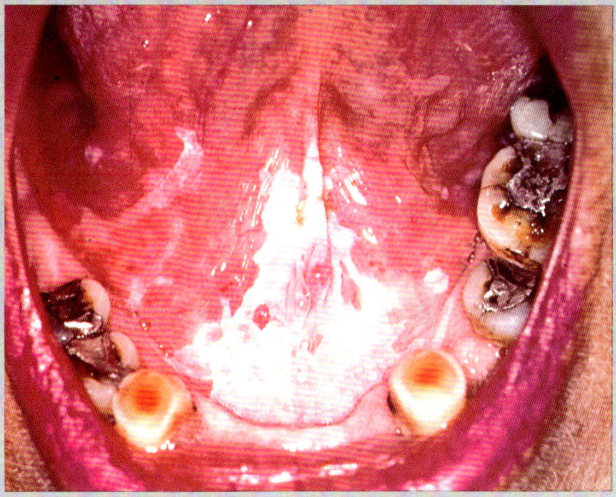

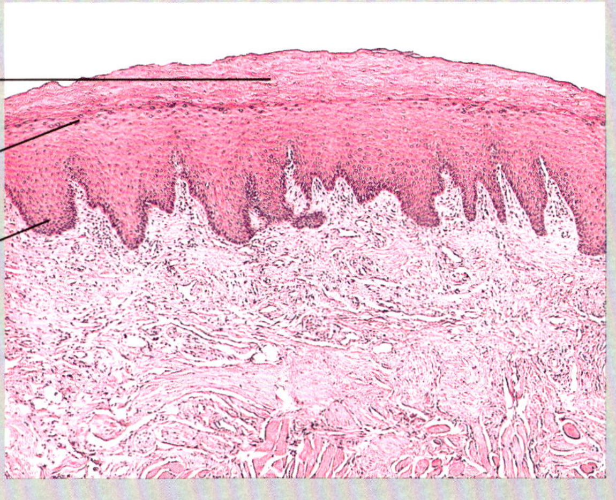

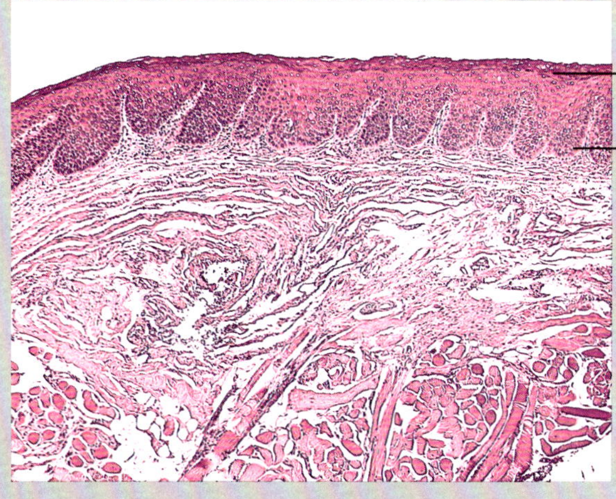

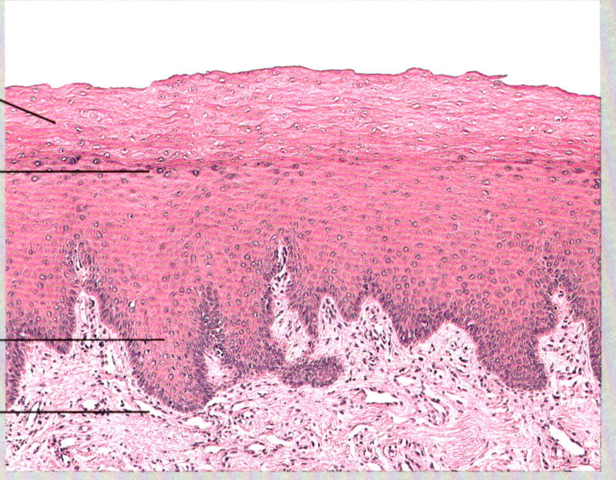

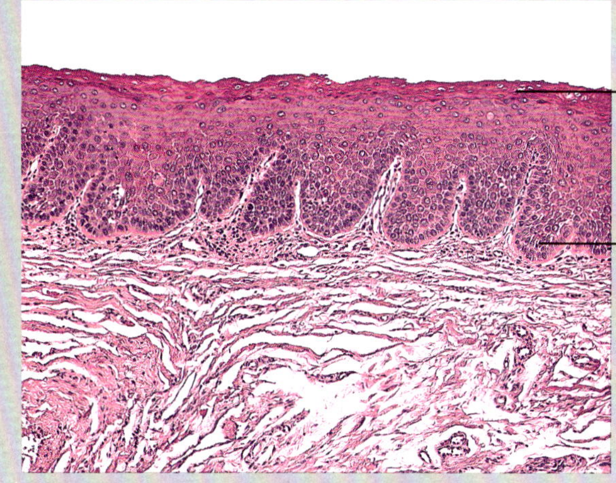

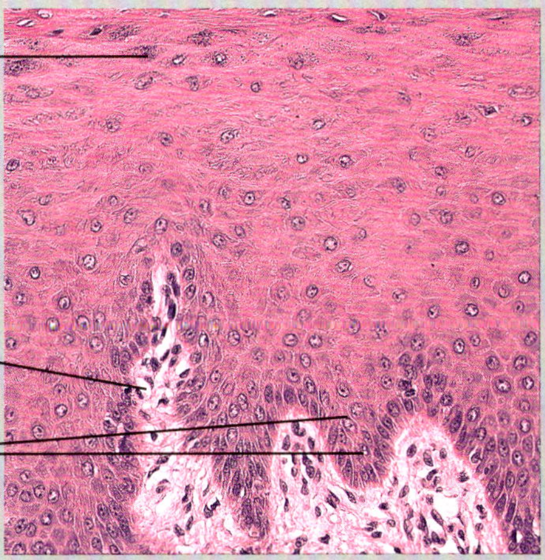

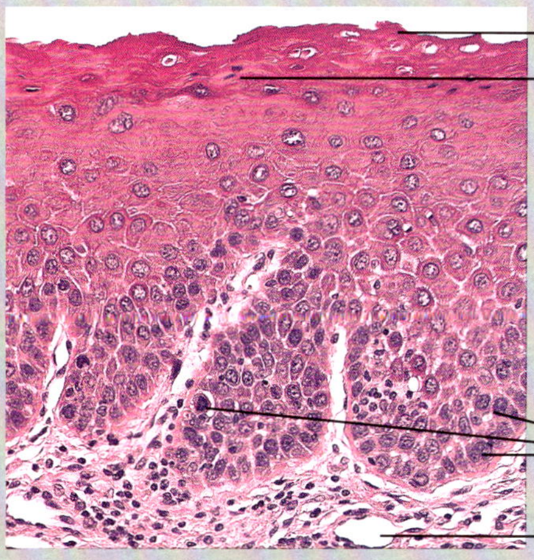

LEUKOKERATOSIS and leukoplakia are white, slightly elevated nonindurated lesions of the mucosae (especially of the mouth, but also of the vagina and other areas) that have histopathologic features in common, namely, hyperkeratosis, a thickened epithelium, and an infiltrate of mononuclear cells. The white color (leuko-) in both leukokeratosis and leukoplakia results from abnormal production and maceration of cornified cells.

The main difference between these two conditions lies in atypicality of the keratinocytes (large, hyperchromatic, and pleomorphic nuclei with mitotic figures) in leukoplakia and absence of atypicality in leukokeratosis. We advocate the use of the term leukoplakia for those white lesions on mucous membranes that are characterized by the histopathologic changes enumerated in the preceding list, and not as a clinical diagnosis for any white lesion on those sites. Leukoplakia is the mucous membrane analogue of solar keratosis, radiation keratosis, and arsenical keratosis, namely, a proliferation of atypical keratinocytes with characteristic clinical and histopathologic features. Like solar keratosis, radiation keratosis, and arsenical keratosis, leukoplakia is an early stage in the evolution of squamous-cell carcinoma. The cause of oral leukoplakia is elusive, but smoking and chewing of tobacco surely are factors in many instances. Another white lesion of mucous membranes that may present a problem of differential diagnosis clinically is candidiasis. The cornified layer of such a lesion teems with hyphae.

The importance of making a definite diagnosis of leukoplakia is that a neglected lesion may eventuate in a squamous-cell carcinoma large enough and deep enough to be destructive locally and to metastasize.

In contrast, leukokeratosis oris is a wholly benign condition that may revert to normal mucous membrane when its cause is removed. The most common cause of leukokeratosis oris is persistent trauma or friction by dentures, maloccluded teeth, or habitual biting of the lips or buccal mucosa. In short, leukokeratosis is simply hyperkeratotic lichen simplex chronicus on mucous membranes.

The atypical nuclei in leukoplakia, like those in its cutaneous analogues, reside in the lower portion of the epithelium. In contradistinction, in squamous-cell carcinoma in situ, i.e., erythroplasia of Queyrat, atypical nuclei are present throughout most or all of the thickened epithelium. As long as the atypical keratinocytes are confined to thickened epithelium of mucous membranes and to epidermis as they are in leukoplakia, solar keratosis, radiation keratosis, arsenical keratosis, erythroplasia, and Bowen's disease, the process is benign biologically, i.e., it cannot and does not metastasize. Nevertheless, each of those proliferations of atypical keratinocytes should be removed completely in order to prevent eventuation of embryonic squamous-cell carcinomas into ones with capability for metastasis. No clinician and no histopathologist, by morphologic signs alone, can predict which rare lesion of leukoplakia or solar keratosis will metastasize eventually.

Some clinical lesions of leukoplakia have red areas interspersed among whitish zones, and still other lesions are mostly red. The name erythroplakia has been given to those mostly red lesions on mucous membranes that, like leukoplakia, are characterized histopathologically by atypical keratinocytes in the lower part of the epithelium and that, if left untreated, may progress to fatal squamous-cell carcinoma. In brief, leukoplakia, erythroplakia, and erythroplasia are evolving squamous-cell carcinomas on mucous membranes. Just as solar keratoses may be mostly white or red clinically depending on the amount of cornification associated with them, so, too, their analogues on mucous membranes may be mostly white (i.e., leukoplakia) or red (i.e., erythroplakia) for the same reason.

Parenthetically, when a lesion of leukoplakia is rubbed persistently, features of leukokeratosis are likely to be superimposed upon it. In those instances, atypical keratinocytes, a thickened epithelium, hypergranulosis, and both parakeratosis and compact orthokeratosis will be seen together.

29. Seborrheic Keratosis, Acanthotic Type *vs.* Eccrine Poroma

Seborrheic Keratosis, Acanthotic Type	*Eccrine Poroma*
1. Sessile exo-endophytic neoplasm	1. Polypoid or sessile predominantly endophytic neoplasm
2. Orthokeratosis in delicate basket-woven and laminated pattern	2. Parakeratosis alternates with orthokeratosis in compact pattern
3. Thin granular zones	3. Thick granular zones
4. Thick anastomosing tracts of mostly basaloid cells are continuous with the epidermis and confined to a thickened papillary dermis	4. Interconnected lobules of poroid or cuticular cells are continuous with the epidermis but often extend far into the reticular dermis
5. Basaloid cells merge with spinous cells of the epidermis and of infundibular epithelium, including that around "horn pseudocysts"	5. Poroid or cuticular cells at the periphery of a neoplasm are demarcated sharply from contiguous spinous cells of normal epidermis
6. No cuticular cells at all	6. Cuticular cells in variable numbers
7. "Squamous eddies" common	7. No "squamous eddies"
8. Mitotic figures few or absent	8. Mitotic figures may be numerous
9. Melanin in basaloid cells usually	9. Melanin in poroid cells uncommon
10. No necrotic cells usually	10. Many necrotic cells, solitary and en masse
11. "Horn pseudocysts" usual	11. "Horn pseudocysts" exceptional
12. No ductal structures	12. Ductal structures often
13. No separation of neoplasm from adjacent stroma	13. Neoplasm separated by clefts from adjacent stroma occasionally
14. No granulation tissue-like stroma in the thickened papillary dermis	14. Stroma composed of granulation tissue often; sometimes mucinous
15. Other variants of seborrheic keratosis (e.g., verrucous, adenoid) present in the same lesion sometimes	15. Other types of poromas (e.g., hidroacanthoma simplex, dermal duct tumor, and poroid hidradenoma) present sometimes

Seborrheic Keratosis, Acanthotic Type

Eccrine Poroma

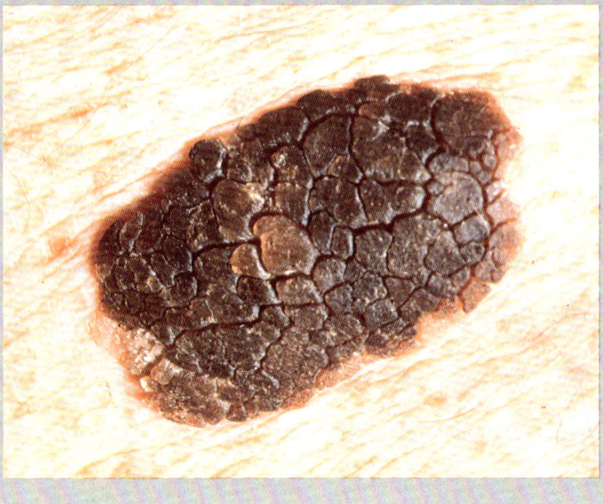

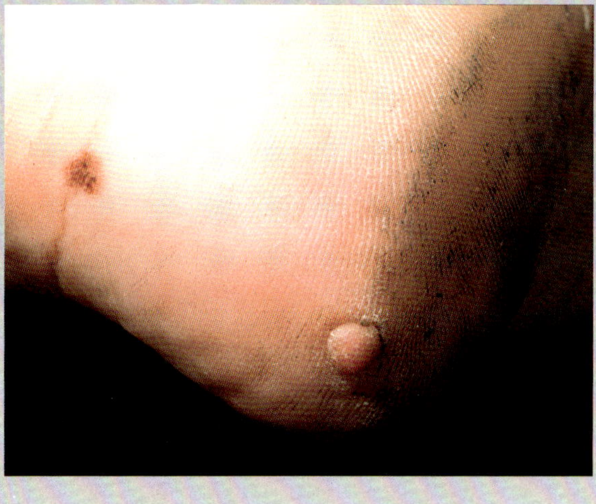

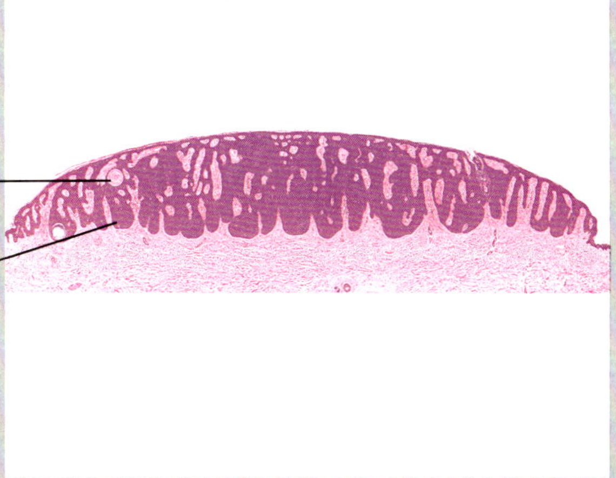

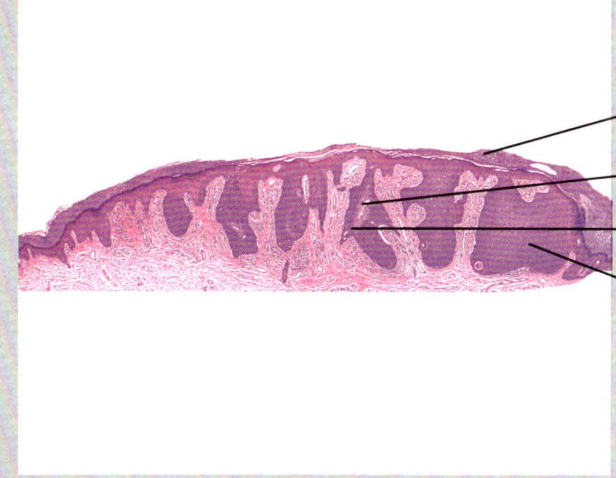

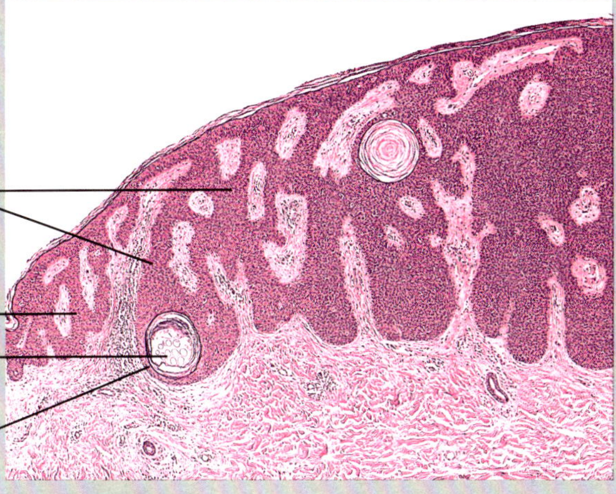

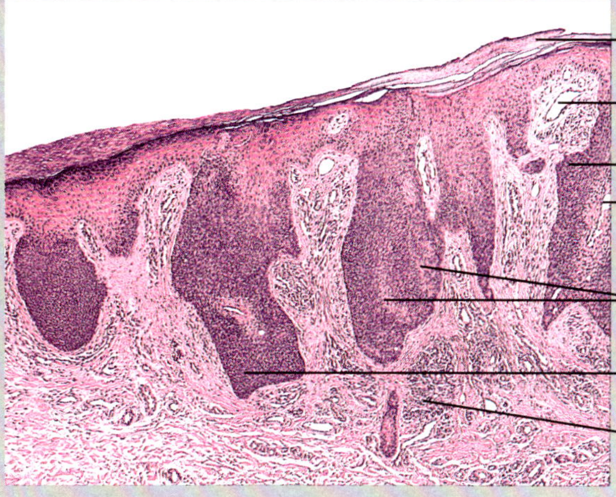

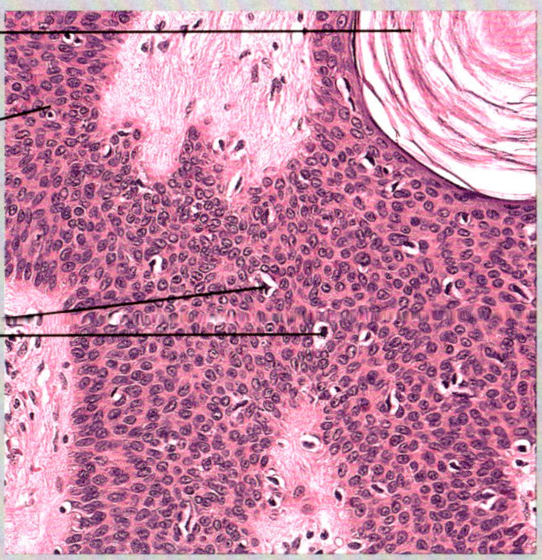

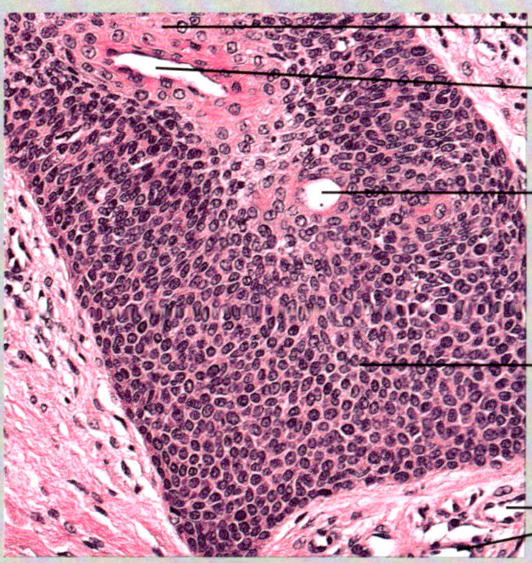

SEBORRHEIC keratosis of the acanthotic type and eccrine poroma are both benign, epithelial, exo-endophytic neoplasms comprised mostly of small, round (basaloid) cells. Melanocytes may be scattered among keratinocytes in both conditions.

Seborrheic keratoses are common lesions that tend to present themselves, sometimes in large numbers, on the skin of older persons, especially on the face, scalp, and trunk. They are relatively soft and have a surface that varies from flat to verrucous, and a color that ranges from light tan to black. Because seborrheic keratoses are traumatized readily, often artifactually, by a person who bears them, a variety of histopathologic changes develop in them. Those range from formation of "squamous eddies" to development of nuclear atypia that may simulate the kind seen in squamous-cell carcinoma. Of the three major patterns of seborrheic keratoses, namely, acanthotic, adenoid (reticulated), and verrucous, only the acanthotic type presents a problem in differential diagnosis from eccrine poroma.

Eccrine poroma is a relatively uncommon neoplasm compared to seborrheic keratosis. Although it has some predilection for palms and soles, it may arise anywhere on the integument. Clinically, eccrine poroma usually presents itself as a solitary firm lesion that may be flat-topped, or more commonly sessile or pedunculated. Abundant granulation tissue associated with some of these neoplasms conveys a clinical appearance like that of pyogenic granuloma. The neoplasm differentiates in the direction of acrosyringeal segments of eccrine ducts and, therefore, consists of cells that line those ducts (cuticular cells), the cells immediately peripheral to lining cells (poroid cells), and tubules themselves. Most eccrine poromas extend from the epidermis into the reticular dermis, and some even stretch into the subcutaneous fat. Intradermal neoplasms whose cells are identical to those of eccrine poroma, but that seem to be separated from the epidermis and arranged in discrete aggregations, have been termed "dermal duct tumors." In actuality, when step sections are cut through dermal duct tumors, nearly always continuity between aggregations and epidermis can be demonstrated and, therefore, they are part of a spectrum of poroid neoplasms that includes eccrine poroma, dermal duct tumor, hidroacanthoma simplex (intra-epidermal nests of cuticular and poroid cells), and poroid hidradenoma (a cystic neoplasm in the dermis constituted of cuticular and poroid cells).

Pathologists tend to speak and write of adnexal neoplasms that "arise from" particular structures such as an eccrine pore or a dermal duct. In our view, there is no compelling evidence that eccrine poroma arises from cells that line the intra-epidermal eccrine pore, or that dermal duct tumor arises from cells of the dermal duct. Those neoplasms differentiate toward eccrine ducts; their site of origin is not known.

Prior to the original description of eccrine poroma by Pinkus in 1956, that neoplasm was misinterpreted histopathologically as an acanthotic type of seborrheic keratosis. From time to time, eccrine poromas and seborrheic keratoses continue to pose problems in histopathologic differential diagnosis—conundra that usually can be resolved if the criteria tabulated here are employed. Seborrheic keratosis is a neoplasm that seems to be composed of epidermal and infundibular keratinocytes. Distinctive tunnels filled with corneocytes ("horn pseudocysts") in seborrheic keratoses are formed by follicular infundibula. The "eddies" of squamous cells found commonly in traumatized seborrheic keratoses represent spirals of sebaceous ducts through the neoplasm. In contrast, eccrine poroma consists of cells like those of the acrosyringium and therefore is devoid of "horn pseudocysts" and "squamous eddies."

30. Sebaceous Hyperplasia *vs.* Nevus Sebaceus of Jadassohn

Sebaceous Hyperplasia	*Nevus Sebaceus of Jadassohn*
1. Dome-shaped papule with a central cell	1. Relatively flat-topped plaque in early stage; papillated or digitated plaque in fully developed and later stages; no dell
2. Basket-weave pattern in the cornified layer	2. Laminated and compact pattern in the cornified layer
3. Papillomatosis either absent or slight	3. Papillomatosis prominent in fully developed lesions
4. Several large sebaceous lobules in a solitary, well-circumscribed conglomerate	4. Few scattered small sebaceous lobules in early lesions; many large sebaceous lobules in clusters across a broad front in fully developed and late lesions
5. Several sebaceous lobules attached to a single sebaceous duct	5. Sebaceous lobules open to a short tubule that serves as both sebaceous duct and infundibulum
6. Sebaceous ducts open into one or several widely dilated follicular infundibula	6. Sebaceous ducts enter a single follicular infundibulum-like structure, often without a distinct intervening sebaceous duct
7. Normal sebaceous follicles or vellus follicles are present within the section	7. No or few normal folliculo-sebaceous units are present within the section usually; alopecic
8. No apocrine glands within the lesion	8. Apocrine glands and ducts, frequently numerous, in the dermis of some lesions
9. Solar elastosis common	9. Solar elastosis rare and then only in late lesions
10. No follicular germs and papillae	10. Follicular germs and papillae present often
11. No associated hamartomas or neoplasms with adnexal differentiation	11. Other hamartomas (e.g., syringocystadenoma papilliferum), benign neoplasms with adnexal differentiation (e.g., trichoblastoma), and rarely malignant neoplasms (e.g., sebaceous carcinoma) may be present in late lesions

Sebaceous Hyperplasia

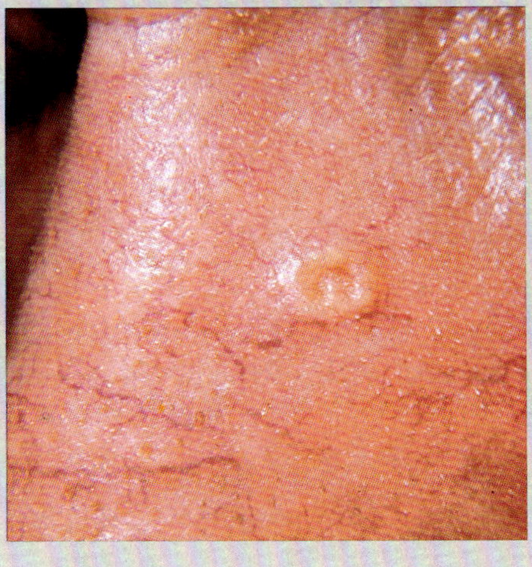

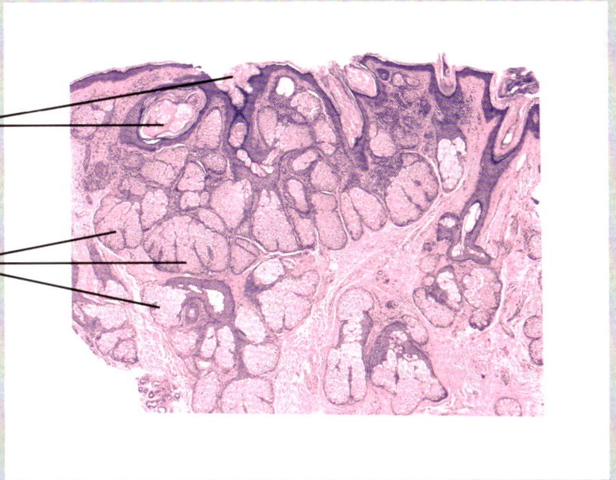

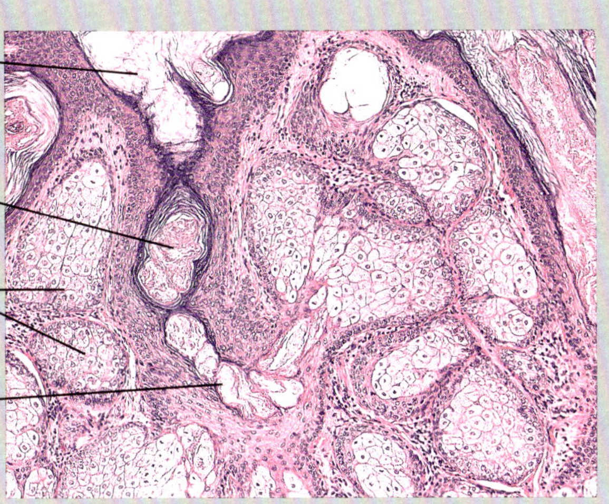

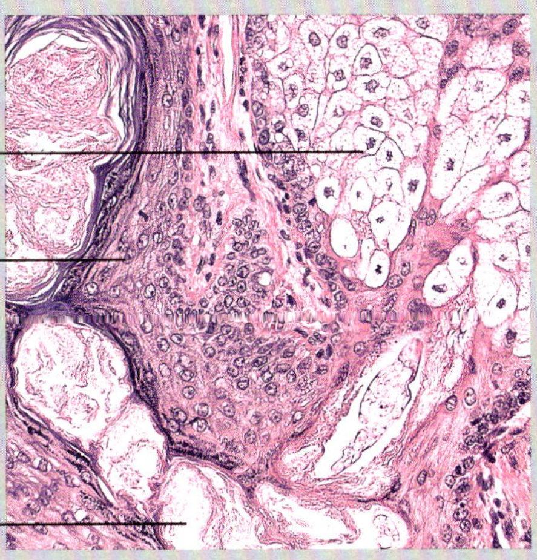

Nevus Sebaceus

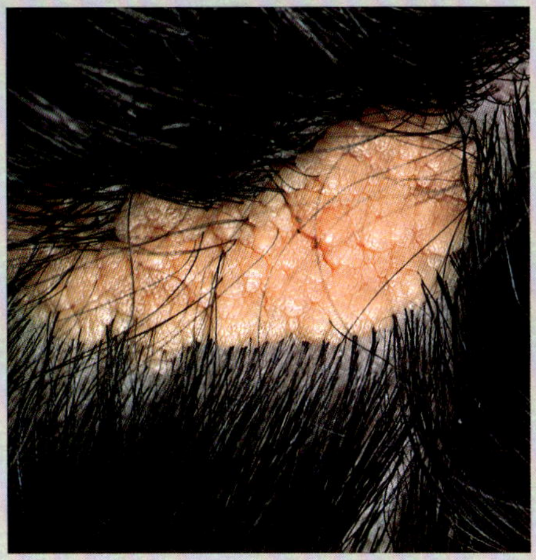

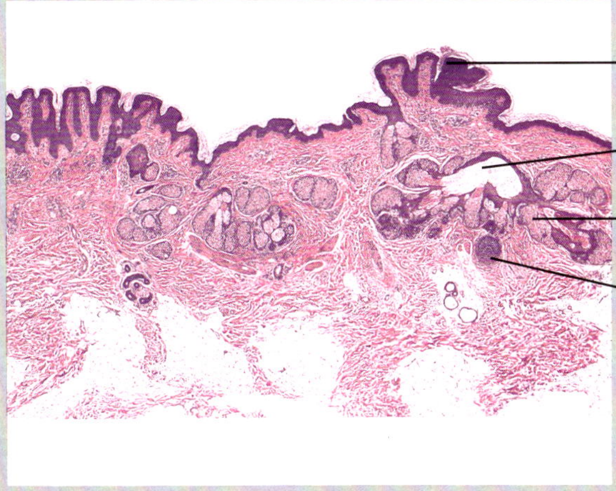

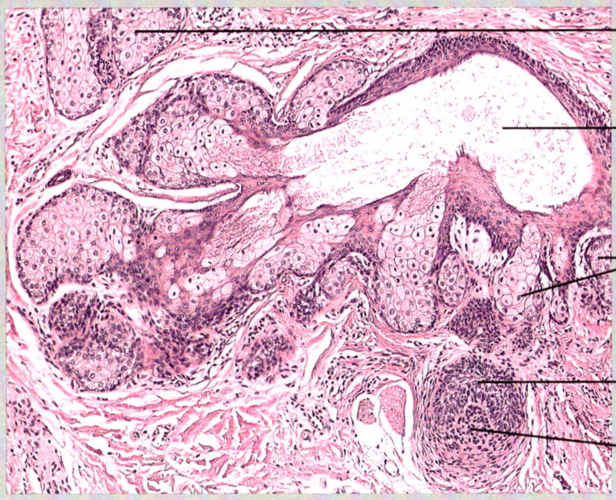

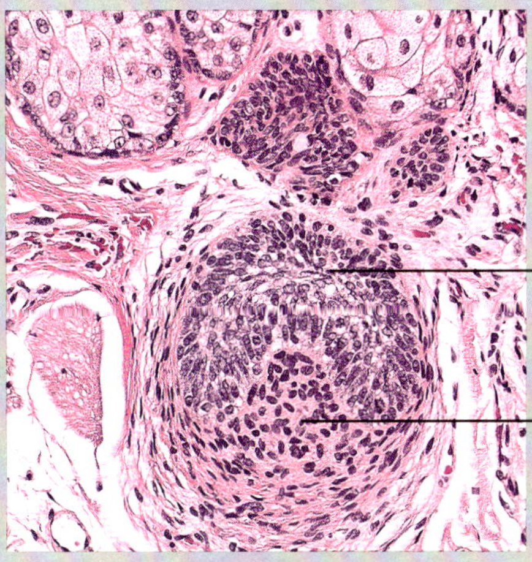

BOTH sebaceous hyperplasia and nevus sebaceus of Jadassohn consist of abnormalities of sebaceous glands. Sebaceous gland hyperplasia is a condition that affects sebaceous units and follicular infundibula mostly, whereas nevus sebaceus is a hamartoma that involves not only sebaceous units, but other adnexal epithelial structures, the epidermis, the dermis, and the subcutaneous fat.

Stereotypical lesions of sebaceous hyperplasia are numerous, small, slightly yellowish papules with delicate rims and central depressions situated on the forehead, cheeks, and nose of middle aged and older persons. A particular solitary lesion of sebaceous hyperplasia may be misinterpreted clinically as a basal-cell carcinoma because both conditions have slightly elevated borders and central dells. In basal-cell carcinoma, however, the central depression usually represents an erosion or ulceration, whereas in sebaceous hyperplasia it is an ostium of a dilated follicular infundibulum or of contiguous infundibula.

Sebaceous hyperplasia also must be differentiated histopathologically from sebaceous adenoma. Sebaceous hyperplasia is a caricature of a normal sebaceous follicle in which large lobules retain their original architecture and composition. In sebaceous adenoma, in contrast, the general architectural pattern of sebaceous lobules is preserved, but those distorted lobules are composed of an increased number of non-vacuolated immature sebocytes, as well as vacuolated mature ones. In a truly normal sebaceous lobule, non-vacuolated cells are positioned in a single row at the periphery. In the abnormal lobules of sebaceous adenoma, they constitute more than just a single row, and not all of them need be stationed at the periphery of a lobule. In sebaceous hyperplasia, well-defined sebaceous ducts serve as conduits between sebaceous lobules and distinct follicular infundibula. As a rule, neither ducts nor infundibula are delineated precisely in sebaceous adenoma.

Commonly, seborrheic keratosis-like changes overlie a lesion of sebaceous hyperplasia and, uncommonly, a verruca, usually a plane one, may surmount it. The same is true also for nevus sebaceus.

Nevus sebaceus, named eponymically for Jadassohn, is usually a solitary lesion that develops during prenatal life and is apparent from its presence at birth or early in neonatal life. Clinically and histopathologically, lesions of nevus sebaceus may be staged roughly as early (pre-pubertal), fully developed (pubertal), and late (post-pubertal). Early lesions are smooth, relatively flat-surfaced, tan to brown, hairless plaques on the scalp, forehead, face, or neck. In time, they increase in size and mass in parallel with the growth of persons who bear them. Their surfaces often become cobblestone-like or warty. As sebaceous glands enlarge at puberty, the hamartoma takes on a yellow-orange color that reflects abundant lipid in numerous sebaceous lobules of different sizes and shapes. In late lesions, many other abnormalities may become manifest in nevus sebaceus, especially syringocystadenoma papilliferum, various benign and malignant neoplasms of sebaceous, eccrine, apocrine, or follicular differentiation, and follicular and apocrine cysts and cystic hamartomas.

Despite the absence of any obvious abnormalities in dermal connective tissue in nevus sebaceus, that tissue must be faulty because so many epithelial abnormalities are present within and above the lesion. Biochemical alterations in the connective tissue probably induce the numerous and varied aberrations of epithelial structures that occur within the distinctive hamartoma.

The presence of nevus sebaceus may presage congenital abnormalities of other systems, for example, the skeletal and cardiovascular ones. In this context, nevus sebaceus is one part of a multisystem disease.

31. Keratoacanthoma *vs.* Squamous-Cell Carcinoma

Keratoacanthoma	*Squamous-Cell Carcinoma*
1. Ulcerated rarely	1. Ulcerated commonly
2. Exo-endophytic neoplasm with a central crater formed by contiguous, dilated infundibula filled with corneocytes	2. Predominantly endophytic neoplasm (except for the verrucous type) with no crater
3. Crater covered partially by overhanging "lips" of infundibular epithelium	3. No enclosing epithelial "lips"
4. Abundant pale-staining cytoplasm of keratinocytes	4. Pale-staining cytoplasm of keratinocytes uncommon
5. Tongues of atypical epithelial cells between collagen bundles in the reticular dermis and oriented somewhat parallel to the skin surface	5. No tongues of atypical epithelial cells between bundles of collagen and parallel to the skin surface
6. Intra-epithelial abscesses within the neoplasm common	6. Intra-epithelial abscesses within the neoplasm uncommon
7. Acantholytic cells within the intra-epithelial abscesses often	7. Acantholytic cells, when present, not associated with discrete abscesses as a rule
8. Gland-like formations within the neoplasm rare	8. "Pseudoglandular" formations often
9. Aggregations of acutely necrotic keratinocytes in resolving lesions	9. No acutely necrotic neoplastic keratinocytes
10. Lymphocytes early; neutrophils, eosinophils, and histiocytes, some of them multinucleated, later	10. Lymphocytes and plasma cells predominant throughout the course
11. Granulation tissue appears prior to resolution	11. No prominent granulation tissue unless beneath an ulcerated neoplasm
12. Granulomatous inflammation around extruded cornified cells in resolving lesions	12. No granulomatous inflammation
13. Fibrosis in a broad zone beneath the epithelial component of resolving neoplasms	13. Fibrosis, when present, is desmoplastic around individual aggregations of neoplastic cells; the neoplasm does not resolve

Keratoacanthoma | *Squamous-Cell Carcinoma*

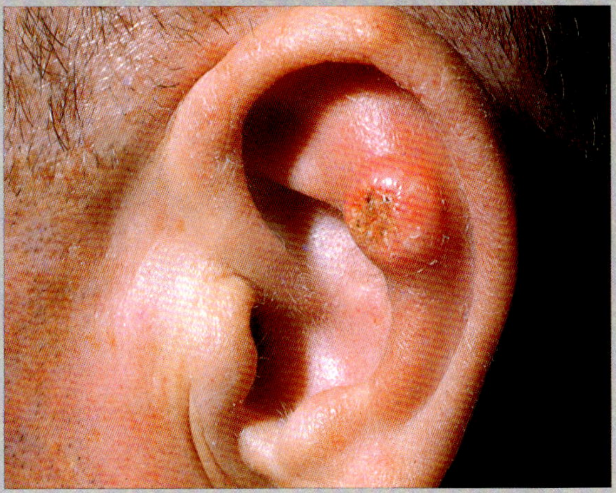

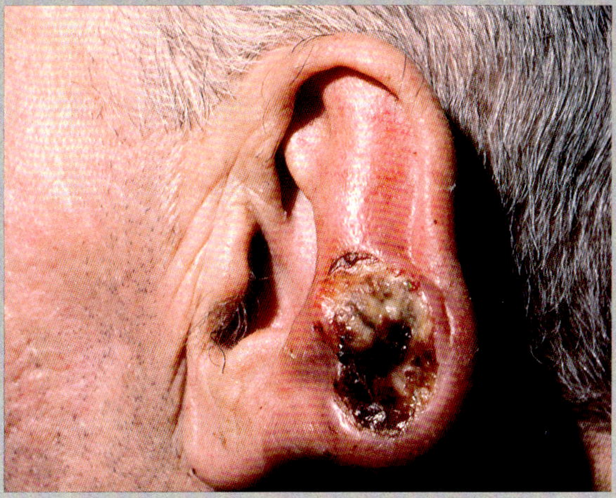

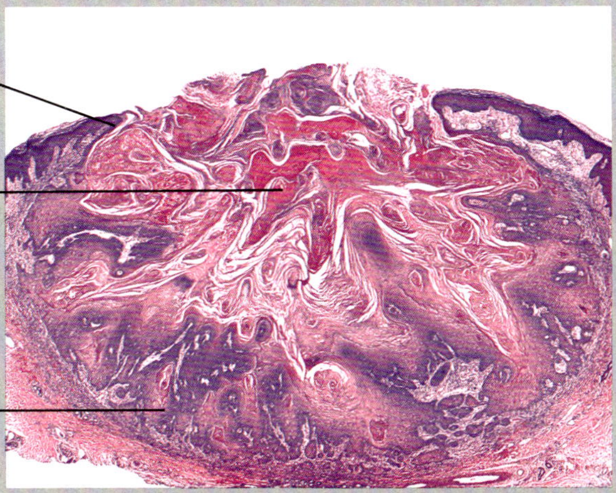

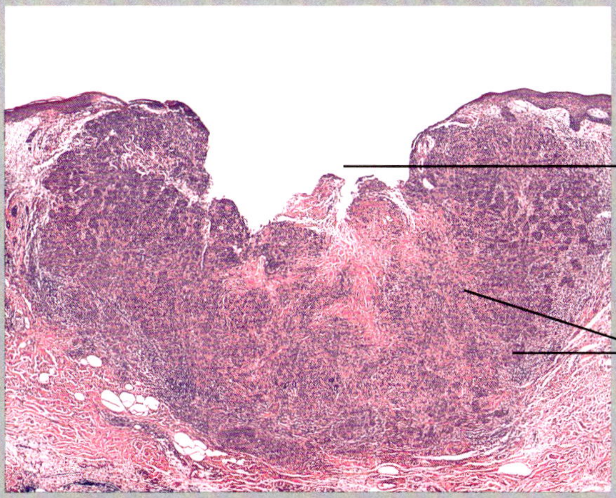

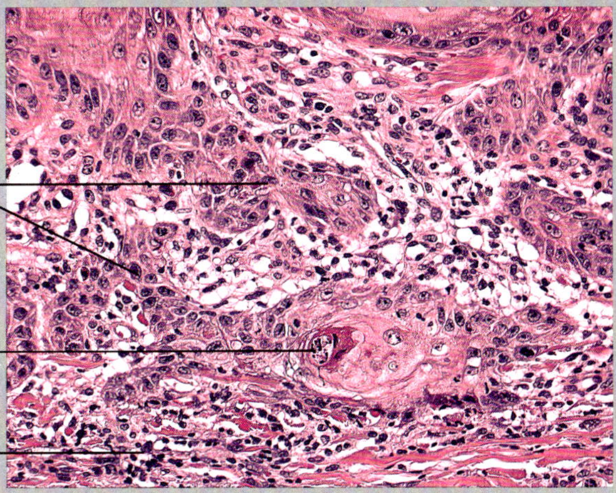

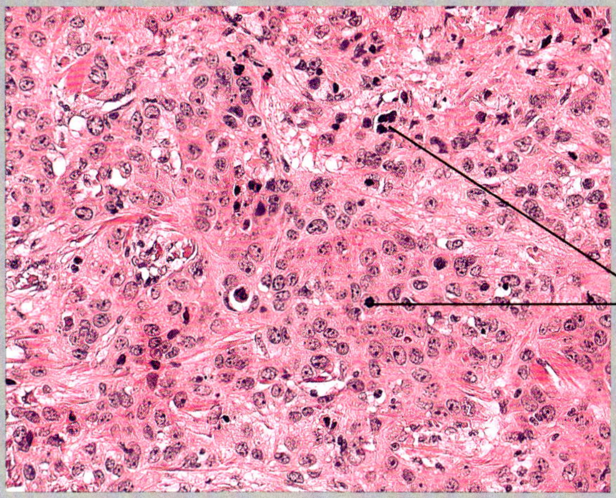

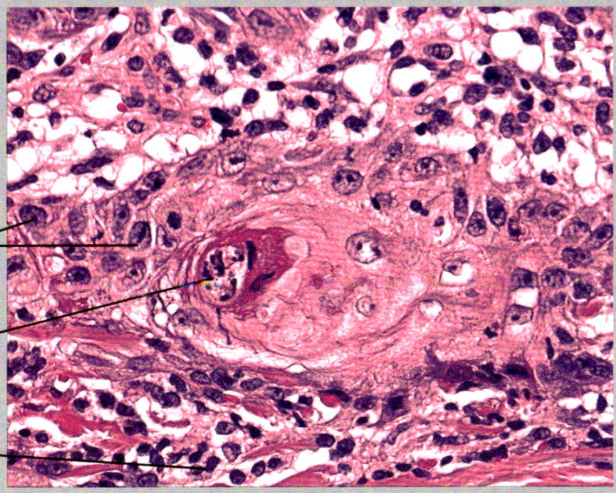

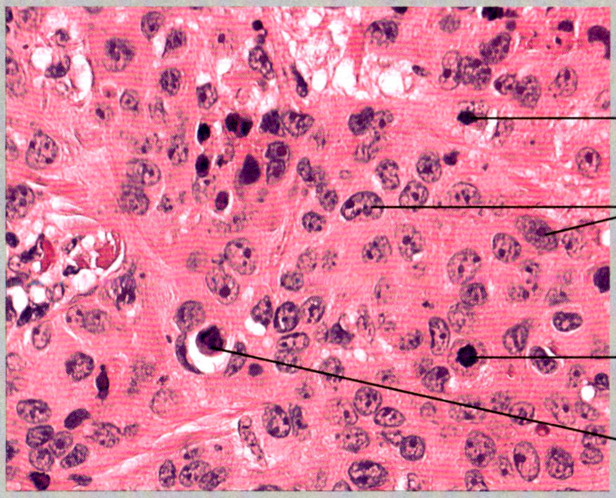

BOTH keratoacanthoma and squamous-cell carcinoma are neoplasms of keratinocytes that have the following histopathologic features in common: atypical keratinocytes with large, hyperchromatic and pleomorphic nuclei, increased numbers of mitotic figures, dyskeratotic cells, infiltrates of inflammatory cells, and solar elastosis. Solar keratoses, basal-cell carcinomas, and even malignant melanomas may be noted episodically in adjacent skin.

The major histopathologic feature that distinguishes keratoacanthoma from squamous-cell carcinoma is architectural pattern and, in particular, silhouette. A proper biopsy is necessary for accurate histopathologic diagnosis which, in turn, is predicated on revelation of that silhouette, something that punch and shave techniques fail to do consistently. Cytologic features, such as nuclear atypia, are not helpful in distinguishing keratoacanthoma from squamous-cell carcinoma. Extraordinary mitotic figures may be found in some keratoacanthomas, just as they may in some squamous-cell carcinomas. In brief, keratoacanthomas cannot be differentiated from squamous-cell carcinomas by cytologic criteria alone. If, however, a proper biopsy specimen is taken, accurate identification of a keratoacanthoma as distinct from a squamous-cell carcinoma may be accomplished in almost every case by attention to their entirely different silhouettes.

Clinically, the type of keratoacanthoma under discussion here usually presents itself as a solitary lesion, most commonly on sun-exposed skin of older individuals. Infrequently, more than one lesion may develop in the same person. A typical "solitary" keratoacanthoma proceeds roughly through two stages. First, there is rapid evolution over a few months of a firm, dome-shaped papule that tends to become a nodule and, sometimes, a tumor characterized by a central crater stuffed with horny material. Then, in another few months, the papule, nodule or tumor gradually resolves, leaving in its wake an irregularly shaped depressed scar. Rarely, a keratoacanthoma may grow for many months and even years to gigantic proportions and be markedly destructive locally. Even these "giant" keratoacanthomas tend, in time, to regress completely without therapy.

The name "keratoacanthoma" has been given to four different neoplasms characterized by crateriform shapes and proliferations of keratinocytes, namely, "solitary" (which is not always solitary), eruptive, familial, and subungual. Biologically, the four types are very different from one another. For example, the "solitary" type almost always regresses in months without treatment; the subungual type does not regress at all. On the contrary, it destroys a distal phalanx eventually.

Squamous-cell carcinoma may arise de novo anywhere on the skin or mucous membranes, but most often develops on sun-damaged skin as a continuous progression of atypical keratinocytes, i.e., a tiny solar keratosis that becomes bigger and bigger and is termed a "squamous-cell carcinoma" when it becomes large enough. There are no repeatable criteria, however, for determination of when a solar keratosis has become a squamous-cell carcinoma, the reason being that a solar keratosis *is* an embryonic squamous-cell carcinoma. Squamous-cell carcinomas in skin that has not been exposed to sunlight, such as those that arise in radiodermatitis or in scars from burns, tend to behave in a biologically malignant fashion and to metastasize more readily than do those that arise in skin damaged severely by sunlight. The latter metastasize only rarely. Clinically, squamous-cell carcinoma of the skin appears commonly as an ulcer surrounded by a firm border, but its surface occasionally may be verrucous, smooth, or adorned by a horn.

The history of rapid growth of a crateriform papule, nodule, or tumor typified histopathologically by proliferation of atypical keratinocytes should alert a microscopist to the probability of keratoacanthoma, rather than of squamous-cell carcinoma (although the latter may grow rapidly in patients who are immunosuppressed). It is imperative that clinicians provide histopathologists not only with adequate biopsy specimens of such lesions, but accurate historical information as well.

In closing, a few lines should be written about the question of the true nature of a "solitary keratoacanthoma," namely, is it something other than a squamous-cell carcinoma? The neoplasm termed "solitary" keratoacanthoma is acknowledged to regress without therapy in the vast majority of instances, an observation that has led most commentators to conclude that the neoplasm is not a carcinoma, but an acanthoma as the name denotes. It also must be acknowledged, however, that seemingly indubitable examples of keratoacanthomas have metastasized, albeit extremely rarely. If those observations are correct, and they appear to be, then "solitary" keratoacanthoma fulfills the single most important criterion for malignancy, i.e., capability for metastasis, and therefore must be considered one of several types of squamous-cell carcinoma. Subungual keratoacanthoma surely is a squamous-cell carcinoma because its growth is relentless and it is destructive.

In sum, the title of this chapter "keratoacanthoma vs. squamous-cell carcinoma" is an oxymoron because keratoacanthoma is interpreted best as a squamous-cell carcinoma, i.e., the type of squamous cell carcinoma that usually regresses, possibly because it is caused by papillomavirus that disappears first.

32. Pagetoid Bowen's Disease *vs.* Extramammary Paget's Disease

Pagetoid Bowen's Disease	*Extramammary Paget's Disease*
1. Parakeratosis usual	1. Orthokeratosis usual
2. No atypical pale cells within the stratum corneum	2. Atypical pale cells within the stratum corneum often
3. Cells with atypical nuclei and pale cytoplasm arranged as solitary units, but more often in nests, at all levels of the epidermis equally	3. Cells with atypical nuclei and pale cytoplasm arranged as solitary units and in nests, predominantly in the lower part of the epidermis
4. Nests of atypical cells merge with keratinocytes in the adjacent epidermis at some points	4. Nests of atypical cells demarcated sharply from keratinocytes in the adjacent epidermis
5. Intercellular bridges visible between pale cells arranged in nests	5. Intercellular bridges not visible between pale cells arranged in nests
6. Epidermal cells between nests of pale cells have atypical nuclei usually	6. Epidermal cells between nests of pale cells have normal nuclei
7. Atypical epidermal cells multinucleated sometimes	7. No multinucleated epidermal cells
8. Dyskeratotic cells within the intra-epidermal lesion	8. No dyskeratotic cells within the intra-epidermal lesion
9. No acinar structures within the epidermis	9. Acinar structures within the epidermis occasionally
10. Cells of the basal layer not flattened by nests of atypical cells; they often appear as a distinct row of columnar keratinocytes arranged in a palisade	10. Cells of the basal layer often flattened by nests of atypical cells
11. Atypical cells spare epithelial structures of adnexa usually	11. Atypical cells extend far down follicular infundibula and eccrine ducts

Pagetoid Bowen's Disease

Extramammary Paget's Disease

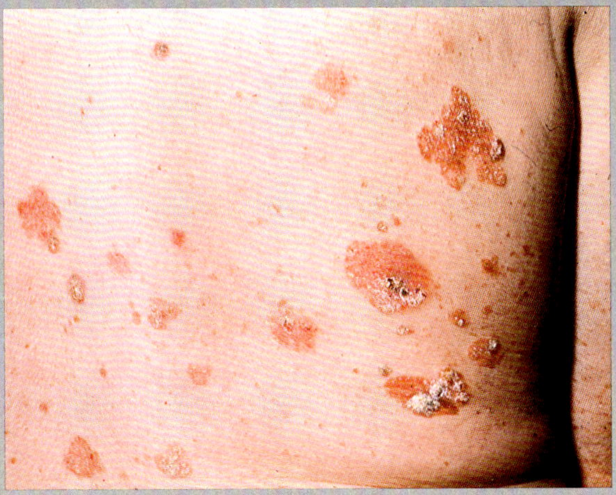

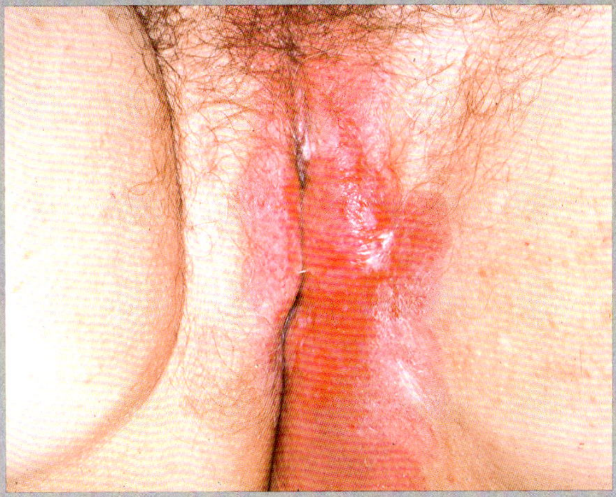

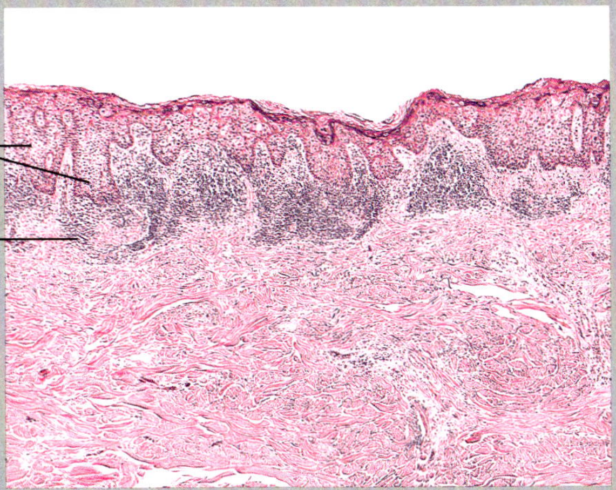

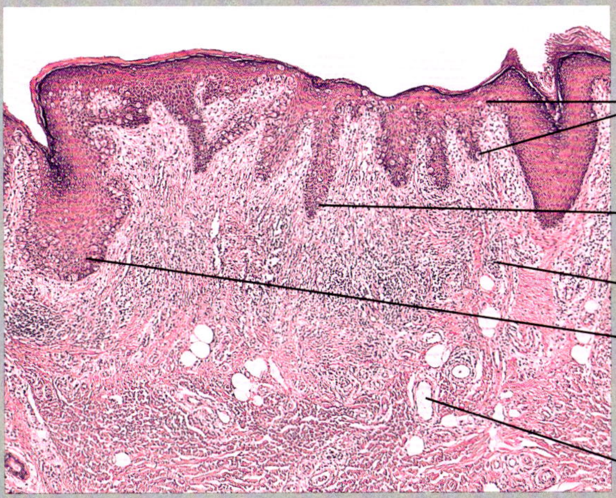

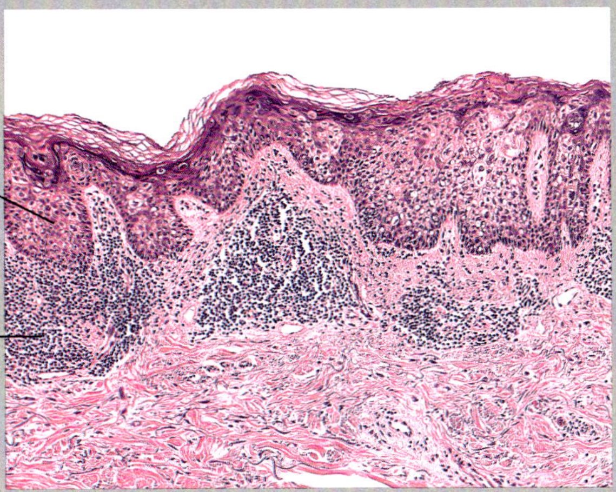

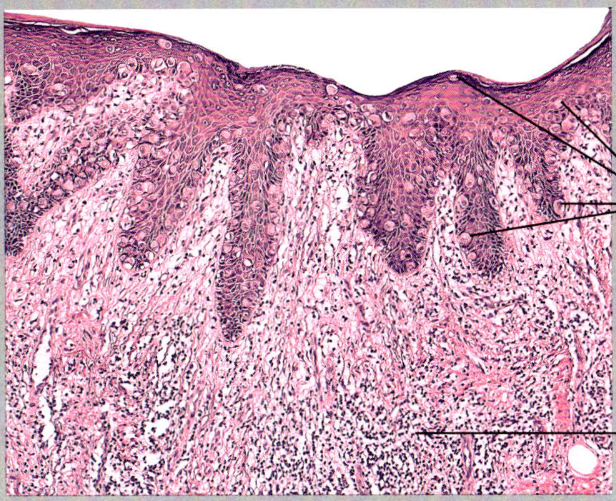

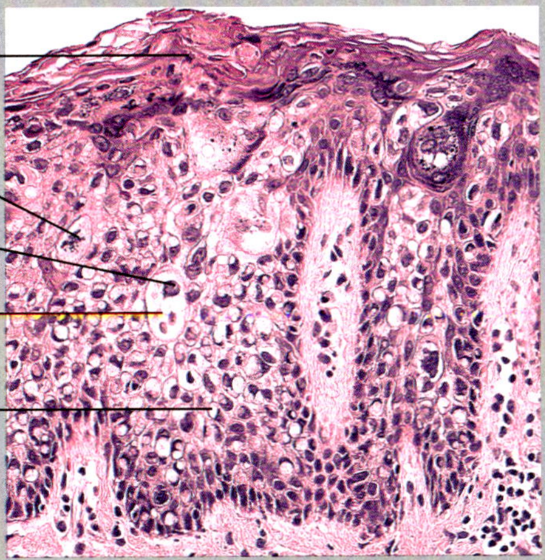

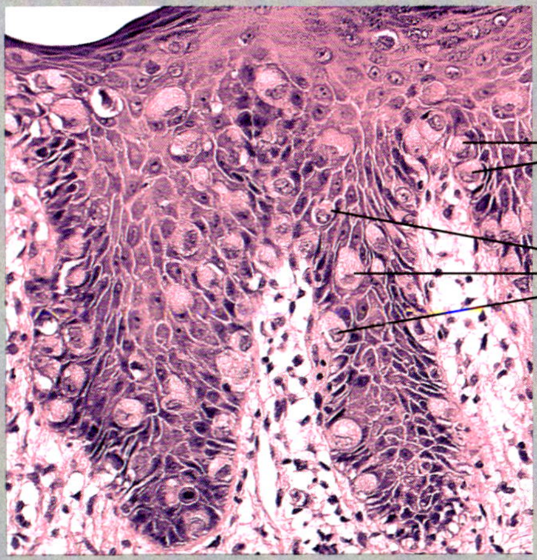

BOTH pagetoid Bowen's disease and extramammary Paget's disease are intra-epidermal carcinomas. Whereas Bowen's disease is a carcinoma in situ with squamous differentiation (it cornifies), extramammary Paget's disease is a carcinoma in situ with glandular differentiation (it attempts to form apocrine epithelium). Despite the tabulated histopathologic differences between them, pagetoid Bowen's disease and extramammary Paget's disease have numerous features in common, namely, atypical cells with abundant, pale-staining cytoplasm, mitotic figures in atypical cells, and atypical pale cells arranged as solitary units and in nests within a thickened epidermis. Neoplastic cells, in time, may extend from the epidermis into the dermis. An infiltrate of inflammatory cells is present in the upper part of the dermis.

Ordinarily, Bowen's disease is not confused histopathologically with extramammary Paget's disease because Bowen's disease is not usually organized in nests of atypical keratinocytes, but instead involves the entire thickness of the epidermis in confluent fashion. In pagetoid Bowen's disease, however, intra-epidermal aggregations of atypical pale cells mimic the nests of extramammary Paget's disease.

The histopathologic distinctions between pagetoid Bowen's disease and extramammary Paget's disease are made readily when the aforementioned criteria are utilized in the interpretation of sections stained merely by hematoxylin and eosin. Specialized stains serve only to confirm a diagnosis made in sections stained by hematoxylin and eosin. In extramammary Paget's disease, the pale cytoplasm of atypical cells contains PAS-positive neutral mucosubstances that are not removed by diastase, whereas PAS-positive material, when present in the cytoplasm of atypical cells in pagetoid Bowen's disease, is removed completely by diastase. Furthermore, the cytoplasm of cells in extramammary Paget's disease is positive with colloidal iron and mucicarmine stains, an indication that acid mucosubstances are present; the neoplastic keratinocytes of pagetoid Bowen's disease are devoid of acid mucosubstances.

Bowen's disease is one of several forms of intra-epidermal squamous-cell carcinoma. It may occur anywhere on the skin and presents itself as a single lesion or as many lesions. The lesions usually are sharply marginated, brown-red plaques covered by scales and crusts. Bowen's disease on mucous membranes, especially on genitalia, is termed erythroplasia of Queyrat. Parenthetically, in our experience, there is no increased incidence of internal malignant neoplasms in patients who have Bowen's disease. Bowenoid papulosis refers to numerous condylomata acuminata on genitalia of young adults which, in time, show all the histopathologic features of Bowen's disease, i.e., squamous-cell carcinoma in situ. In short, bowenoid papulosis has the silhouette of a condyloma and the cytologic attributes of a squamous-cell carcinoma in situ.

Extramammary Paget's disease is an intra-epidermal adenocarcinoma that occurs particularly in the anogenital and axillary regions. The disease consists stereotypically of a solitary, asymmetrical, irregularly shaped, often eroded plaque that varies in color from white to red and extends centrifugally as an ill-defined scalloped border. There is but one authentic form of the disease, namely, an adenocarcinomatous process that originates in the epidermis. A simulator of extramammary Paget's disease extends into the epidermis from a contiguous adenocarcinoma of the genitourinary (e.g., the cervix) or the gastrointestinal (e.g., the rectum) tracts. It is a simulator of, rather than true, extramammary Paget's disease because it actually is a carcinoma of another organ and not a primary adenocarcinoma of the skin. The neoplastic cells in extramammary Paget's disease spread first horizontally within the epidermis and then vertically down epithelial structures of adnexa (in a manner like atypical melanocytes in malignant melanoma). The neoplastic process usually is confined to those epithelia (adenocarcinoma in situ) for the lifetime of a patient. In some instances, however, neoplastic cells of extramammary Paget's disease extend from the epithelium into the dermis from whence they may metastasize, albeit rarely.

Extramammary Paget's disease is a wholly different pathologic process from mammary Paget's disease in which neoplastic cells of an adenocarcinoma originate in lactiferous ducts and ascend those ducts to reach the epidermis where they are arranged in a pattern similar to that of extramammary Paget's disease. The adenocarcinomatous cells of mammary Paget's disease contain little or no acid mucosubstances, whereas those of extramammary Paget's disease are so replete with them that "signet-ring cells" form commonly.

Pagetoid Bowen's disease and extramammary Paget's disease also must be differentiated histopathologically from pagetoid malignant melanoma in situ because some examples of melanoma in situ, especially those situated on the trunk and extremities, are characterized by atypical pagetoid melanocytes distributed in pagetoid pattern within the epidermis and adnexal epithelia. Distinction between them is especially difficult in those unusual circumstances in which the pagetoid cells of Bowen's disease and the pagetoid cells of extramammary Paget's disease contain melanin in their cytoplasm. Some pagetoid cells of melanoma in situ are present always at the dermo-epidermal junction, whereas Paget cells of extramammary Paget's disease are situated in or above the basal layer of the epidermis, not at the dermo-epidermal junction itself.

33. Trichoepithelioma *vs.* Basal-Cell Carcinoma, Nodular Type

Trichoepithelioma	*Basal-Cell Carcinoma, Nodular Type*
1. Ulceration infrequent	1. Ulceration frequent
2. Neoplasm symmetrical	2. Neoplasm asymmetrical
3. Neoplasm well-circumscribed with smooth margins	3. Neoplasm poorly circumscribed, often with jagged margins
4. Follicular differentiation in the form of germs and papillae; less often as bulbs, outer and inner sheaths, and even rudimentary hairs	4. Indubitable follicular differentiation extremely rare
5. Cribriform pattern of neoplastic basaloid cells	5. No cribriform pattern of neoplastic basaloid cells
6. Necrotic neoplastic cells few and usually as solitary units	6. Necrotic neoplastic cells numerous and often en masse
7. No melanin in germinative cells usually	7. Melanin in germinative cells often
8. Acid mucosubstances unusual within aggregations of epithelial cells or in the stroma	8. Acid mucosubstances usual within aggregations of epithelial cells and in the stroma
9. No clefts between aggregations of neoplastic cells and stroma; clefts within the stroma itself and between stroma and the adjacent normal dermis	9. Clefts common between aggregations of neoplastic cells and stroma; no clefts between stroma and the adjacent normal dermis
10. Cornification of neoplastic epithelial cells (i.e., "cysts" that contain corneocytes) common	10. "Cysts" that contain corneocytes uncommon
11. Foreign-body granulomas common around cornified cells from ruptured "cysts"	11. No granulomatous inflammation as a rule
12. Stroma highly fibrocytic like that of perifollicular connective tissue sheaths	12. Stroma not like that of perifollicular sheaths
13. No edema of stroma	13. Edema of stroma
14. Infiltrates of inflammatory cells unusual	14. Infiltrates of inflammatory cells usual

Trichoepithelioma

Nodular Basal-Cell Carcinoma

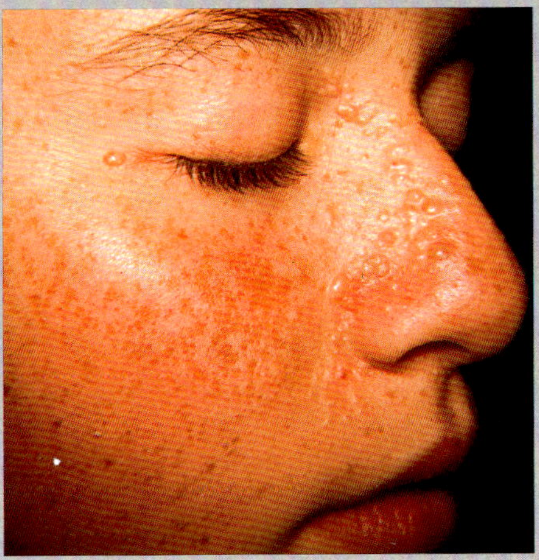

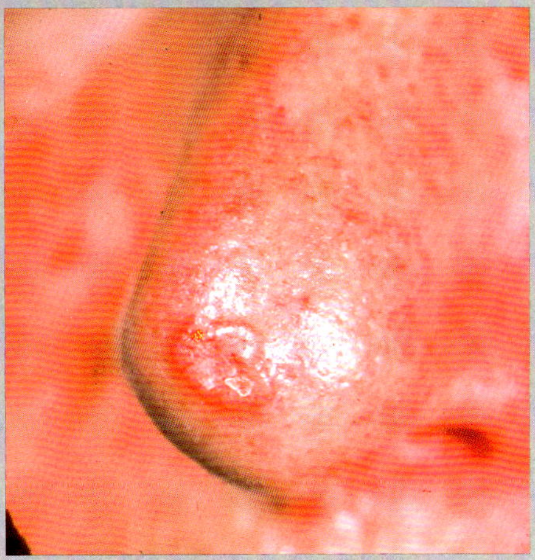

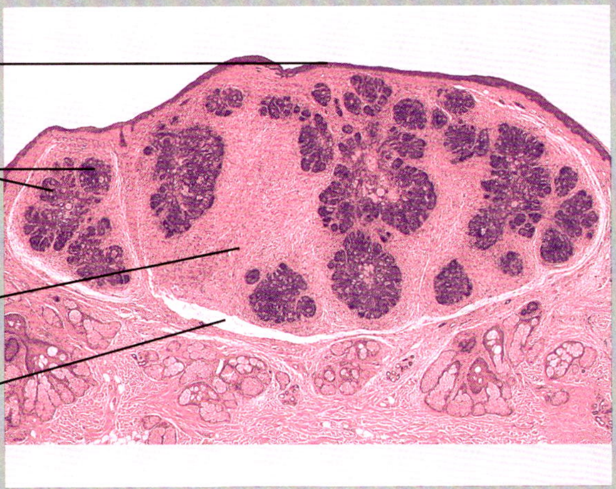

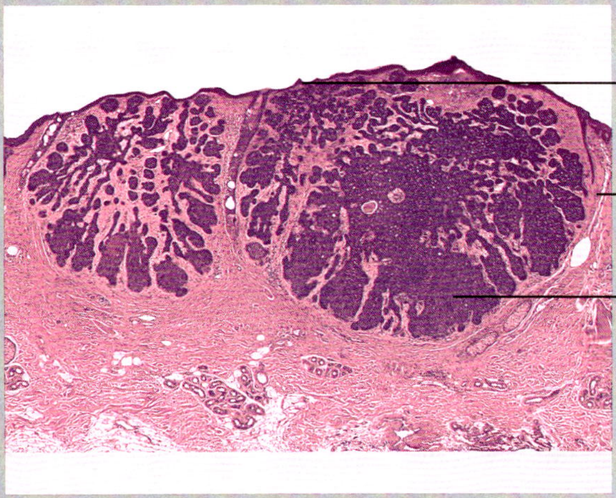

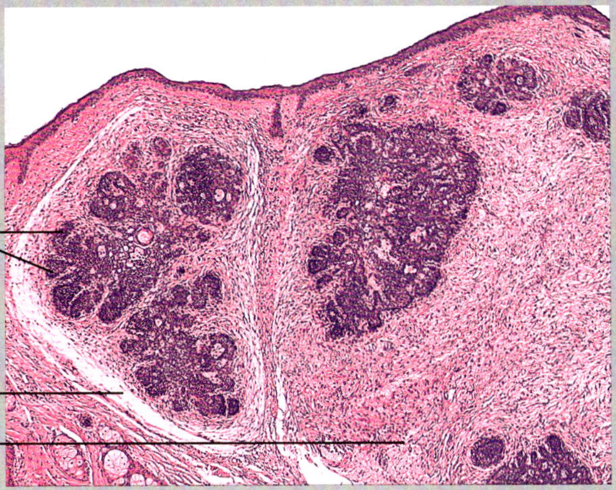

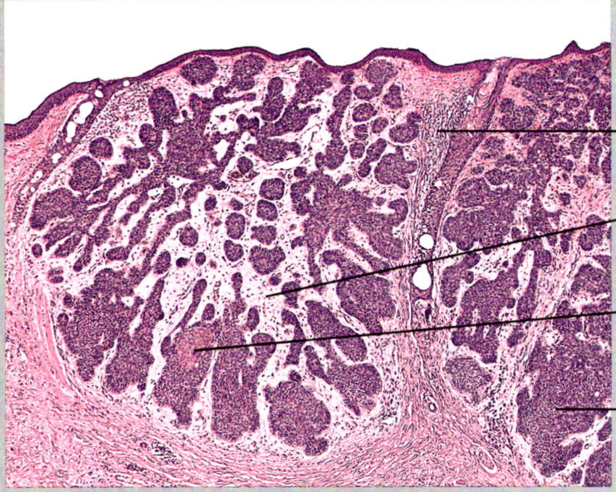

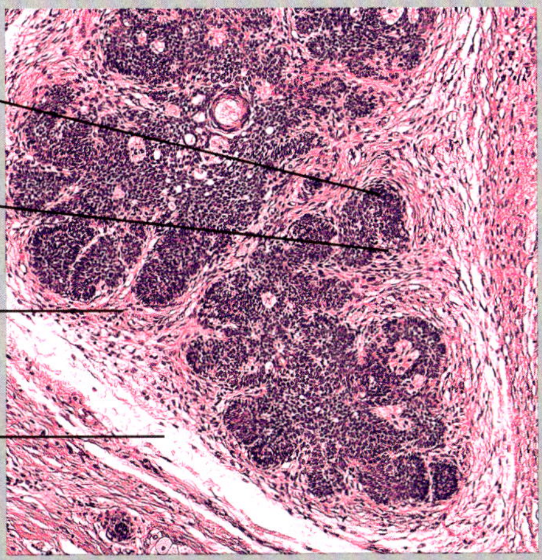

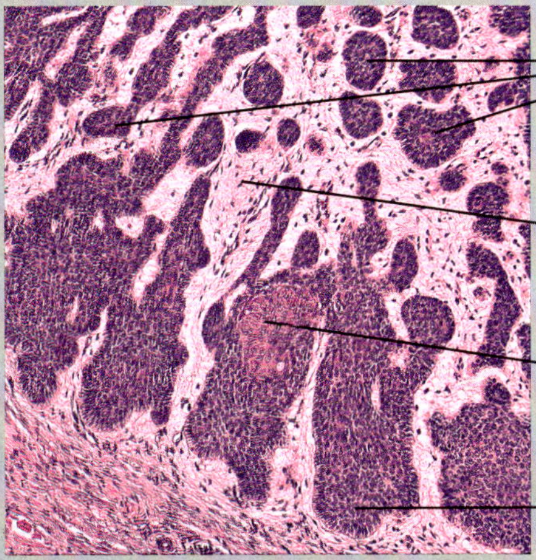

TRICHOEPITHELIOMAS and nodular basal-cell carcinomas are epithelial neoplasms with the following histopathologic features in common:

1. Dome-shape
2. Aggregates of basaloid (germinative) cells
3. Cells at the peripheries of aggregations of neoplastic epithelial cells aligned in palisades usually
4. Necrotic cells present within epithelial aggregations commonly
5. Amyloid deposits in the stroma commonly.

Generally, these two neoplasms of basaloid cells with completely different biologic behavior may be distinguished histopathologically from one another with confidence if the tabulated criteria are applied. This is especially true when a biopsy specimen of an entire neoplasm is submitted for examination by conventional microscopy. In some infrequent instances, however, differentiation between them may be nearly impossible. In still others, histopathologic features of both trichoepithelioma and of basal-cell carcinoma may be present in the same specimen.

Clinically, trichoepitheliomas may occur as numerous lesions on a face, but more commonly the neoplasm presents itself as a solitary papule or nodule there. Trichoepitheliomas are skin-colored and frequently are traversed by telangiectases. In cases of numerous trichoepitheliomas, inheritance is through an autosomal dominant trait. Solitary trichoepithelioma is not inherited. Epithelioma adenoides cysticum is another, older, and antiquated appellation for numerous trichoepitheliomas. An interesting association of benign neoplasms with adnexal differentiation is the concurrence, episodically, of trichoepitheliomas and cylindromas in the same patient. This association implies that cylindroma is a neoplasm with apocrine, rather than eccrine, differentiation (follicular, sebaceous, and apocrine structures form a unit in utero and thereafter).

Conventionally, trichoepithelioma is considered to be a wholly different neoplasm than trichoblastoma, but, in actuality, it is one of the various expressions of trichoblastoma because it fulfills the requisite histopathologic criteria, namely, a benign neoplasm constituted mostly of follicular germinative cells.

So-called desmoplastic trichoepithelioma consists of columns and cords of epithelial cells, cornifying cyst-like structures that tend to calcify, and a collagenous stroma in which rims of collagen bundles form around columns and cords of epithelial cells. Desmoplastic trichoepithelioma is not truly a trichoepithelioma because it usually does not exhibit indubitable follicular differentiation as a rule, and it is not really desmoplastic because there is no prominent fibroplasia. In about 10% of all specimens of desmoplastic trichoepithelioma, cells of a melanocytic nevus are present within its substance. In brief, desmoplastic trichoepithelioma bears no relationship, clinically or histopathologically, to the benign neoplasm with follicular differentiation that is one of the two major subjects of this chapter.

Nodular basal-cell carcinoma refers to that type of basal-cell carcinoma which is constituted of small or large aggregations of neoplastic basaloid cells. It usually occurs as a single lesion on sun-damaged skin of individuals with fair complexions. Such persons, however, may have several basal-cell carcinomas. Basal-cell carcinoma is generally a malignant neoplasm of middle-aged or older individuals, except in the systemic condition known as nevoid basal-cell carcinoma syndrome in which children are affected by scores, and sometimes hundreds, of these carcinomas. Basal-cell carcinomas may develop in a variety of atrophic scars, such as those caused by radiotherapy, vaccinations, burns, lupus vulgaris, and discoid lupus erythematosus.

Besides the nodular type, there are only four other major types of basal-cell carcinoma based upon clinico-pathologic correlation, namely, superficial, infundibulo-cystic, morphea-like, and fibroepitheliomatous. The histopathologic patterns of basal-cell carcinoma, however, are numerous, e.g., cystic, microcystic, adenoid cystic, adenoid, trabecular, fenestrated, labyrinthine, and cribriform. Basal-cell carcinomas of all types may be pigmented by melanin.

34. Metastatic Carcinoma From a Breast *vs.* Morphea-like Basal-Cell Carcinoma

Metastatic Carcinoma from a Breast

1. Strands, cords, and columns of neoplastic cells within the dermis
2. Differentiation is frequently tubular
3. Columns of neoplastic cells do not branch
4. Neoplastic cells may be entirely within the deep part of the dermis
5. Neoplastic cells are found within lymphatics often
6. Neoplastic cells are not basaloid, i.e., their cytoplasm is abundant
7. Nuclei of neoplastic cells are pleomorphic
8. Nucleoli are prominent
9. Numerous mitotic figures in neoplastic cells
10. Collagen bundles that surround the neoplastic cells are thickened and brightly eosinophilic; the number of fibrocytes often is decreased
11. No elastotic material often

Morphea-like Basal-Cell Carcinoma

1. Cords and columns of neoplastic cells within the dermis; no strands as a rule
2. Differentiation is rarely tubular
3. Columns of neoplastic cells tend to branch
4. Neoplastic cells are never entirely within the deep part of the dermis
5. Neoplastic cells are not housed within lymphatics
6. Neoplastic cells are basaloid, i.e., their cytoplasm is scant
7. Nuclei of neoplastic cells are monomorphic
8. Nucleoli are not noticeable usually
9. Few mitotic figures in neoplastic cells
10. Collagen bundles that surround the neoplastic cells are fibrillar and amphophilic; the number of fibrocytes is increased
11. Extensive elastotic material often

Metastatic Carcinoma from the Breast

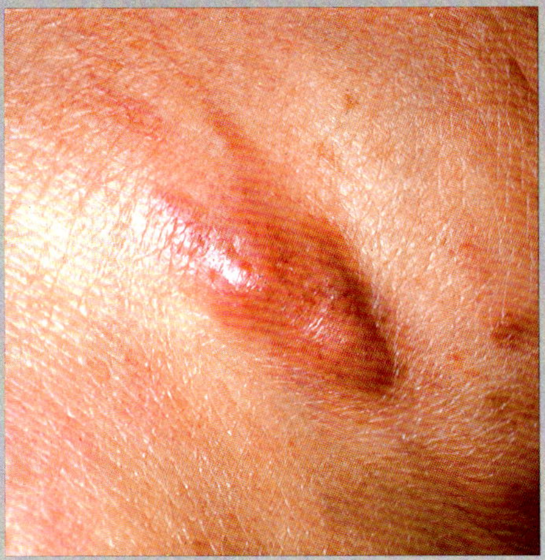

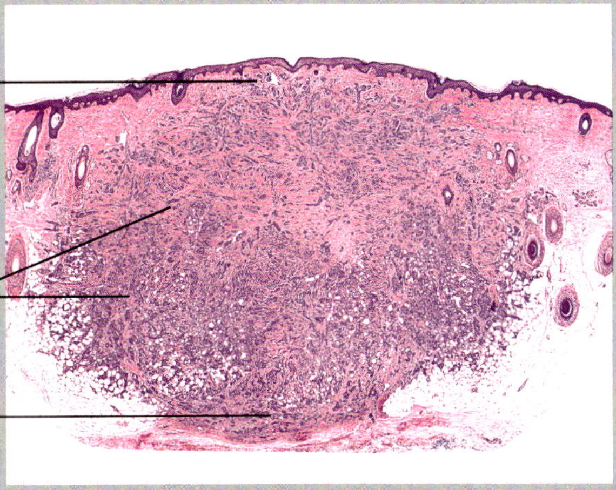

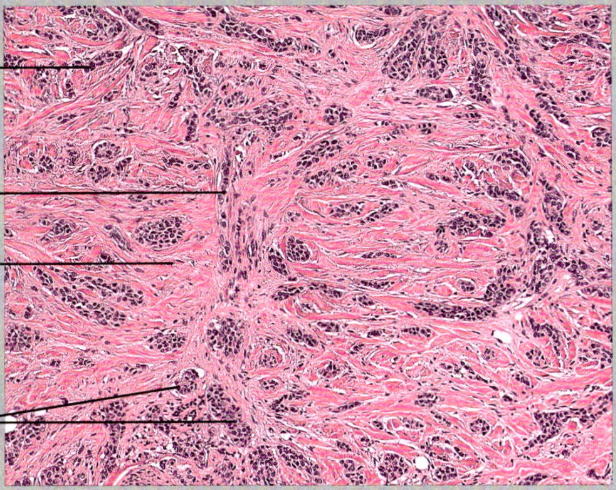

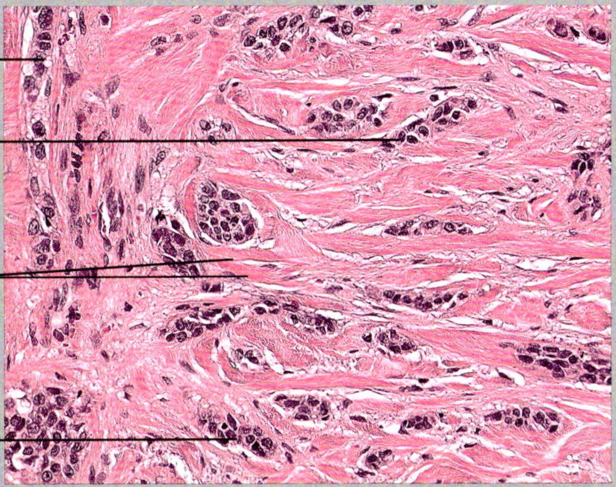

Morpheiform Basal-Cell Carcinoma

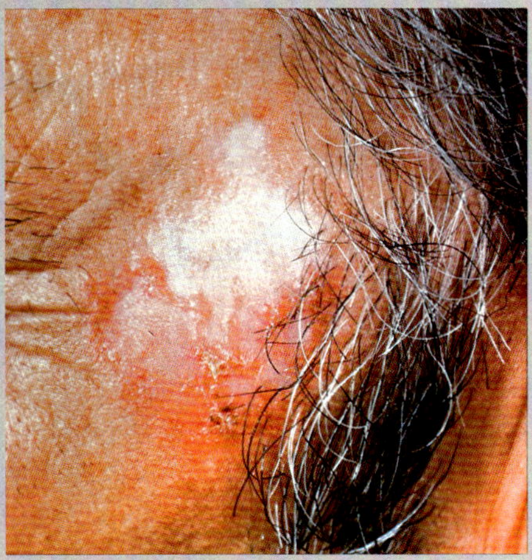

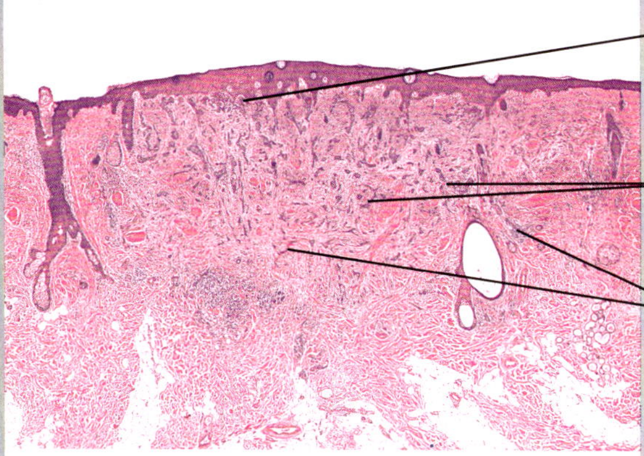

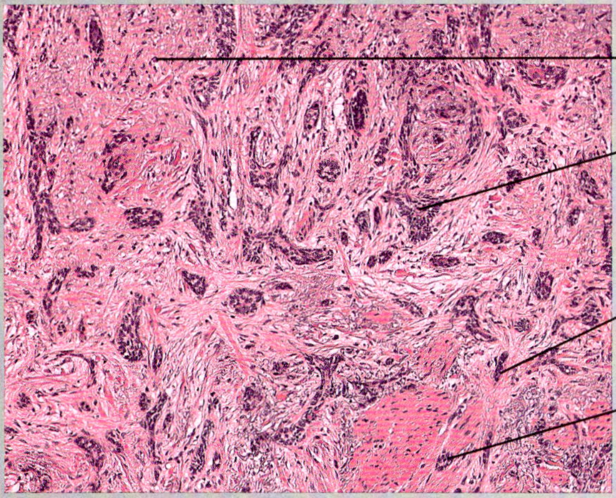

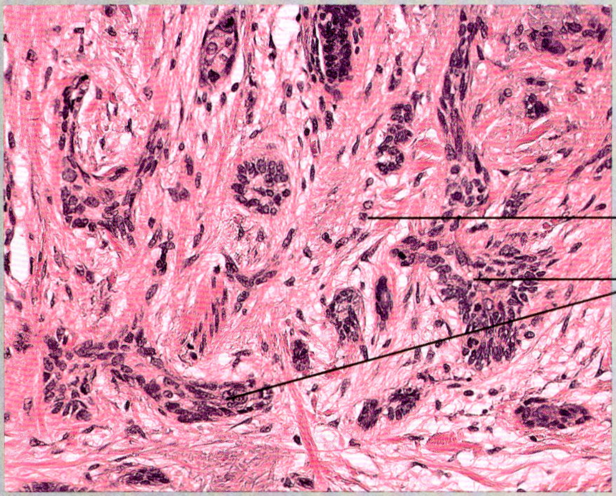

In general, neoplasms metastatic to the skin present little difficulty in differential diagnosis from neoplasms that are primary in the skin. Carcinoma of the breast is an exception. Metastatic carcinoma from the breast may be mistaken for a wholly inflammatory skin condition if there are but a few neoplastic cells and numerous inflammatory cells scattered diffusely among bundles of collagen. As a rule, when difficulties arise in differentiating metastatic carcinoma to the skin from carcinoma primary in the skin, morphea-like basal-cell carcinoma is the primary carcinoma at issue. Other synonyms for morphea-like basal-cell carcinoma are morpheiform basal-cell carcinoma, fibrosing basal-cell carcinoma, sclerosing basal-cell carcinoma, and syringomatous basal-cell carcinoma.

Metastatic carcinoma from the breast and morphea-like basal-cell carcinoma have several histopathologic features in common such as:

1. Epithelial cells arranged in columns and cords
2. Linear orientation between bundles of collagen
3. Embedment of neoplastic cells in a fibrotic stroma
4. Appearance of hyperchromatic nuclei, and
5. Presence of inflammatory cells.

Metastatic carcinoma to the skin from the breast may present itself in four different clinical forms as follows:

1. Inflammatory: red, edematous, and indurated (similar to that in erysipelas) because of obstruction of lymphatics by the neoplastic cells
2. Telangiectatic: purple papules, nodules, and hemorrhagic patches and plaques that resemble vascular neoplasms
3. Nodular: deep-seated nodules that appear in mastectomy scars especially
4. Cancer en cuirasse: diffuse, firm, brawny, tan plaque.

Metastases from carcinoma of a breast occur most often by way of lymphatics, but occasionally they travel by blood vessels. The scalp is the most common end of a journey for metastases by hematogenous routes, but any site on the skin may be affected by metastatic carcinoma from the breast.

Morpheiform basal-cell carcinoma presents itself clinically as an indurated yellow-tan or whitish patch or plaque across which course telangiectases. The surface of the skin usually is intact, but rarely may be ulcerated.

Syringoma may be confused histopathologically with metastatic carcinoma from a breast and with morpheiform basal-cell carcinoma. Syringomas also are comprised of columns and cords of epithelial cells, tubules, and collagenous stroma. The tubular structures of syringomas, however, unlike those in metastatic adenocarcinoma, often show comma-like extensions that have been compared to the shape of tadpoles. Cornifying cysts and calcification are common features of syringoma, but not, as a rule, of metastases from carcinoma. Clinically, syringomas are small, yellowish-tan papules on lower eyelids, but the lesions may occur in other areas of the skin such as the cheek, axillae, abdomen, and chest. Syringomas tend to affect women more commonly than men.

Desmoplastic trichoepithelioma also must be distinguished histopathologically from metastatic carcinoma to the skin and from morpheiform basal-cell carcinoma. The crucial feature in this differentiation is tendency of the cords of cells in desmoplastic trichoepithelioma to be surrounded by rims of collagen bundles, to be associated with cysts that contain cornified cells that calcify, and to harbor, episodically, cells of a melanocytic nevus.

35. Simple Lentigo *vs.* Solar Lentigo

Simple Lentigo	*Solar Lentigo*
1. Laminated orthokeratotic cornified layer contains abundant melanin often	1. Compactly orthokeratotic cornified layer contains relatively little melanin usually
2. Thin elongated rete ridges	2. Slightly bullous elongated rete ridges
3. No nubbins of epithelium at right angles to thin rete ridges; no signs of seborrheic keratoses	3. Nubbins of epithelium sometimes at bases of bulbous rete ridges and at right angles to them; resemble hockey sticks and represent eventuation into reticulated seborrheic keratosis
4. Marked hyperpigmentation throughout the entire thickness of the epidermis	4. Slight to moderate hyperpigmentation of the epidermis, most apparent in the basal layer
5. Marked increase in number of melanocytes arranged as solitary units at the dermo-epidermal junction	5. Slight increase in number of melanocytes dispersed as solitary units at the dermo-epidermal junction
6. Melanocytes, in time, form small nests at bases of rete ridges (junctional nevus)	6. Melanocytes do not form nests
7. Large globules of melanin (giant melanosomes) within some melanocytes occasionally	7. No giant melanosomes within melanocytes
8. Solar elastosis uncommon and incidental	8. Solar elastosis present always and essential pathogenetically
9. Collagen bundles in the papillary dermis in concentric and lamellar arrangement often	9. No concentric or lamellar arrangement of collagen bundles
10. Numerous melanophages usually	10. Few melanophages usually

Simple Lentigo	*Solar Lentigo*

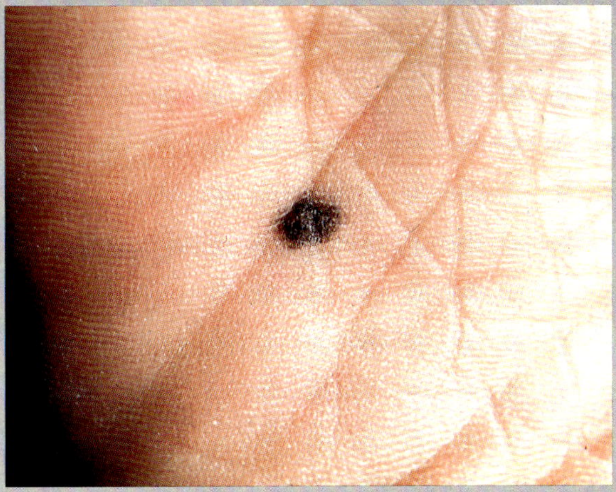

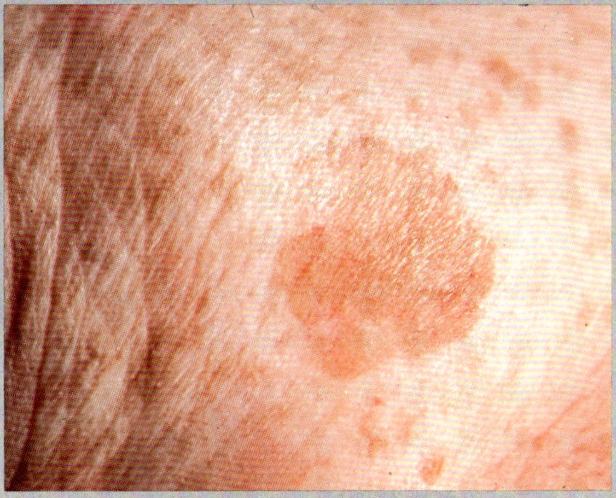

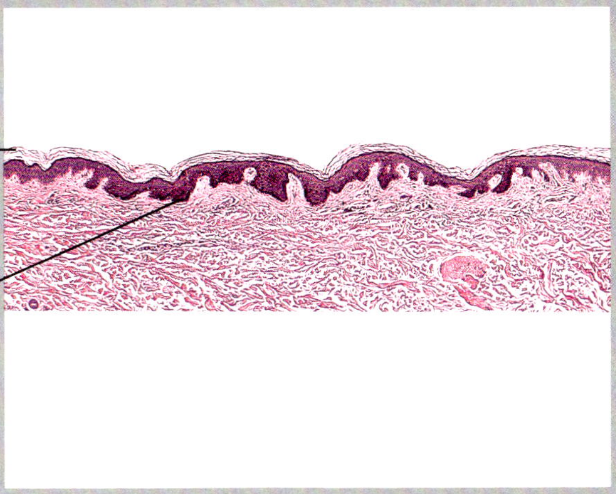

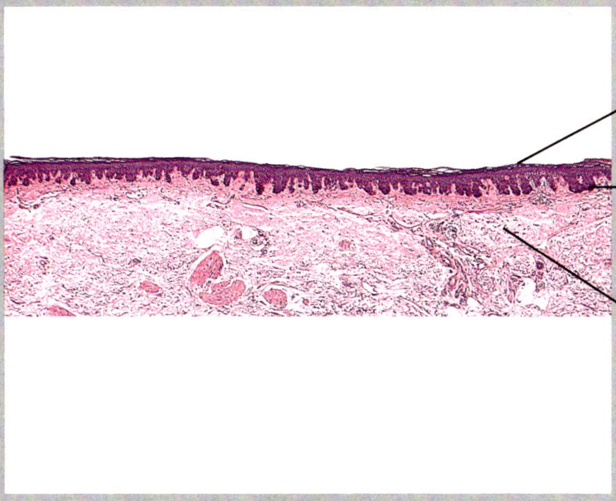

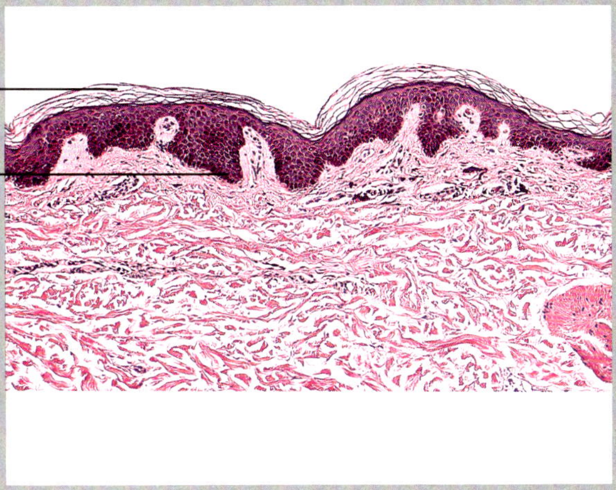

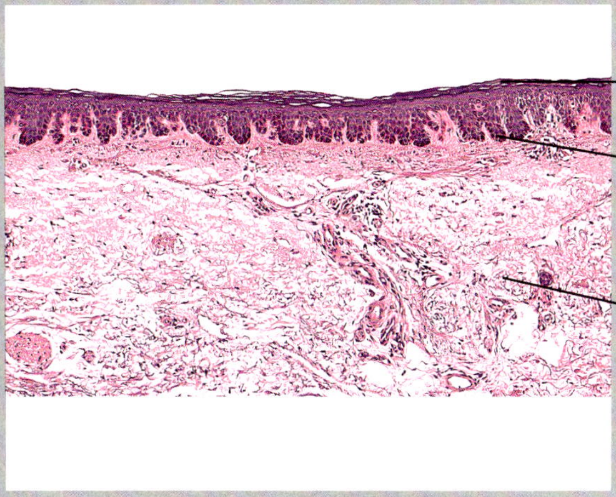

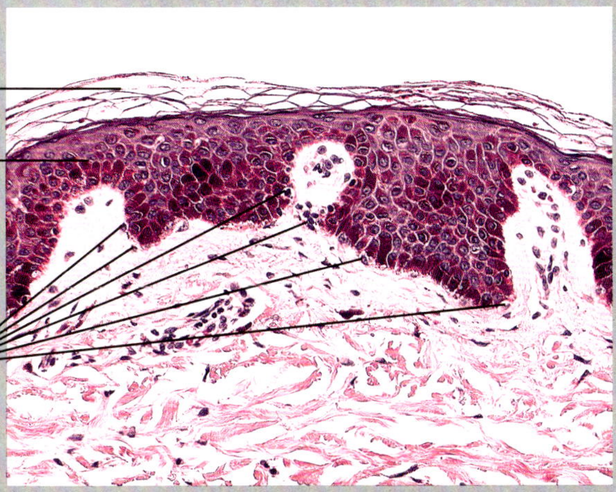

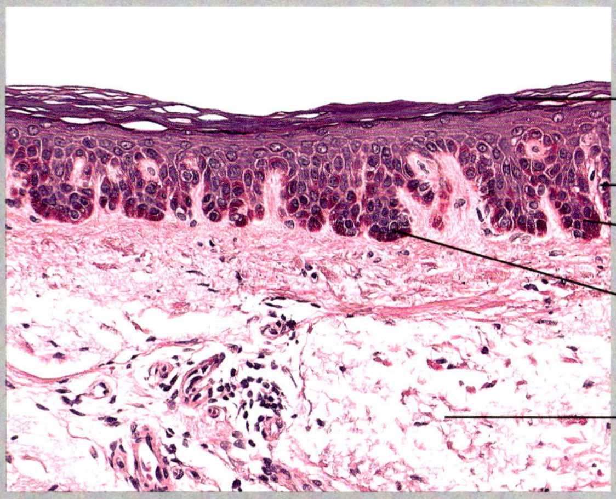

SIMPLE lentigo (also known as juvenile lentigo) and solar lentigo (also called senile lentigo) are common, wholly benign, pigmented lesions that share histopathologic features. Both are characterized, in most examples, by elongated rete ridges, hyperpigmentation, and melanophages in the upper part of the dermis. Both have an increased number of monomorphous melanocytes within the epidermis arranged as solitary units and situated only in the basal layer. They differ principally in the shape of the rete ridges (thin in simple lentigo and relatively broad in solar lentigo) and in the number of melanocytes (many more in simple lentigo than in solar lentigo). In brief, simple lentigo is fundamentally a proliferation of melanocytes with concurrent alterations in keratinocytes and collagen bundles in the papillary dermis, whereas solar lentigo is basically a proliferation of keratinocytes with associated changes in melanocytes and no ostensible modifications in collagen bundles.

Clinically, simple lentigines are small, round to oval, dark brown to black macules that often have strikingly reticulated peripheries. They occur anywhere on the skin surface of young individuals especially, but not exclusively. Simple lentigines may appear at almost any age, and are not related causally to sun exposure. By adulthood they tend to become less pigmented.

Solar lentigines, in contrast, are relatively large, irregularly shaped, mottled, tan to brown, macular and subtly papular, slightly scaly lesions that develop only on parts of the skin that have been exposed to sunlight for long periods of time. For that reason, they are found most often on older individuals, especially on the face and dorsa of the hands and forearms. They generally begin to appear after the age of 40, increasing progressively in number with age. Solar lentigines, as their name implies, always are induced by long-standing exposure to sunlight and therefore always are associated histopathologically with solar elastosis. In common parlance, solar lentigines are known as "liver spots."

Simple lentigines represent an early stage in the evolution of junctional nevi. Evidence for that continuum is the presence frequently of nests of melanocytes within thin rete ridges of simple lentigines. When nests of melanocytes form in a simple lentigo, the lesion is termed a junctional nevus conventionally, and by me some years ago, playfully, for purposes of teaching, a "jentigo." In time, a lesion with typical histopathologic features of a simple lentigo may exhibit nests of melanocytes not only within the epidermis, but in the papillary dermis, too. That lesion is designated, in standard parlance, a compound nevus, but was referred to by us in former time, in the same spirit as "jentigo," as "compendigo." In short, a simple lentigo is merely the earliest stage in what is likely to become a junctional, compound, and intradermal nevus of Clark's (so-called dysplastic) type. To our knowledge, a simple lentigo does not eventuate in an Unna's, Miescher's, or Spitz's nevus.

Simple lentigines are to junctional, compound, and intradermal stages of Clark's nevi what solar lentigines are to seborrheic keratoses of reticulated, and sometimes other, types. Virtually all reticulated types of seborrheic keratosis begin as solar lentigines. It is a continuous single pathologic process that has been given two different names. In actuality, simple lentigo is a junctional nevus and solar lentigo is a seborrheic keratosis, just as solar keratosis is a squamous-cell carcinoma.

Simple and solar lentigines are differentiated easily histopathologically from ephelides (freckles) in which rete ridges have normal shapes and normal complements of melanocytes but only slight hyperpigmentation, which is barely noticeable in the basal layer. Clinically, freckles, like solar lentigines, appear consequent to exposure to ultraviolet light, but that exposure need merely be brief and the lesions that result are smaller, never scaly, and relatively evanescent.

Labial lentigo differs from simple lentigo and solar lentigo. It occurs mostly on an oral lip, but also occurs on a vulvar lip and on the penis. Labial lentigo is characterized by an increased number of dendritic melanocytes in a markedly pigmented epithelium. All of the melanocytes are situated at the junction of epithelium and lamina propria. Sometimes the dendrites extend upward to beyond the mid portion of the epithelium. Labial lentigo is differentiated histopathologically from melanosis of the genitalia by more melanocytes, longer dendrites of melanocytes, and more melanin in the epithelium, and clinically by smaller size, uniform pigmentation, and no resemblance to melanoma.

So-called lentigo maligna (Hutchinson's freckle) is completely unrelated to simple lentigo, solar lentigo, and freckle. It is a melanoma in situ that occurs in severely sun-damaged skin, usually of the head and neck of persons with light complexions. Histopathologically, it sometimes may be mistaken for a junctional nevus. The contrasting features of these two very different conditions are listed and discussed in the next chapter.

36. Junctional Nevus *vs.* Melanoma in Situ on Sun-Damaged Skin of a Face

Junctional Nevus	*Melanoma in situ on Sun-Damaged Skin of a Face*
1. Symmetric	1. Asymmetric
2. Sharp circumscription of the intra-epidermal melanocytic component	2. Poor circumscription of the intra-epidermal melanocytic component
3. Epidermis normal or slightly thickened	3. Epidermis thinned usually
4. Preservation of the normal pattern between rete ridges and dermal papillae	4. Loss of the normal pattern between rete ridges and dermal papillae
5. Nests of melanocytes predominate over melanocytes arrayed as solitary units	5. Atypical melanocytes within the epidermis arrayed mainly as solitary units in some high-power fields
6. Nests of melanocytes relatively equidistant from one another	6. Nests of melanocytes not equidistant from one another
7. Margins of nests of melanocytes smooth	7. Margins of nests of melanocytes jagged sometimes
8. Nests of melanocytes vary little in size and shape	8. Nests of melanocytes vary considerably in size and shape
9. Nests of melanocytes well-circumscribed and discrete	9. Nests of melanocytes usually poorly circumscribed and often confluent
10. Melanocytes arrayed as solitary units confined to the dermo-epidermal junction	10. Some melanocytes arrayed as solitary units above the dermo-epidermal junction in many instances
11. Infiltrate of lymphocytes sparse to moderately dense as a rule	11. Infiltrate of lymphocytes moderately dense to dense often
12. Few melanophages usually	12. Many melanophages usually
13. Little solar elastosis in the dermis usually (and then incidental)	13. Extensive solar elastosis in the dermis always (and important pathogenetically)

Junctional Nevus

Melanoma in Situ on Sun-Damaged Skin of the Face

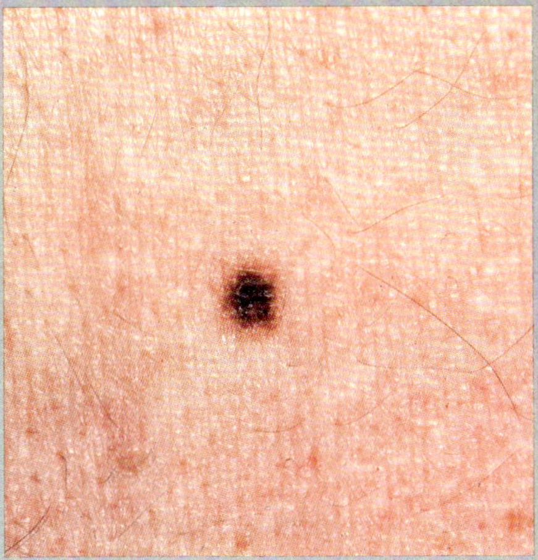

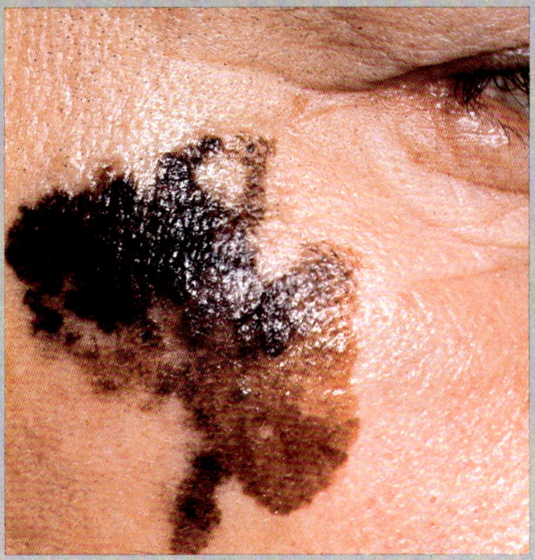

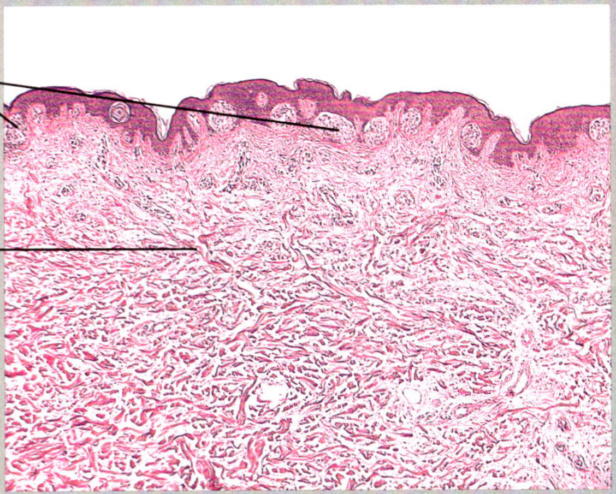

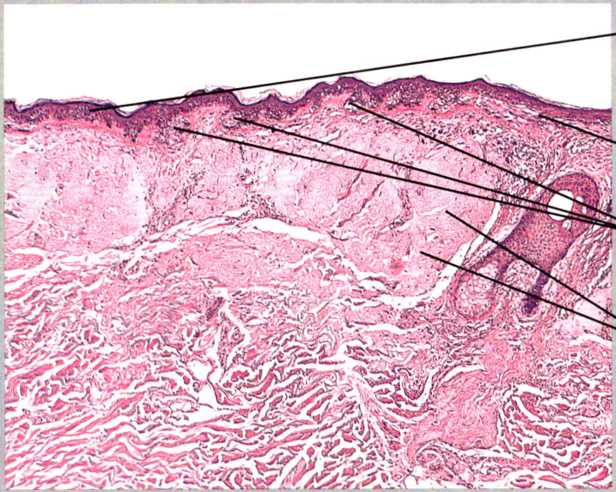

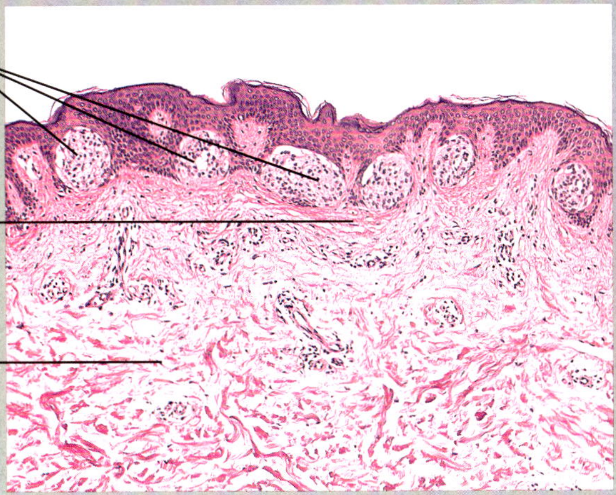

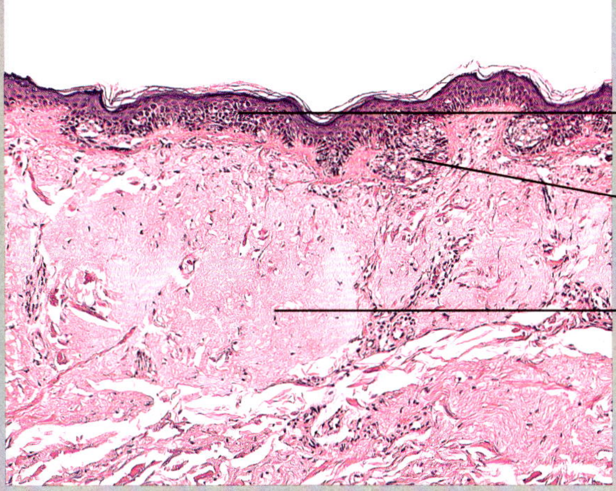

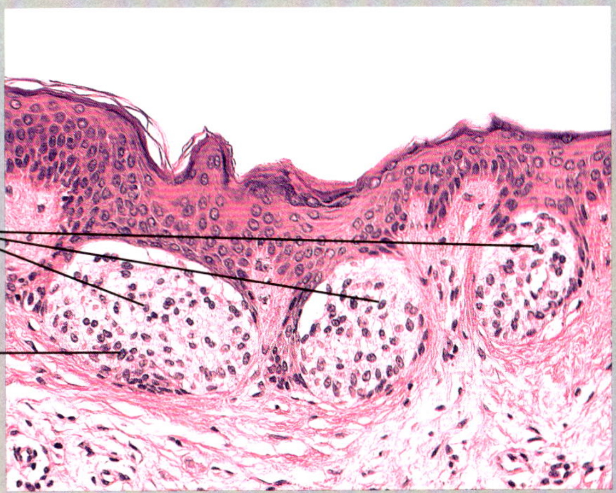

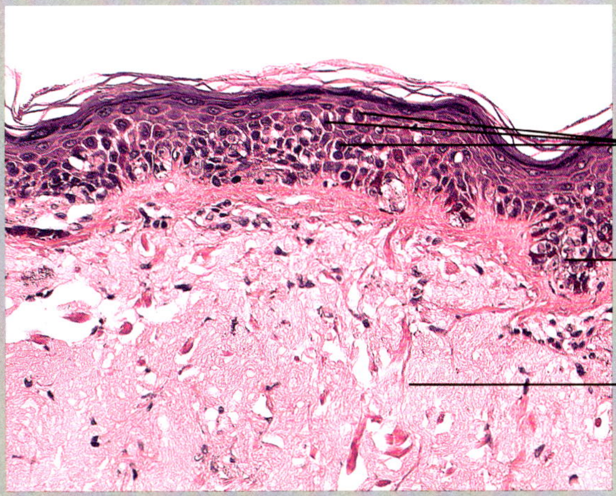

JUNCTIONAL nevus and malignant melanoma in situ on sun-damaged skin of a face especially (lentigo maligna) are both melanocytic proliferations in which nests of melanocytes tend to form within a hyperpigmented epidermis, and melanophages accumulate in a thickened papillary dermis.

Acquired junctional nevi of all types present themselves clinically as macules or very slightly elevated papules that are sharply circumscribed, relatively uniform in pigmentation, and smooth-surfaced. They vary in color from tan to brown to pink, and range in size from less than a millimeter to more than a centimeter. Junctional nevi usually appear during the first decade of life, but sometimes arise much later than that.

Melanocytic nevi of junctional type tend to become compound and eventually entirely intradermal. It was once widely believed that junctional nevi, especially those said to be "active" or those on palms, soles, and sites of irritation, were precursors of malignant melanomas. In fact, junctional nevi at all these sites now are acknowledged to be completely benign. It is exceptional for malignant melanoma to develop upon a pre-existing junctional nevus; the vast majority arise de novo and those that do not begin in nevi of compound or intradermal types. Furthermore, the concepts of "junctional activity" and "active junctional nevus" evade the obligatory judgment in diagnosis of benign or malignant nature, and should be abandoned because they obscure and confuse, rather than enlighten. The same is true for the opaque term "dysplasia."

The cells that form nests in a junctional nevus are melanocytes, i.e., they make melanin and have all the ultrastructural and biochemical characteristics of melanocytes. To refer to them or their intradermal relations as "nevus cells" beclouds their identity. In actuality, those cells conventionally termed "nevus cells," "nevocytes," and "nevomelanocytes" are melanocytes.

Lentigo maligna (Hutchinson's freckle, melanosis circumscripta precancerosa of Dubreuilh) is a euphemism for melanoma in situ on skin, especially on a face, that has been damaged badly by sunlight. It begins clinically as a light-brown macule that gradually becomes darker as it extends centrifugally. Over several years, the flat neoplasm may attain several square centimeters or even inches in an irregular outline. A patch of well-developed lentigo maligna usually has gradations of color from light brown to black within it. Not every macule of melanoma on sun-battered skin of a face eventuates in a patch. Some progress to papules and even to nodules and tumors. The same may be said for macules of melanoma on every anatomic site.

The histopathologic sequence of changes in lentigo maligna, as in melanoma in situ on all anatomic sites, begins with proliferation of individual melanocytes whose nuclei are typical, proceeds to proliferation of melanocytes with atypical nuclei, and eventuates in formation of nests of atypical melanocytes within the epidermis and adnexal epithelium. After several years, usually between 10 and 20, atypical melanocytes from the epidermis descend into the dermis. As the neoplastic melanocytes descend further, they gain potential for metastasis. The first clinical evidence of descent into the dermis is a small papule which, in time, may become nodular. The entire process, from the outset, is that of malignant melanoma.

Malignant melanoma in situ on sun-damaged skin of a face, like the patch stage of Kaposi's sarcoma and the patch stage of mycosis fungoides (e.g., parapsoriasis en plaques), is not life-threatening. Only when papulation or nodularity supervenes (dermal involvement by atypical melanocytes) does melanoma have the potential to metastasize and cause death.

Morphologically, if only the lesion itself of so-called lentigo maligna or lentigo maligna melanoma is studied, no single clinical or histopathologic feature or constellation of features enables it to be differentiated from a melanoma on any other cutaneous site. Clinically, all melanomas on all anatomic sites are, more or less, asymmetric, poorly circumscribed, and variegated in colors of brown mostly. Histopathologically, all are asymmetric, poorly circumscribed, and characterized by atypical melanocytes arranged both as solitary units and in nests. These nests are not equidistant from one another, they vary in size and shape, and they tend to become confluent. Melanocytes that are arranged as solitary units predominate over nests of melanocytes in some high-power fields, and some melanocytes are scattered above the dermo-epidermal junction. Clues to diagnosis of malignant melanoma situated specifically on sun-damaged skin of the face are not found in the melanoma itself, but in the rest of the section, namely, numerous large sebaceous glands associated with vellus hair follicles and abundant solar elastosis.

It is now appreciated that melanomas on skin of a face damaged severely by sunlight behave in about the same fashion biologically as melanomas on all other anatomic sites. It also is apparent that junctional nevi rarely develop in skin injured severely by sunlight. Last, melanomas on skin that has been injured badly by sunlight rarely arise in pre-existing melanocytic nevi of any kind. Nearly all arise de novo.

37. Spitz's Nevus, Compound Type *vs.* Malignant Melanoma

Spitz's Nevus, Compound Type	*Malignant Melanoma*
1. Lesion symmetric	1. Lesion asymmetric
2. Sharp circumscription of the neoplasm	2. Poor circumscription of the neoplasm
3. Maturation of melanocytes (decrease in nuclear size) with progressive descent	3. No maturation of melanocytes with progressive descent into the dermis usually
4. Nests of melanocytes relatively uniform	4. Nests of melanocytes vary markedly
5. Nests of melanocytes within the epidermis elongated and perpendicular often	5. Nests of melanocytes within the epidermis neither elongated nor perpendicular usually
6. Melanocytes in nests cohesive	6. Melanocytes in "nests" not cohesive sometimes
7. Clefts between nests of melanocytes and adjacent keratinocytes are the rule	7. Clefts, sometimes broad, beneath nests at the dermo-epidermal junction episodically
8. Nests of epidermal and dermal melanocytes tend to be discrete	8. Nests of epidermal and dermal melanocytes tend to become confluent; the latter may form sheets of cells
9. Melanocytes at the base of the neoplasm are arranged as single cells commonly	9. Melanocytes at the base of the neoplasm are not arranged as single cells usually
10. No pagetoid melanocytes usually	10. Pagetoid melanocytes often
11. Mitotic figures near base of lesion uncommon	11. Mitotic figures near base of lesion common
12. Dull pink globules arranged as solitary units and in clusters within the epidermis	12. No dull pink globules within the epidermis as a rule
13. Hyperkeratosis prominent; hypergranulosis and marked spinous-cell hyperplasia usual	13. Hyperkeratosis not prominent; no hypergranulosis usually; little epidermal hyperplasia
14. No evidence of regression	14. Foci of regression sometimes
15. Infiltrate of lymphocytes around blood vessels throughout the neoplasm	15. Infiltrate of lymphocytes mostly beneath the neoplasm

Spitz's Nevus, Compound Type

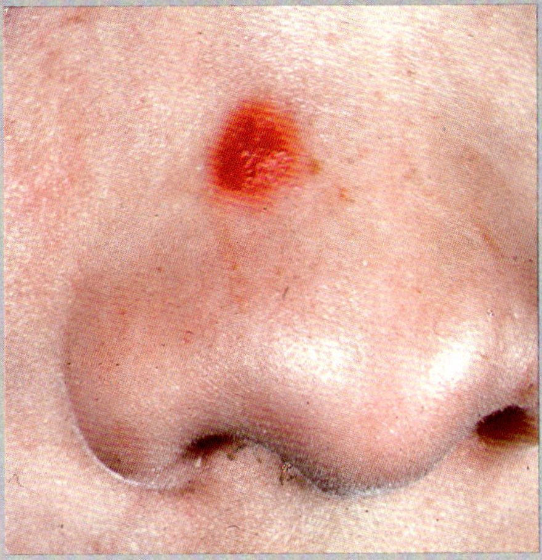

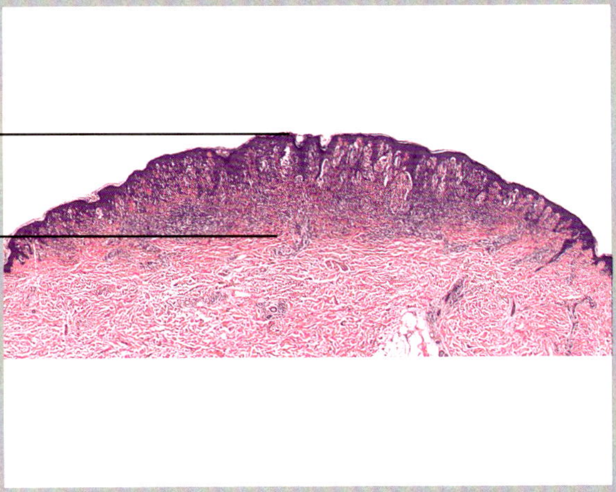

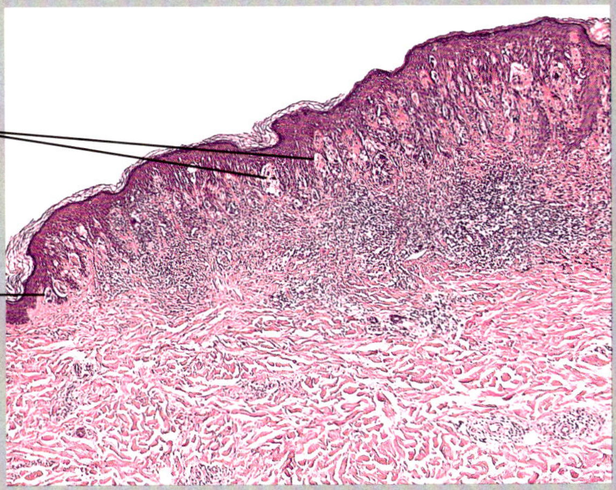

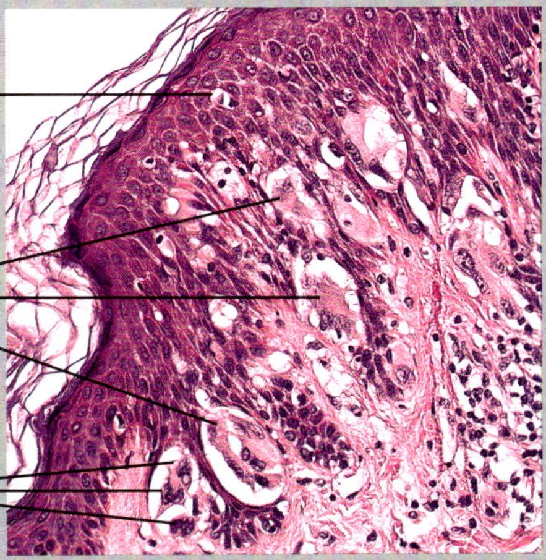

Malignant Melanoma on the Trunk or Proximal Extremities

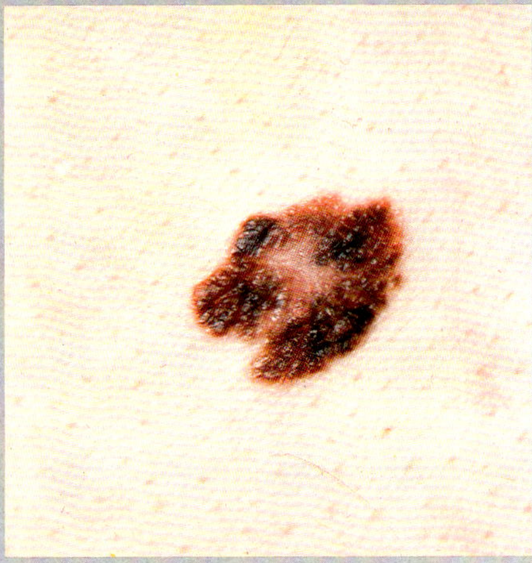

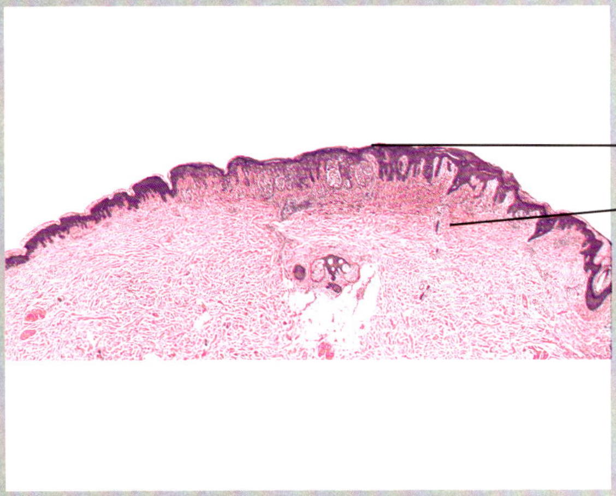

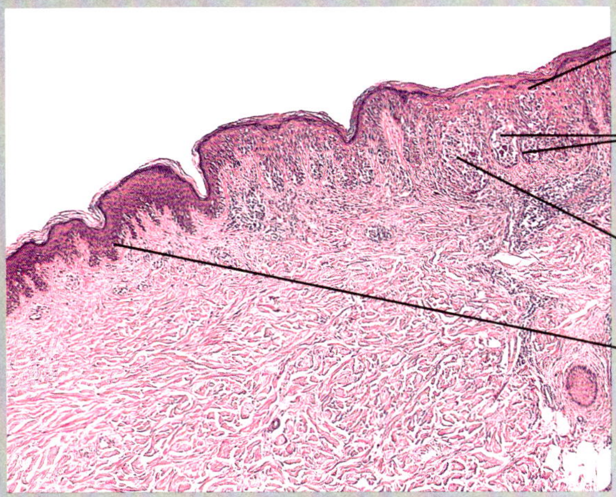

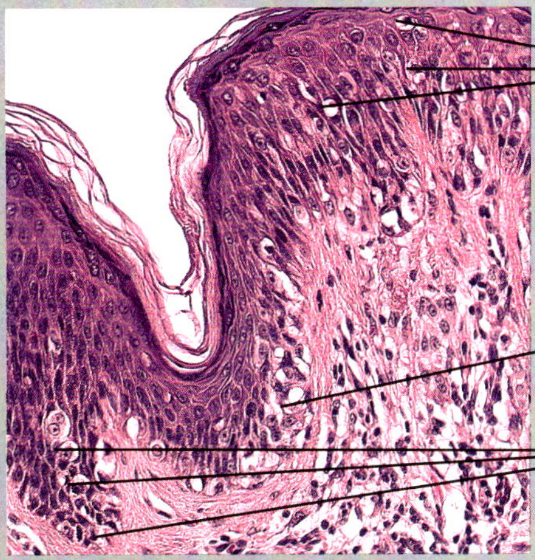

A compound type of Spitz's nevus and a malignant melanoma have several features in common including nests of atypical melanocytes within the epidermis (scattered often above the dermo-epidermal junction and sometimes at all levels of the epidermis) and the dermis, some neoplastic melanocytes in mitosis, and an infiltrate of lymphocytes in the dermis. In actuality, nuclear atypia of melanocytes may be more striking in some Spitz's nevi than in many malignant melanomas.

Spitz's nevus occurs in both children and adults and, clinically, may be darkly pigmented or entirely devoid of pigment. The non-pigmented manifestation presents itself typically as an orange-red, smooth-surfaced, or papillomatous papule or nodule. The pigmented expression of Spitz's nevus is a well-circumscribed, oval or oblong, tan, brown, or even black papule, often with a plateau-like surface. A lesion of Spitz's nevus, in most instances, is situated on the head or extremities (very commonly on legs of women), but sometimes on the trunk. A desmoplastic variant occurs in long-standing lesions of Spitz's nevus in adults. The prominent fibroplasia may cause a Spitz's nevus to be misinterpreted, clinically and histologically, as a dermatofibroma or as a desmoplastic melanoma. The presence of large, often polygonal melanocytes dispersed as solitary units and in small nests within a fibrotic stroma enables differentiation of the melanocytic neoplasm from the inflammatory dermatofibroma. The silhouette of desmoplastic Spitz's nevus (symmetry and sharp circumscription) and the absence of neurotropism enable differentiation of the benign neoplasm from desmoplastic melanoma.

The large size of some of the melanocytes, i.e., large nuclei and abundant cytoplasm, is the common denominator of nearly all forms of Spitz's nevi, the exception being the pigmented spindle (oval)-cell variant. Another important feature of Spitz's nevus is the shapes of the melanocytes. Most commonly they are oval, round, and polygonal, and less commonly spindled or dendritic. Multinucleated melanocytes, sometimes in large numbers, are expected findings in Spitz's nevi, although they need not be present in every specimen. In short, Spitz's nevus is merely one type of melanocytic nevus and, like all the others, behaves in a benign fashion biologically. Therefore, the notion of "metastasizing Spitz's nevus" is illogical and without foundation. A Spitz's nevus purported to have metastasized was, in truth, a melanoma from the outset.

Malignant melanoma may develop anywhere on the integument, but most frequently it appears on the legs of women and on the trunks of men. Clinically, melanoma is characterized by asymmetry, variegation in color (nuances of brown especially, but also hues of gray, black, and blue), irregularity of borders, and unevenness of surface. Prognosis in melanoma depends, in part, upon the depth of extension of the neoplastic melanocytes into the dermis and beneath it, but there are many other, probably even more decisive, factors in regard to prognosis yet to be identified.

Virtually all melanomas primary in the skin arise within the epidermis and extend horizontally within it for varying periods before neoplastic melanocytes descend into the dermis. In brief, all primary melanomas in skin are at first "superficially spreading." Although cytologic features of atypical melanocytes in the epidermis of melanomas vary somewhat on different anatomic sites (for example, those on the head and neck usually are oval or round, those on the trunk and extremities usually pagetoid, and those in early lesions on the palms and soles predominantly dendritic), any of these cytopathologic variants of melanocytes, as well as ballooned, polygonal, spindled, and multinucleated ones, may be seen in melanomas on any anatomic site. Furthermore, combinations of cytopathologic variants of melanocytes may appear together in the same melanoma. The criteria for differentiation of malignant melanomas from Spitz's nevi tabulated at the outset of this chapter apply to melanomas in general, irrespective of anatomic site.

Pagetoid melanocytes are seen commonly in melanomas, especially those that develop on the trunk and on proximal extremities. They hardly ever are found, however, in Spitz's nevi. Balloon cells are observed in melanomas, albeit rarely, but balloon cells do not appear in Spitz's nevi.

In sum, the crucial features for histopathologic differentiation of the two neoplasms of atypical melanocytes under discussion here are the same ones that apply in distinguishing benign from malignant neoplasms in general, namely, architectural pattern, and silhouette in particular. Too much concern for cytologic detail can lead a histopathologist to "overdiagnose" a Spitz's nevus as a melanoma. Such errors occur because melanocytes in some Spitz's nevi have strikingly atypical nuclei, many of them may be in mitosis, and an occasional mitotic figure even may be abnormal. Careful heed to architectural pattern can minimize those errors.

38. Pyogenic Granuloma, Fully Developed Lesion *vs.* Kaposi's Sarcoma, Nodular Stage

Pyogenic Granuloma, Fully Developed Lesion	*Kaposi's Sarcoma, Nodular Stage*
1. Exophytic growth predominantly	1. Endophytic growth predominantly
2. Collarette of adnexal epithelium invariable	2. Collarette of adnexal epithelium occasional
3. Granulation tissue constitutes the lesion	3. Granulation tissue present only beneath ulcerated lesions
4. Muscle-containing "feeder" blood vessel spirals through the reticular dermis to the base of the lesion	4. No "feeder" blood vessel in the dermis
5. Oval cells (endothelial cells and fibrocytes) not arranged in an organized pattern	5. Spindle cells (neoplastic endothelial cells) arranged in interlacing fascicles
6. Erythrocytes present mostly within dilated endothelium-lined spaces	6. Erythrocytes present mostly in slits between spindle cells
7. No hyaline globules within endothelial cells	7. Hyaline globules within some neoplastic endothelial cells
8. Extravasation of erythrocytes and deposits of hemosiderin within the stroma focally	8. Extravasation of erythrocytes and deposits of hemosiderin among spindle cells diffusely
9. Fibrous septa intersect vascular elements with formation of lobules	9. No fibrous septa
10. Moderately dense, mixed infiltrate of inflammatory cells dispersed throughout the stroma	10. Sparse mononuclear infiltrate of inflammatory cells in non-ulcerated lesions; variably dense mixed-cell infiltrate beneath ulcers

Pyogenic Granuloma	*Kaposi's Sarcoma, Nodular Stage*

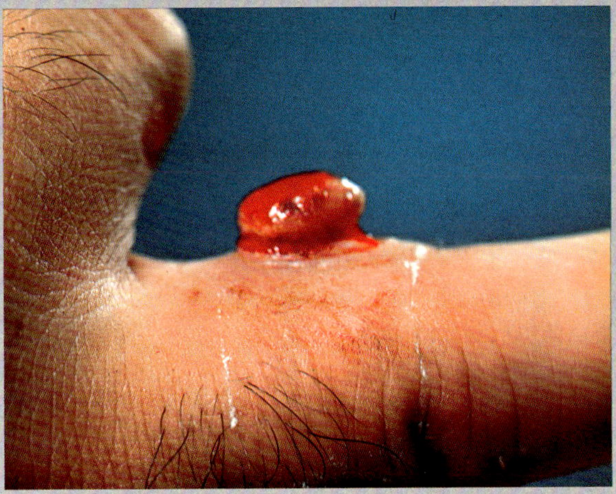

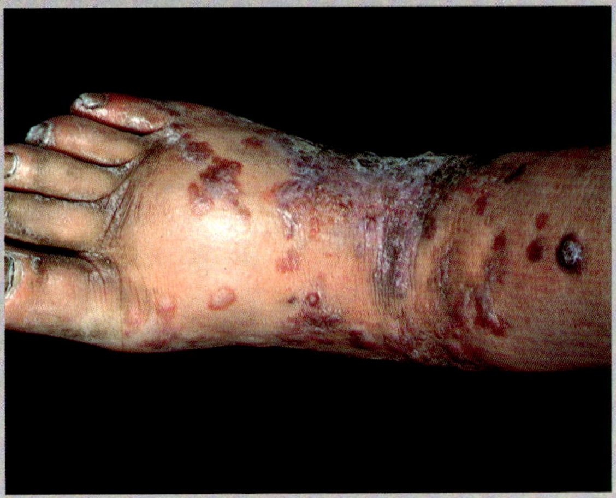

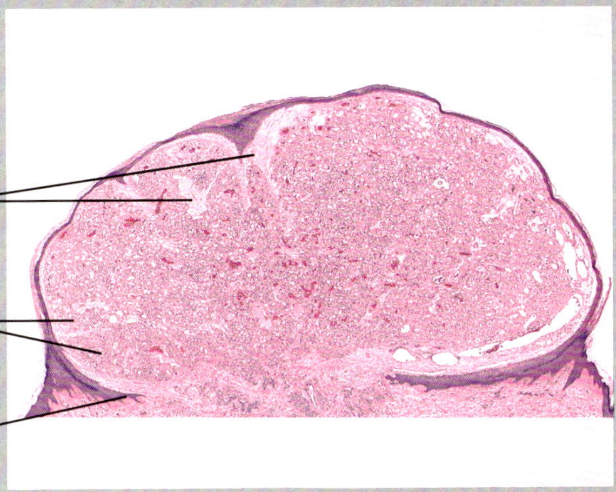

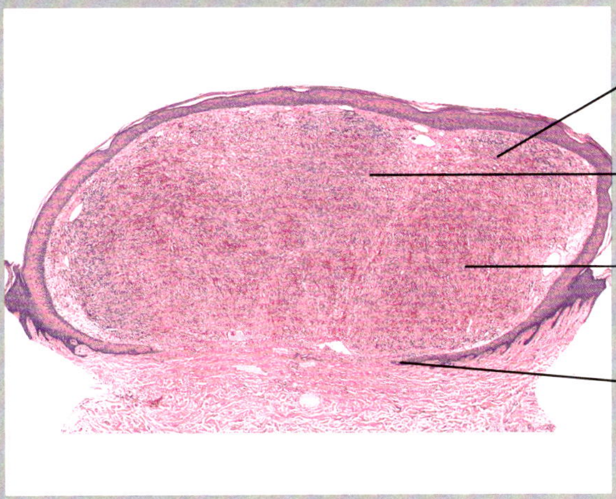

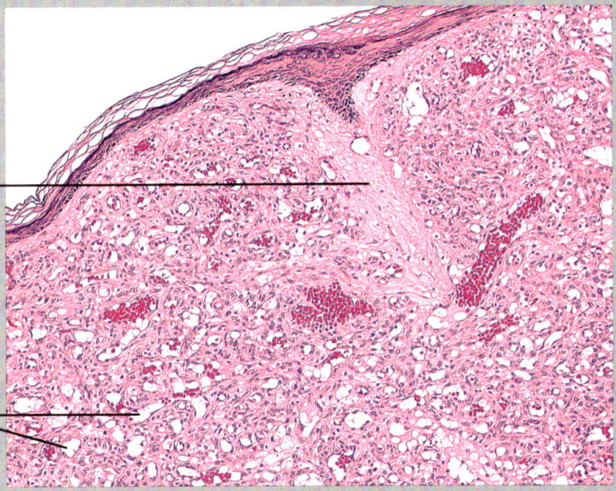

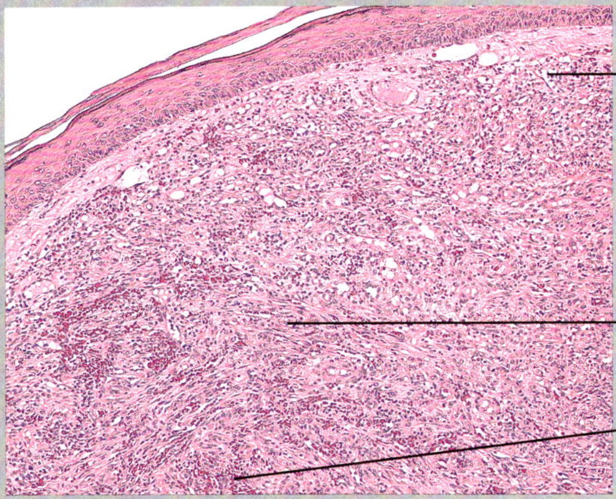

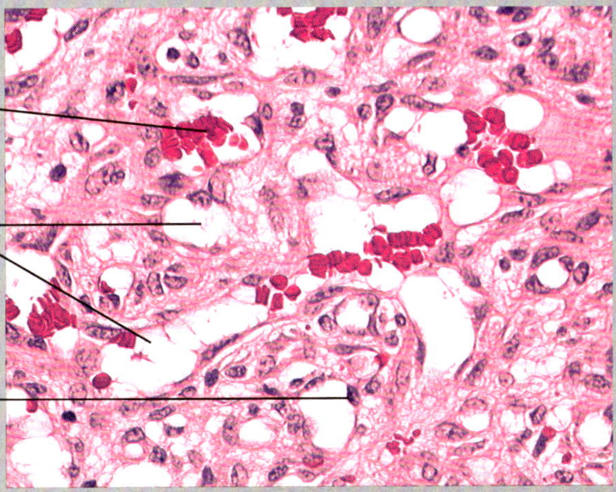

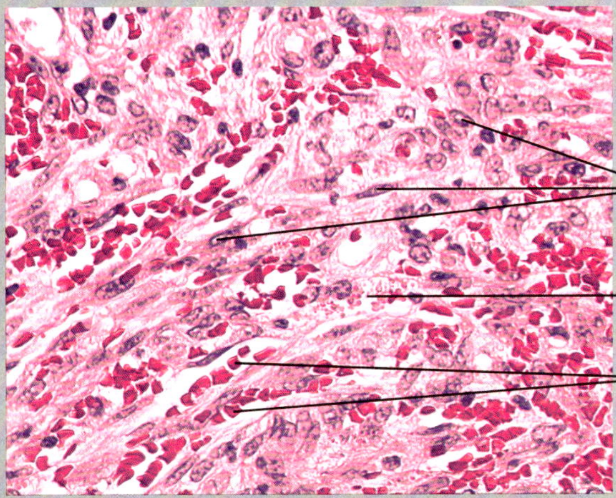

BOTH pyogenic granuloma and Kaposi's sarcoma consist of proliferations of endothelial cells, but the former is a hyperplasia and the latter a neoplasia. In most instances, papular and nodular lesions of Kaposi's sarcoma are differentiated easily by conventional microscopy from fully developed lesions of pyogenic granuloma. Problems of differential diagnosis arise, however, when lesions of Kaposi's sarcoma ulcerate and granulation tissue forms exuberantly beneath the ulcer. In those cases, the preceding tabulated criteria are helpful in distinguishing the hyperplastic process from the neoplastic one. The histopathologic features listed for Kaposi's sarcoma apply only to papules, nodules, and tumors, and not to earlier patches and plaques, which are not a problem in differentiation from pyogenic granuloma.

Clinically, pyogenic granuloma and Kaposi's sarcoma are found predominantly in the skin of the extremities. The hands, fingers, and face (all highly vascular regions) are more commonly affected by pyogenic granulomas, usually in the form of a solitary, reddish-orange to brown, translucent, ulcerated papule or nodule, and rarely as numerous lesions. In contrast, lesions of Kaposi's sarcoma tend to be numerous, usually are purple to dark brown, and assume various sizes and shapes. Occasionally, Kaposi's sarcoma may present itself as a solitary lesion and no other lesions may appear for an extended time. Pyogenic granuloma affects men and women equally, whereas Kaposi's sarcoma affects men much more frequently than women.

Pyogenic granuloma and Kaposi's sarcoma may be divided roughly into three stages of evolution. A pyogenic granuloma follows trauma, often a penetrating injury, grows rapidly as "proud flesh" that consists histopathologically of exuberant granulation tissue beneath an ulcer and, in time, resembles a hemangioma, clinically and histopathologically. In resolution, an ulcerated pyogenic granuloma re-epithelializes, develops thick, fibrous septa that intersect the angiomatous elements and, last, involutes by progressive fibrosis.

Kaposi's sarcoma begins as a macule or patch that is characterized histopathologically by an increased number of endothelium-lined spaces with jagged outlines that form around normal venules of the pre-existing superficial vascular plexus. Those normal venules are surrounded by a sparse to moderately dense infiltrate of lymphocytes and plasma cells. Gradually, as plaques emerge, numerous foci of proliferation of thin-walled, bizarre-shaped blood vessels and of oval cells scattered interstitially appear throughout the dermis, accompanied there by extravasated erythrocytes, siderophages, and an increasing number of plasma cells. As nodules develop, Kaposi's sarcoma consists of a neoplasm comprised of fascicles of oval and spindle cells that involve the entire reticular dermis and, in some lesions, the subcutaneous fat. Erythrocytes, either as solitary units or as clusters, are found in interstices (slits) between the closely packed spindle cells. When erythrocytes are ingested by endothelial cells and undergo degeneration as pink globules of various sizes, they are known as "hyaline globules." Those globules represent erythrophagocytosis and are virtually pathognomonic of Kaposi's sarcoma.

Kaposi's sarcoma is purported to occur in three distinct populations: (1) Ashkenazi Jews and Mediterranean peoples, especially Italians, (2) black Africans in the south of Africa, and (3) persons who are immunosuppressed overtly. It may be that all patients afflicted by Kaposi's sarcoma are immunosuppressed, many only covertly. The histopathologic findings in Kaposi's sarcoma in these three populations are the same irrespective of "population."

Whereas pyogenic granuloma occurs only in the skin and on mucous membranes, Kaposi's sarcoma also may involve internal organs, especially lymph nodes, lungs, and the gastrointestinal tract in 10% or more of patients. Furthermore, patients with Kaposi's sarcoma have a greater incidence of lymphoreticular disorders such as Hodgkin's disease and lymphocytic leukemia. Although not in itself lethal, patients with Kaposi's sarcoma may die of bleeding from gastrointestinal or pulmonary lesions, from infections superimposed upon massively edematous ulcerated lower extremities, or from associated lymphoreticular diseases.

Is Kaposi's sarcoma a sarcoma? It is not because it does not fulfill criteria for a malignant neoplasm, namely, capability to cause death either by metastasis or by local destruction of tissue.

39. Angiolymphoid Hyperplasia with Eosinophilia *vs.* Angiosarcoma

Angiolymphoid Hyperplasia with Eosinophilia	*Angiosarcoma*
1. Dome-shaped papules, nodules, and tumors	1. Patch or plaque usually
2. Ulceration rare	2. Ulceration common
3. Well-circumscribed lesion composed of relatively few thick-walled blood vessels	3. Poorly circumscribed neoplasm composed of innumerable thin-walled vessels
4. Involves the dermis alone and/or the subcutaneous fat	4. Involves both the dermis and the subcutaneous fat in most instances; compromises deeper structures in some instances
5. A single pattern throughout each lesion, namely, discrete, muscle-containing blood vessels that resemble small veins which vary in size and shape	5. Two patterns often present in the same lesion: (1) bizarre-shaped, irregularly anastomosing, vascular channels and (2) solid areas with little or no suggestion of vascular differentiation
6. No projections into vascular lumina	6. Bulbous, villous, or frond-like projections of neoplastic cells from walls of vessels into lumina often
7. Cells with large, relatively monomorphous nuclei line vascular channels; none in mitosis	7. Cells with atypical nuclei line vascular channels, i.e., cells with large hyperchromatic and pleomorphic nuclei; many nuclei are in mitosis, some of them abnormal
8. Endothelial cells protrude into lumina, but do not appear to lose contact with walls of vessels or with one another	8. Atypical endothelial cells that protrude into lumina frequently appear to lose contact with vessel walls and with one another, giving the impression of floating free within a space
9. Erythrocytes wholly within vascular channels	9. Erythrocytes both inside and outside of vascular channels
10. Eosinophils may be numerous	10. Eosinophils few or absent
11. Lymphoid follicles present episodically	11. No lymphoid follicles as a rule
12. Acid mucosubstances abundant in the stroma	12. No acid mucosubstances within the stroma

Angiolymphoid Hyperplasia with Eosinophilia

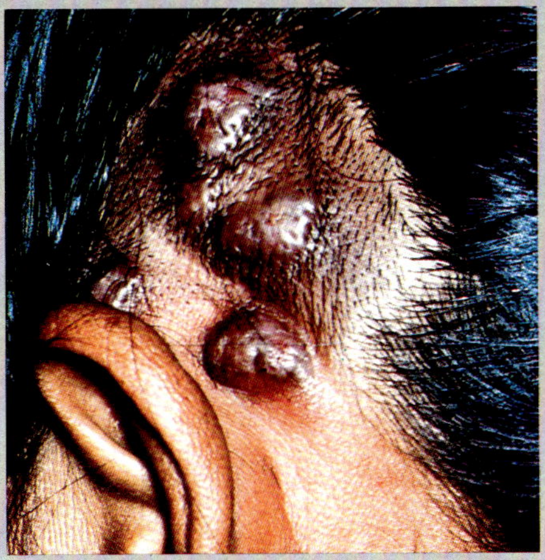

Angiosarcoma

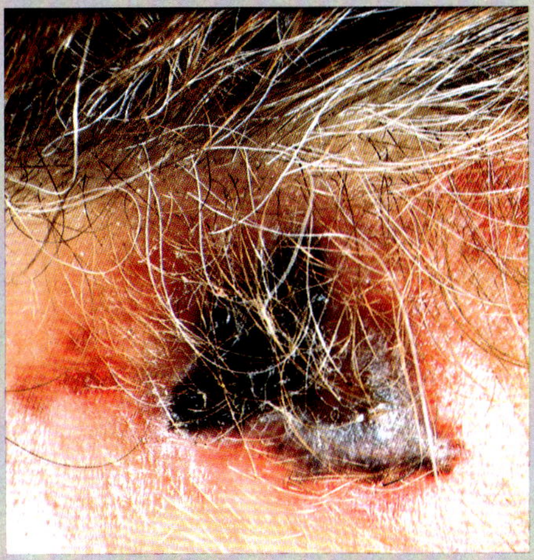

patchy infiltrate of lymphocytes and eosinophils

aberrant blood vessels

base of wedge-shaped lesion

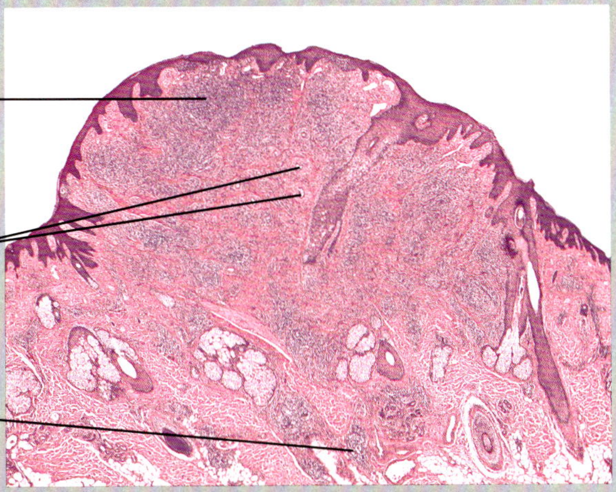

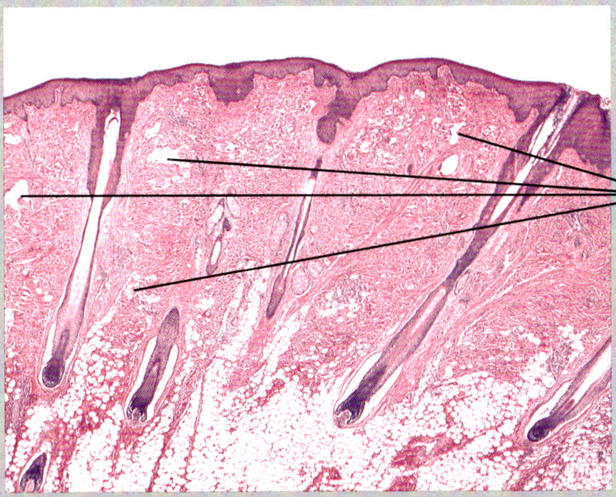

bizarrely shaped endothelium-lined spaces with jagged outlines

infiltrates of lymphocytes and eosinophils

distinctive abnormal blood vessels

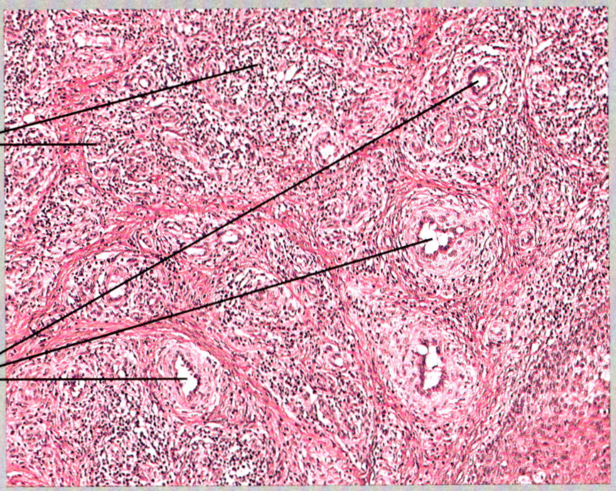

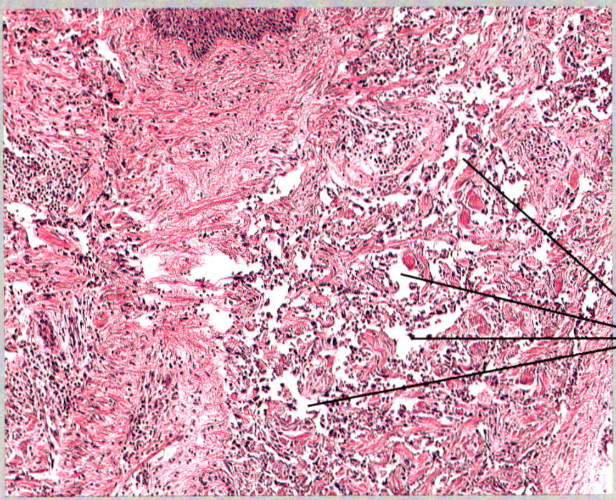

proliferation of bizarrely shaped vessels lined by atypical endothelial cells

lymphocytes

ntracytoplasmic vacuoles in ndothelial cells

plump oval endothelial cells protrude into lumen

perivascular fibroplasia

eosinophils

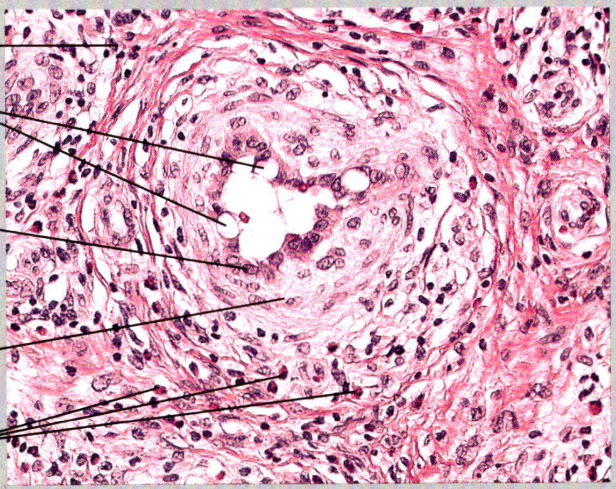

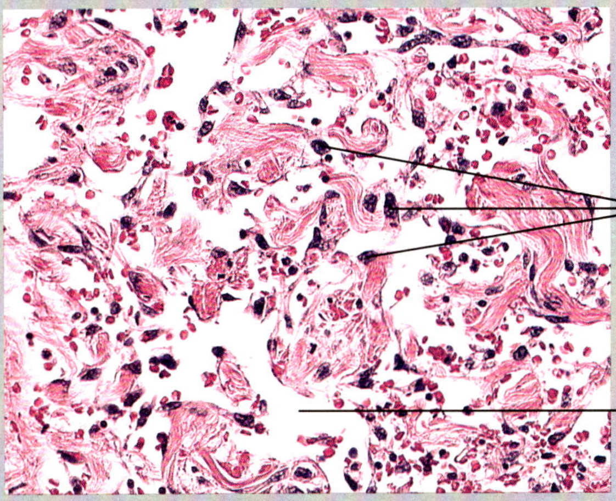

markedly atypical neoplastic endothelial cells

anastomosis of large vascular spaces with jagged outlines

BOTH angiolymphoid hyperplasia with eosinophilia and angiosarcoma are pathologic processes that involve endothelium-lined vessels. Whereas angiolymphoid hyperplasia with eosinophilia is a vascular malformation that results from an arterio-venous shunt, angiosarcoma is a malignant neoplasm. Although clinically and biologically the two conditions are very different from one another, they have several histopathologic findings in common. Both may have prominent vascular channels lined by abnormal endothelial cells that protrude into lumina of those channels. For this reason, histopathologists who are not acquainted with angiolymphoid hyperplasia with eosinophilia may misinterpret it as angiosarcoma unless the aforementioned listed differences are taken into account.

Clinically, angiolymphoid hyperplasia develops as macules that quickly become papules and then nodules on the head, especially around the ears, of younger individuals. The nodules enlarge to become tumors that may range in size from 2 to 5 cm in diameter and then cease to grow. Some nodules and tumors even regress. Angiosarcoma, in contrast, tends to occur on the face, especially on the scalp, of older individuals as firm bluish-purple patches and plaques that extend inexorably in breadth and in depth.

Angiolymphoid hyperplasia behaves in a benign fashion as is expected of a vascular malformation. Angiosarcomas, on the other hand, even when ablated by "wide and deep" excisions, almost always cause death by metastases.

The Stewart-Treves syndrome is angiosarcoma (presumably lymphangiosarcoma) that develops in a lymphedematous arm as a consequence of radical mastectomy (which also includes lymphedema) for carcinoma of the breast. The histopathologic features described here for angiosarcomas in general apply equally to lymphangiosarcomas as described by Stewart and Treve. Synonyms for angiosarcoma are malignant hemangio- or lymphangio-endothelioma.

It should be noted that several variants of angiolymphoid hyperplasia, such as papular angioplasia and pseudopyogenic granuloma, have been described. We consider these simply to be different names for angiolymphoid hyperplasia. Kimura's disease, however, is not a synonym for angiolymphoid hyperplasia. It is an inflammatory process composed invariably of lymphoid follicles and innumerable eosinophils, but not at all of vascular abnormalities.

Histopathologically, angiolymphoid hyperplasia may involve the dermis only, the subcutaneous fat only, or the dermis and the subcutaneous fat together. The condition originally was termed angiolymphoid hyperplasia with eosinophilia because individual lesions were seen to consist of lymphoid follicles and numerous eosinophils, as well as aberrant blood vessels.

As so often is the case in histopathologic differentiation of a malignant neoplasm like angiosarcoma from a simulator of one like angiolymphoid hyperplasia with eosinophilia, a histopathologist is well advised to pay attention strictly to the distinctly different architectural patterns, rather than to give too much credence to cytologic details of them. Not only are the endothelial cells in both angiosarcoma and angiolymphoid hyperplasia marked by abnormal nuclei, but their cytoplasm may contain characteristic, variably sized circular lacunae, signs of vascular differentiation that represent recapitulation of events in formation of vessels in embryonic life. In short, these two conditions of large endothelial cells, so different biologically, are best distinguished from one another by viewing them at scanning, rather than high-power, magnification.

40. Lymphomatoid Papulosis *vs.* Mycosis Fungoides, Plaque Stage

	Lymphomatoid Papulosis		*Mycosis Fungoides, Plaque Stage*
1.	Papules and nodules	1.	Plaques
2.	Erosion and/or ulceration common	2.	No erosion or ulceration usually
3.	Parakeratosis often contains neutrophils	3.	Ortho- and parakeratosis; no neutrophils
4.	Wedge-shaped necrosis and individually necrotic keratinocytes in the epidermis at times	4.	Individually necrotic keratinocytes sometimes; no confluent necrosis
5.	Intra-epidermal vesicles or pustules often	5.	No intra-epidermal vesicles or pustules
6.	Atypical lymphocytes scattered as solitary units within the epidermis	6.	Atypical lymphocytes arranged as solitary units and in collections within the epidermis
7.	Atypical lymphocytes within the epidermis similar in size to those within the dermis	7.	Atypical lymphocytes within the epidermis often larger than those within the dermis
8.	Dermal infiltrate wedge-shaped	8.	Dermal infiltrate not wedge-shaped
9.	Many extravasated erythrocytes within the dermis and the epidermis	9.	Few, if any, extravasated erythrocytes
10.	Edema in the papillary dermis usually; no wiry bundles of collagen there	10.	No edema in the papillary dermis; wiry bundles of collagen there
11.	Mucin increased in the reticular dermis often	11.	Mucin in the dermis not increased
12.	Infiltrate in the reticular dermis interstitial as well as perivascular	12.	Infiltrate in the reticular dermis mostly perivascular
13.	Neutrophils may be numerous	13.	No neutrophils usually
14.	Plasma cells common	14.	Plasma cells uncommon
15.	Bi- and multinulceated atypical lymphocytes that resemble Reed-Sternberg cells in some lesions	15.	Bi- or multinucleated lymphocytes rare
16.	Contiguous lymphocytes of very different sizes	16.	Contiguous lymphocytes of similar size
17.	Many mitotic figures in lymphocytes, some abnormal	17.	Few lymphocytes in mitosis
18.	Nuclear "dust" and evidences of karyophagocytosis common	18.	No nuclear "dust"
19.	Neutrophils in lumina of small blood vessels	19.	No neutrophils in lumina of blood vessels
20.	Blood vessels have thick walls and plump endothelial cells	20.	No alterations in walls of blood vessels as a rule
21.	Vasculitis of small and medium-sized blood vessels in about 10% of specimens	21.	No vasculitis
22.	Degeneration of collagen bundles and necrosis of adnexal epithelium secondary to vasculitis	22.	No degeneration of collagen bundles or necrosis of epithelium
23.	No follicular mucinosis	23.	Follicular mucinosis episodically
24.	Infiltrate in the subcutaneous fat common	24.	Infiltrate in the subcutaneous fat rare

Lymphomatoid Papulosis

Mycosis Fungoides, Plaque Stage

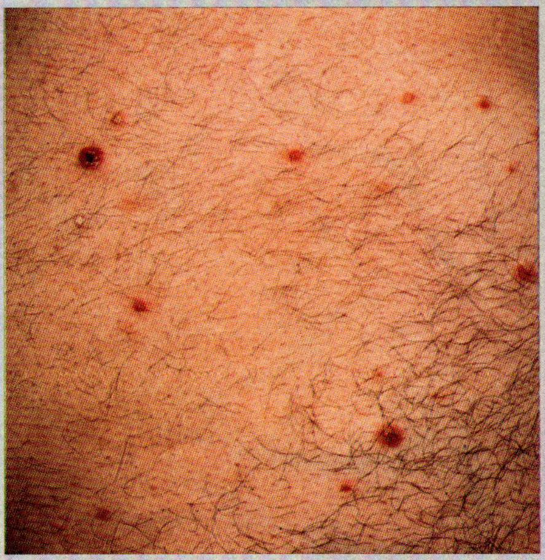

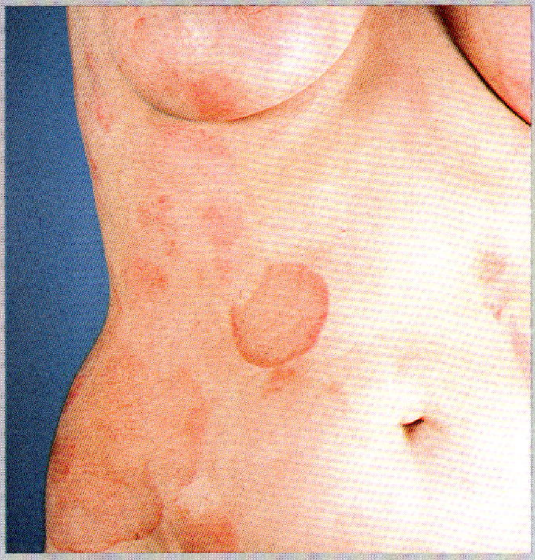

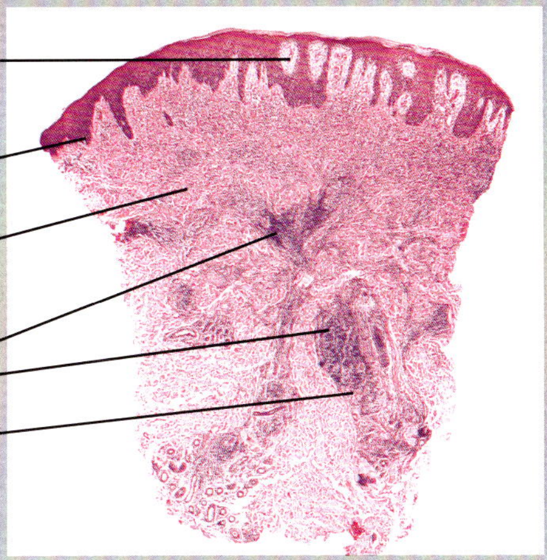

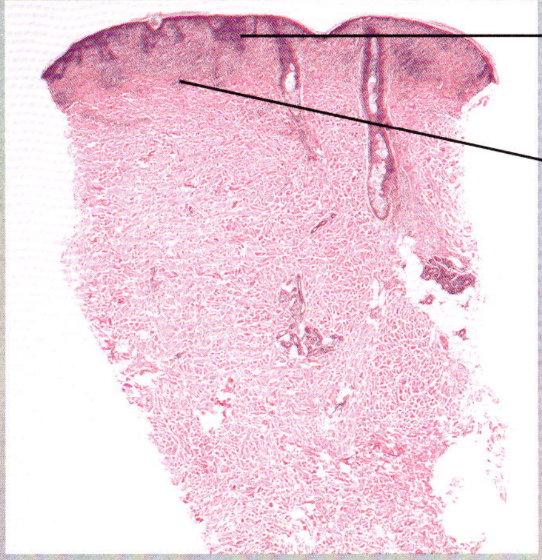

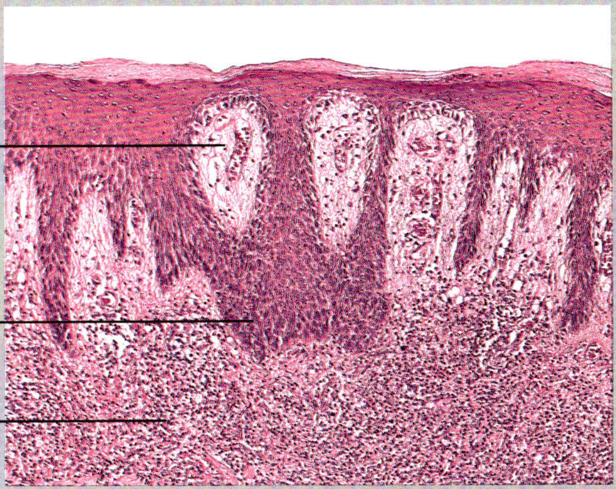

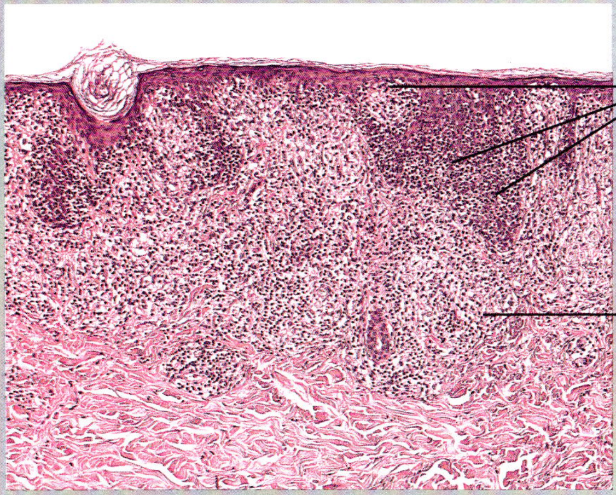

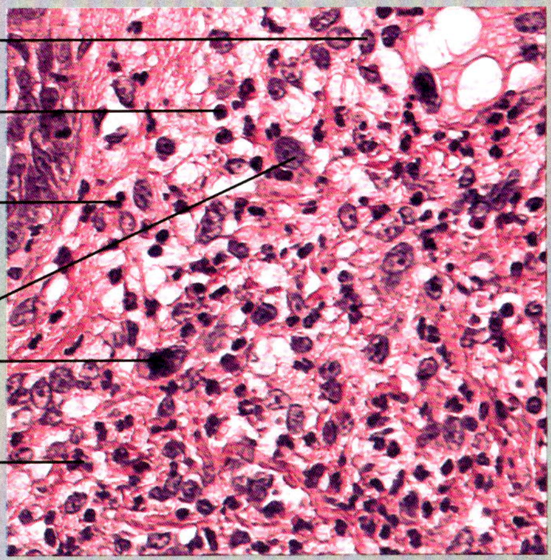

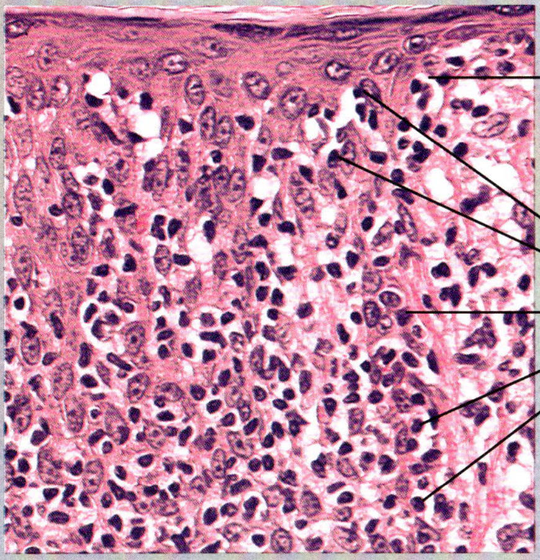

LYMPHOMATOID papulosis and the plaque stage of mycosis fungoides have many histopathologic features in common. In both, a superficial and deep infiltrate may be accompanied by a band-like infiltrate in a papillary dermis that may contain eosinophils and atypical lymphocytes. Many of the atypical lymphocytes have cerebriform nuclei. Mitotic figures may be seen within lymphocytes. For these reasons, distinguishing histopathologically between the two conditions is sometimes extremely difficult, but the differential features just listed help to identify them correctly .

Clinically, lymphomatoid papulosis consists of macules, papules, scaly papules, vesiculopustules, and small ulcers that heal with scars, usually develops in persons over 25 years of age, is more common in women, lasts for years, and is associated with nodules (and sometimes plaques).

Histopathologically, lymphomatoid papulosis usually is characterized by superficial and deep wedge-shaped infiltrates that obscure the dermo-epidermal interface, necrosis and ulceration of the epidermis, edema and hemorrhage in the papillary dermis, a mixed-cell infiltrate within which are atypical lymphocytes, lymphocytes with cerebriform nuclei, and lymphocytes in mitosis. Some lesions are marked by binucleated or multinucleated lymphocytes that resemble those of Hodgkin's disease, evidence of karyophagocytosis, and small vessel vasculitis.

The clinical spectrum of mycosis fungoides ranges from early macules and patches through papules and plaques to nodules and tumors. Some plaques may resolve without treatment and regress to become atrophic patches. All the morphologic expressions of mycosis fungoides may be present concurrently in the same patient. During the patch stage of mycosis fungoides, the cellular infiltrate consists of lymphocytes, practically none of which are atypical in most instances when viewed by conventional microscopy. Even in patches of mycosis fungoides, however, lymphocytes are scattered as solitary units within the epidermis, especially in the basal layer where they tend to be aligned focally. When lymphocytes are sprinkled in the spinous zone, they are accompanied by scant spongiosis and no spongiotic vesiculation. These findings, in the context of wiry bundles of collagen in a thickened papillary dermis, enable accurate diagnosis of mycosis fungoides and differentiation of it from spongiotic dermatitides. In acute spongiotic dermatitides, such as allergic contact dermatitis, nummular dermatitis, and pityriasis rosea, spongiosis is more prominent than in mycosis fungoides, vesicles may eventuate, edema is discernible commonly in the papillary dermis, and there are no wiry bundles of collagen there. As plaques develop in mycosis fungoides, lymphocytes continue to monopolize the lichenoid infiltrate, but in late plaques, eosinophils and even a few plasma cells may join the preponderant lymphocytes, many of which have atypical nuclei. In fully developed plaques of mycosis fungoides, numerous atypical lymphocytes are present within the epidermis, mostly as solitary units and sometimes in collections (Pautrier's) of various sizes and shapes. Atypical lymphocytes within the epidermis of mycosis fungoides tend to be larger than those within the dermis. By the time nodules form, the dense, diffuse, often monomorphous infiltrate of atypical lymphocytes constitutes what formerly was called reticulum-cell sarcoma.

Mycosis fungoides usually begins in adulthood and tends to have a variable but chronic course. The patch stage may persist for many years without symptoms or signs of involvement of internal organs by the disease. As plaques develop, the prognosis worsens and the presence of nodules and tumors presages a grim end because concurrent systemic disease is then inevitable. In actuality, mycosis fungoides seems to be a systemic disease from the outset.

What then is the relationship, if any, between lymphomatoid papulosis and mycosis fungoides on the one hand, and mycosis fungoides and other malignant lymphomas on the other? The atypical lymphocytes with cerebriform nuclei in lymphomatoid papulosis are indistinguishable by conventional and electron microscopy from those in mycosis fungoides. The binucleated and multinucleated lymphocytes seen in other specimens of lymphomatoid papulosis look like cells of Hodgkin's disease. Although most patients with lymphomatoid papulosis have an uneventful course, except for the appearance and disappearance of skin lesions, about 10% of them generate plaques that are similar, clinically and histopathologically, to plaques of mycosis fungoides. Another small percentage of them develop systemic manifestations just like those of Hodgkin's disease. A few patients with lymphomatoid papulosis, after years of short-lived skin lesions, have developed cutaneous nodules and tumors that become ulcerated and, concurrently, have shown evidences of systemic malignant lymphoma, to which some of them succumbed.

One hypothesis holds that immune factors of the host keep the atypical lymphocytes of lymphomatoid papulosis in check. When these factors fail, the atypical cells proliferate unchecked and the result is malignant lymphoma in skin and internal organs. More about the enigmatic process termed lymphomatoid papulosis must be learned before these issues can be resolved.

41. Pseudolymphoma, B-Cell Type *vs.* Malignant Lymphoma, B-Cell Type

Pseudolymphoma, B-cell Type	*Malignant Lymphoma, B-Cell Type*
1. Mixed-cell infiltrate, i.e., plasma cells, eosinophils, or histiocytes, or any combination, in addition to preponderant lymphocytes	1. Monomorphous infiltrate of lymphocytes
2. Density of cellular infiltrate in upper part of dermis equals or exceeds that in lower part ("top-heavy"); infiltrate wedge-shaped at times	2. Density of cellular infiltrate in lower part of dermis often is greater than upper part ("bottom-heavy"); infiltrate not wedge-shaped
3. Small lymphocytes predominate	3. Larger lymphocytes predominate
4. Adnexal structures present	4. Adnexal structures largely absent
5. No lymphocytes in walls of large vessels	5. Lymphocytes in walls of large vessels at times
6. Vasculature prominent; thick-walled blood vessels lined by plump endothelial cells	6. Vasculature not prominent
7. Lymphoid follicles present in about 5% of specimens	7. No lymphoid follicles as a rule
8. Tingible bodies, i.e., lymphocytic nuclear "dust" within macrophages, in germinal centers common	8. No tingible bodies usually
9. Mitotic figures only in germinal centers	9. Mitotic figures everywhere
10. No abnormal mitotic figures	10. Abnormal mitotic figures sometimes
11. No necrosis en masse within cellular infiltrate; few individually necrotic cells	11. Necrosis en masse sometimes within cellular infiltrate; many individually necrotic cells often
12. Histiocytic giant cells episodically	12. No histiocytic giant cells
13. Epidermis hyperplastic sometimes; no ulceration usually	13. Epidermis thinned sometimes; ulceration occasionally

Pseudolymphoma | Malignant Lymphoma, B-Cell Type

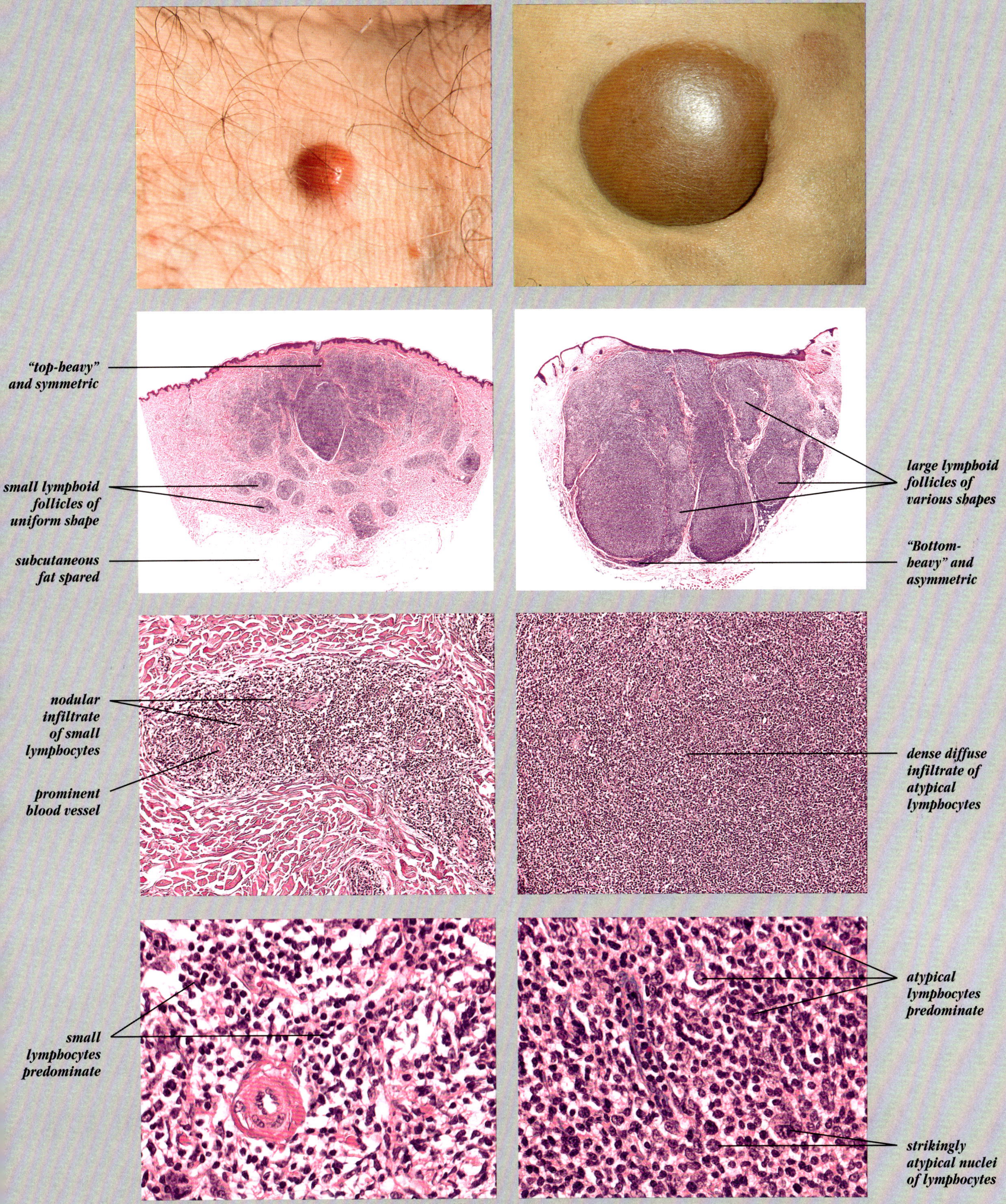

PSEUDOLYMPHOMA, an inflammatory process, and malignant lymphoma, a neoplastic process, have clinical and histopathologic features in common. Clinically, both may be papular, plaque-like, nodular, or tumorous, plum-colored, and firm. Histopathologically, they consist of dense nodular or diffuse infiltrates within which atypical lymphocytes and mitotic figures in lymphocytes may be found in variable numbers. The infiltrates may involve both the dermis and the subcutaneous fat. These shared features make differentiation of pseudolymphomas from malignant lymphomas exceedingly difficult at times, especially when a biopsy specimen has been taken by shave or punch technique. The aforementioned histopathologic differences usually are helpful in resolving the issue (i.e., inflammatory or malignant neoplastic), but inevitably there are instances of mistaken identity. The ultimate criterion for correct identification is biologic behavior, to wit, the course of the process over years. Pseudolymphomas regress in time, whereas malignant lymphomas tend to progress and end fatally.

Lesions of malignant lymphomas in skin usually are numerous and widespread. Although rarely, lymphomas begin in the skin, the vast majority of them arise in internal organs and involve the skin only secondarily. Two major categories of malignant lymphomas are B-cell and T-cell types. These can be subdivided by nuclear size into small, intermediate, and large populations of lymphocytes. T-cell types of lymphomas, of which mycosis fungoides is the paradigm, tend to affect the epidermis (and, episodically, adnexal structures continuous with it) as well as the dermis, whereas B-cell types usually spare the epidermis. The histopathologic criteria proposed here for differentiation of a pseudolymphoma from a malignant lymphoma apply only to B-cell types of lymphoma (more is written about features of T-cell lymphoma in the preceding chapter). Of these criteria, the single most important for diagnosis of B-cell lymphomas is the monomorphous quality of the infiltrate, in contrast to pseudolymphomas which only rarely are comprised entirely of lymphocytes. Parenthetically, lymphocytic leukemias may be indistinguishable histopathologically from B-cell lymphomas.

Pseudolymphomas may simulate malignant lymphomas of both B- and T-cell types. Pseudolymphoma, B-cell type, refers to lesions that, in times past, also were named Spiegler-Fendt sarcoid, lymphocytoma cutis, lymphadenosis benigna cutis, and cutaneous lymphoid hyperplasia, to mention but a few synonyms. These lesions have been reputed to follow trauma, rupture of follicular cysts, insect bites, vaccinations, and hyposensitization injections, although in most instances the causes of pseudolymphomas in general remain obscure. Clinically, pseudolymphoma of the B-cell type presents itself typically as a solitary pink-purple papule, nodule, or plaque on a face. Lesions may be multiple on a face or on any other anatomic site, and tend to be agminated. As a rule, an individual nodule of pseudolymphoma may be impossible to distinguish clinically from one of malignant lymphoma, but a huge tumor almost always signifies lymphoma.

Pseudolymphoma, T-cell type, refers to inflammatory diseases in the skin that resemble mycosis fungoides because of the presence within the epidermis of numerous lymphocytes, mostly arranged as solitary units, but sometimes in clusters that resemble collections of Pautrier. In some spongiotic dermatitides such as allergic contact dermatitis, nummular dermatitis, lichen striatus, and Gianotti-Crosti syndrome, spongiotic foci within which many keratinocytes remain trapped may simulate Pautrier's collections. The nuclei of those often stellate-shaped keratinocytes are much paler than those of lymphocytes, and intercellular bridges are notable between some of them. These two features, and the presence of more marked spongiosis, permit a spongiotic inflammatory process to be distinguished from mycosis fungoides in which spongiosis also is present.

An attempt should be made in the case of every pseudolymphoma to search for a cause of it, and to give it a precise etiologic diagnosis. Only when no cause is evident should the imprecise diagnosis of pseudolymphoma be rendered. Pseudolymphomas of the T-cell type, such as spongiotic simulators of mycosis fungoides, also may be diagnosed with precision in many instances. Terms like pseudolymphoma, pseudosarcoma, pseudocarcinoma, and pseudomelanoma are helpful in alerting pathologists to pitfalls in misinterpretation of benign conditions as malignant, but those terms are nonspecific and, whenever possible, should be avoided in favor of specific diagnoses couched in the language of clinical dermatology.

In conclusion, the criteria listed at the outset of this chapter are helpful in differentiating malignant lymphomas from inflammatory conditions that simulate them, but they are flawed. No matter how rigorously the criteria are applied, there will be instances where they do not enable precise diagnosis of the particular nodular and diffuse, mostly lymphocytic infiltrate under scrutiny.

42. Xanthogranuloma *vs.* Reticulohistiocytic Granuloma

Xanthogranuloma	*Reticulohistiocytic Granuloma*
1. Cytoplasm of histiocytes foamy usually; not granular	1. Cytoplasm of histiocytes finely granular usually; foamy sometimes
2. Cytoplasm of histiocytes pale and devoid of color	2. Cytoplasm of histiocytes amphophilic
3. Touton giant cells (also termed "wreath cells" because a circlet of nuclei separates amphophilic centers from foamy peripheries) numerous usually, but may be absent	3. No Touton giant cells
4. Multinucleated giant cells often prominent	4. Mononuclear giant cells often prominent
5. Mitotic figures in mononuclear cells sometimes numerous	5. Few, if any, mononuclear cells in mitosis
6. Mixed-cell infiltrate of lymphocytes, plasma cells, neutrophils, and eosinophils often	6. Relatively monomorphous infiltrate of characteristic histiocytes; mixture of cells only occasionally

Xanthogranuloma | *Reticulohistiocytic Granuloma*

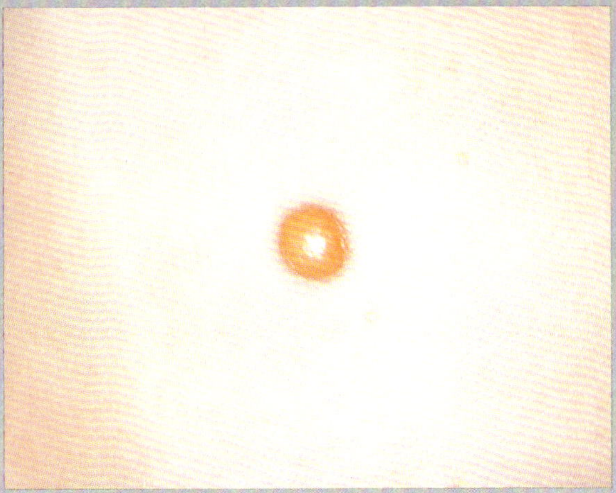

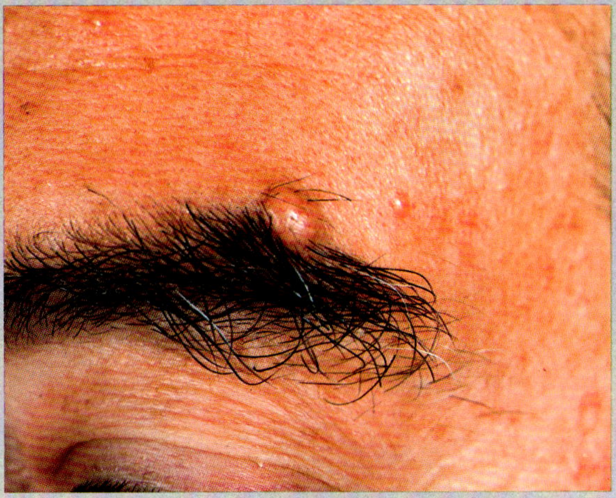

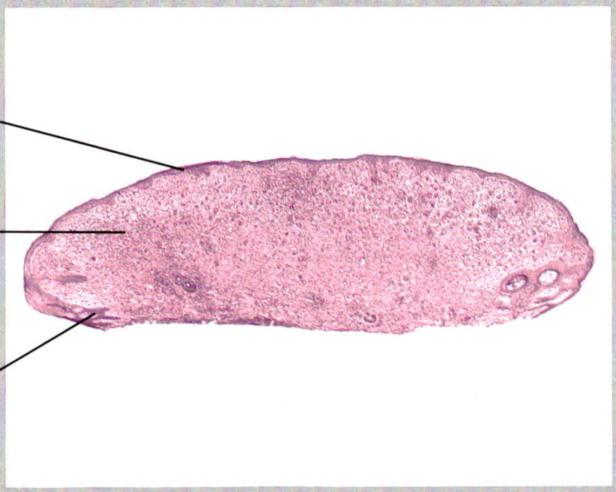

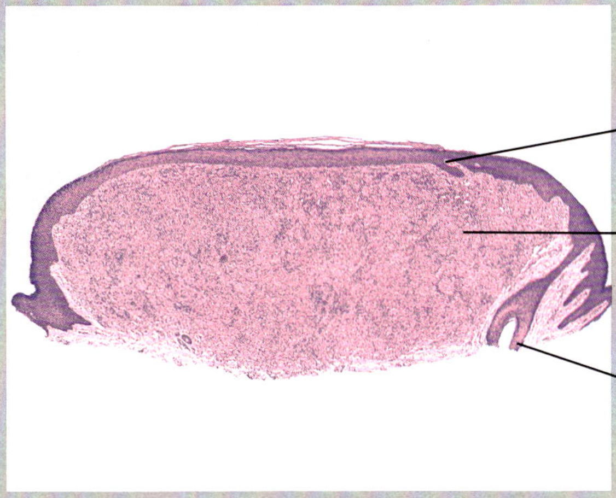

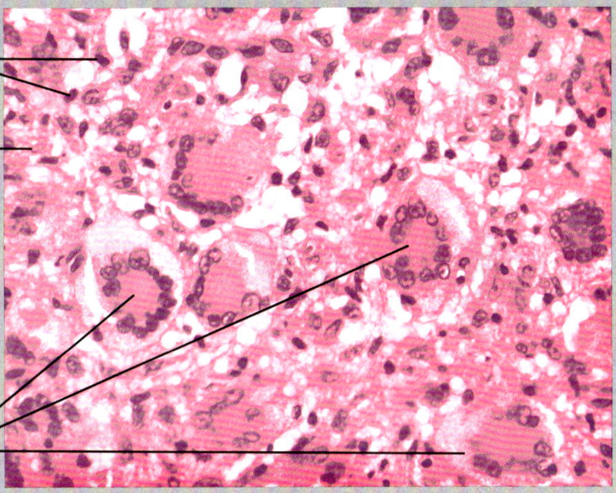

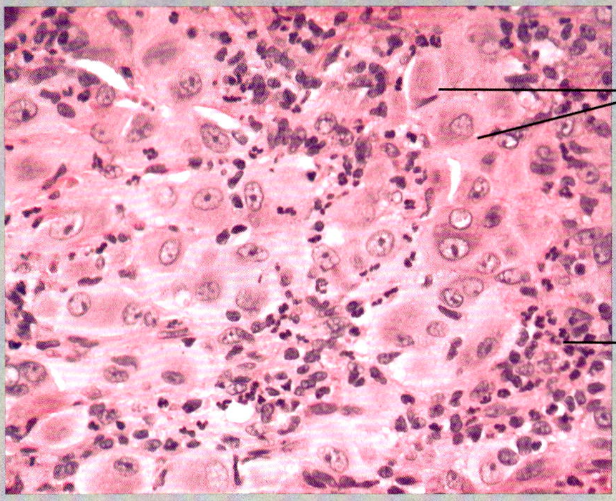

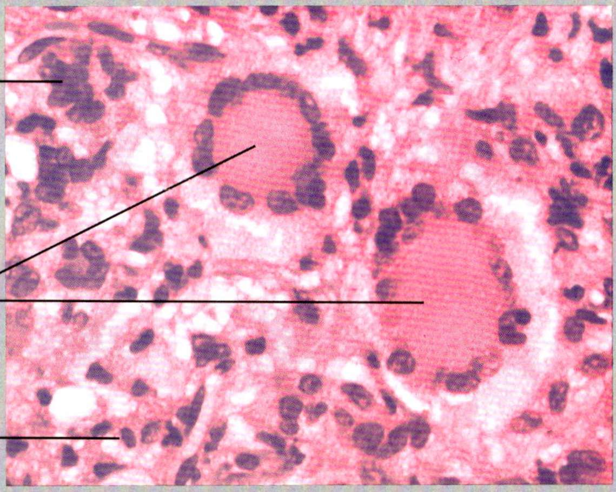

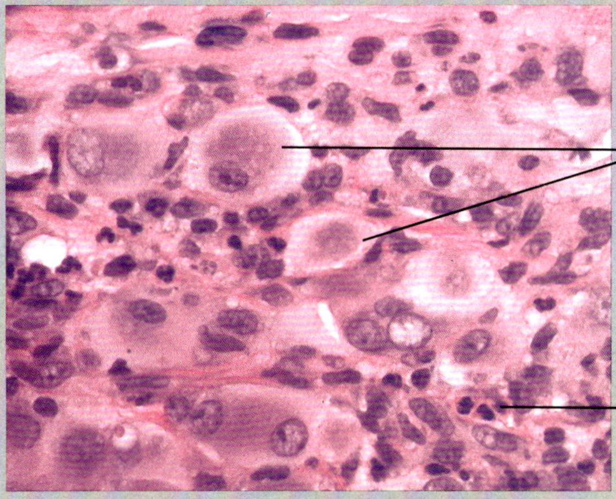

XANTHOGRANULOMAS and reticulohistiocytic granulomas share several histopathologic features, namely, relative circumscription by collarettes of adnexal epithelium, dense, diffuse, predominantly histiocytic infiltrates, mononucleated and multinucleated histiocytic giant cells, and resolution with fibrosis. These similarities not only pose problems in histopathologic differential diagnosis, but they prompt reflection about the possibility that the two seemingly different conditions actually might be related closely or even the same disease.

Clinically, xanthogranulomas are papules or nodules with a yellow, orange, or tan hue. The color results from abundant lipid within histiocytes that comprise the lesion. The condition is better termed xanthogranuloma than nevoxanthoendothelioma, the former designation, which implies incorrectly that it is a nevus partly related to blood vessels.

Although xanthogranulomas may occur at any age, they are more common in infants and young children. In youngsters, they tend to be numerous, to favor the face, and to involve organs besides the skin, such as an eye and the gastrointestinal and genitourinary tracts. Hemorrhage from xanthogranuloma into the anterior chamber of an iris may lead to permanent blindness. The skin lesions of juvenile xanthogranuloma tend to resolve in months without treatment. The clinical differential diagnosis of many lesions of juvenile xanthogranuloma is nodular lesions of urticaria pigmentosa. Morphologically, they may be indistinguishable, but the lesions constituted of mast cells urticate when they are rubbed, a phenomenon known as Darier's sign. A solitary lesion of juvenile xanthogranuloma may be confused clinically with a Spitz's nevus. Each may be an orange, smooth-surfaced papule. In contrast to the juvenile form, xanthogranulomas in adults almost always are solitary, do not involve organs other than the skin, and generally do not resolve without treatment. No abnormalities of serum lipids are found in either children or adults who bear xanthogranulomas.

One histopathologic presentation of a solitary nodule of xanthogranuloma in adults may be misinterpreted as a malignant neoplasm because it is characterized by a dense diffuse infiltrate of cells that extends throughout the reticular dermis and sometimes far into the subcutaneous fat. Some of the cells may have atypical nuclei and many of the nuclei are in mitosis. A clue to the true xanthogranulomatous nature of such an infiltrate is found, sometimes with difficulty, in the form of slightly foamy cells situated often at the periphery of a lesion.

Reticulohistiocytic granuloma may present itself as a single lesion or as widespread ones (multicentric reticulohistiocytosis). Both forms of reticulohistiocytic granuloma occur entirely in adults, and they exhibit similar histopathologic findings. Persons with multicentric reticulohistiocytosis are reputed to have an increased incidence of internal malignancies, especially of carcinomas.

A solitary reticulohistiocytic granuloma typically is a dome-shaped nodule positioned on a face or scalp. Multicentric reticulohistiocytosis also consists of dome-shaped nodules, and they tend to affect the face and hands. Polyarthritis of variable severity is a common accompaniment of the widespread form of reticulohistiocytic granuloma (interestingly named lipoid dermatoarthritis). Sections of biopsy specimens from the involved joints show the same kind of infiltrate as that contained in skin lesions.

The material that gives cytoplasm of reticulohistiocytic granuloma a "ground glass" appearance is PAS-positive and diastase-resistant, an indication that it is a neutral mucosubstance, probably a glycolipid.

Lesions of histiocytosis X are differentiated by conventional microscopy from those of xanthogranulomas and reticulohistiocytic granuloma by their cells with large kidney-shaped nuclei and, by electron microscopy, by their many Langerhans' granules within abundant cytoplasm of cells that house reniform nuclei.

Touton giant cells are not specific for xanthogranulomas. They may be seen in other xanthomas and, commonly, in the histiocytic stage of evolving dermatofibromas. Furthermore, Touton cells are not a sine qua non for diagnosis of xanthogranuloma; foamy histiocytes (no matter how slightly vascuolated) are. Evolving xanthogranulomas may have no Touton cells.

In sum, one reason the list of differentiating findings at the outset of this chapter is so short is that, in reality, reticulohistiocytic granuloma may be a xanthogranuloma. Features such as "ground glass cytoplasm" and "Touton giant cells," reputed to be differentiating, in actuality, may be irrelevant.

43. Dermatofibroma *vs.* Dermatofibrosarcoma Protuberans

	Dermatofibroma	*Dermatofibrosarcoma Protuberans*
1.	Well-circumscribed, small lesion, often contained wholly within a 4.0-mm biopsy specimen	Poorly circumscribed broad lesion, practically never contained wholly within a 4.0-mm biopsy specimen
2.	Epidermal hyperplasia and hyperpigmentation usually; epidermis sometimes thinned centrally	No epidermal hyperplasia or hyperpigmentation; entire epidermis often atrophic
3.	Induction of follicular and sebaceous structures from epidermal basal cells common	No induction of follicular or sebaceous structures above the neoplasn usually
4.	Numerous oval fibrocytes, histiocytes, and coarse bundles of collagen arranged usually in a haphazard pattern	Numerous oval, spindled, and wavy cells and fibrillar bundles of collagen arranged often in short interlacing fascicles
5.	Fibrocytes insinuated between markedly thickened collagen bundles at the periphery of the lesion	Perineural fibrocytes scattered diffusely among normal collagen bundles at the periphery of the lesion
6.	Cellular infiltrate usually mixed (fibrocytes, histiocytes, lymphocytes, and plasma cells)	Cellular infiltrate usually monomorphous, i.e., perineural fibrocytes
7.	Histiocytic giant cells often present	Multinucleated cells not present
8.	Hemorrhage, siderophages, and foam cells common	Hemorrhage rare; no siderophages or foam cells
9.	Cholesterol clefts often	No cholesterol clefts
10.	Foci of sclerosis in long-standing lesions	No foci of sclerosis
11.	Keloidal bundles of collagen within the substance of the lesion episodically	No keloidal bundles of collagen
12.	Epithelial structures of adnexa destroyed by fibrosis	Epithelial structures of adnexa constricted by impingement of neoplastic cells
13.	Acid mucosubstances in connective tissue slightly increased	Acid mucosubstances in connective tissue markedly increased often
14.	Increased number of prominent blood vessels with plump endothelial cells	Blood vessels not prominent
15.	Perivascular lympho-plasmocytic infiltrates	No perivascular infiltrates
16.	Subcutaneous fat involved occasionally and focally	Subcutaneous fat involved usually and diffusely, beginning in fibrous septa
17.	Skeletal muscle spared always	Skeletal muscle may be involved
18.	No melanocytes within the lesion	Melanocytes within the lesion uncommonly (Bednar tumor)

Dermatofibroma

Dermatofibrosarcoma Protuberans

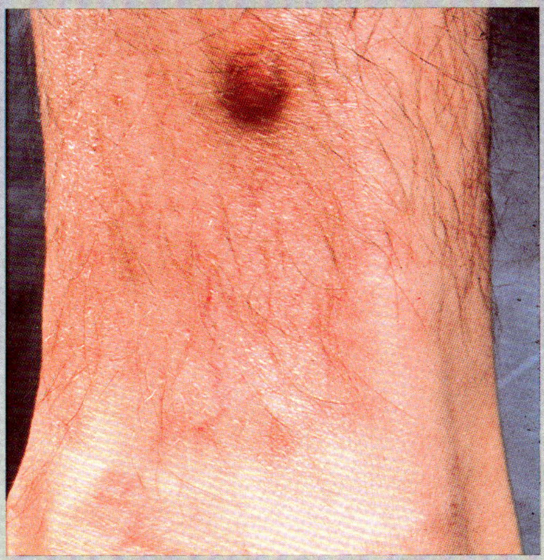

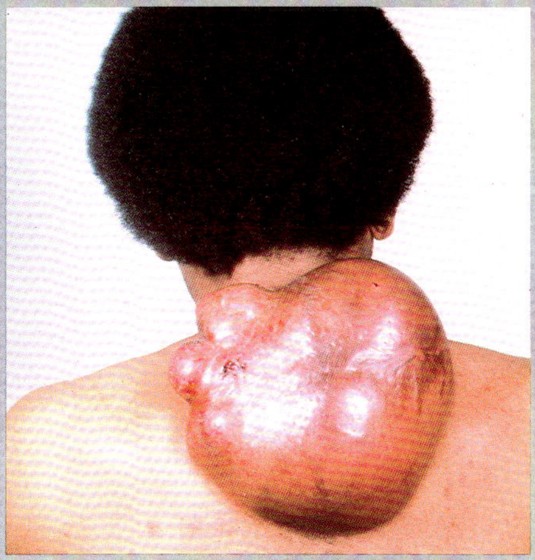

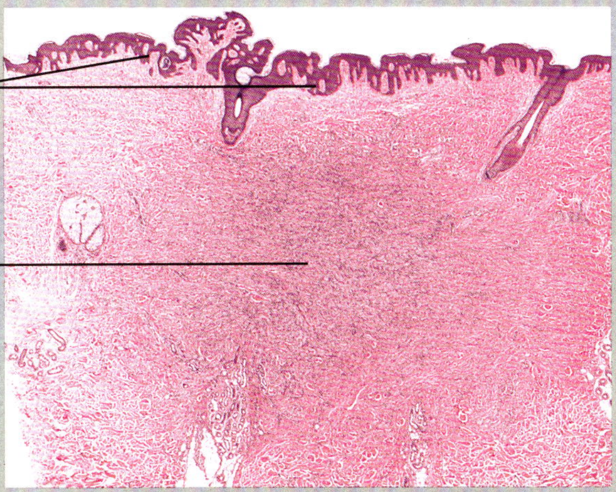

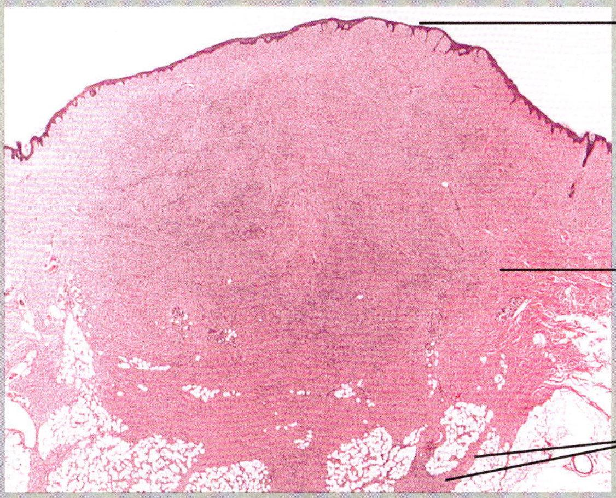

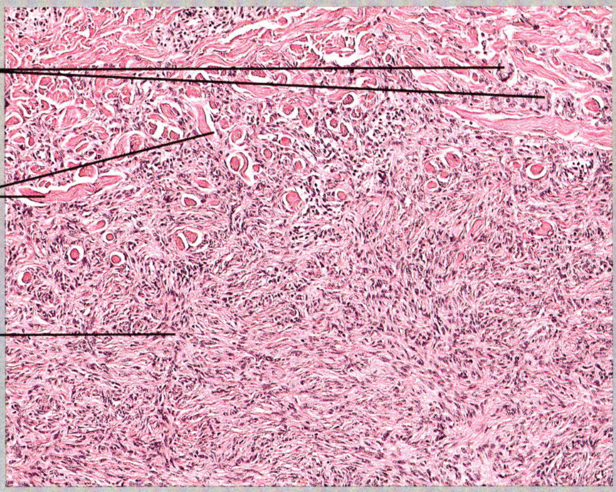

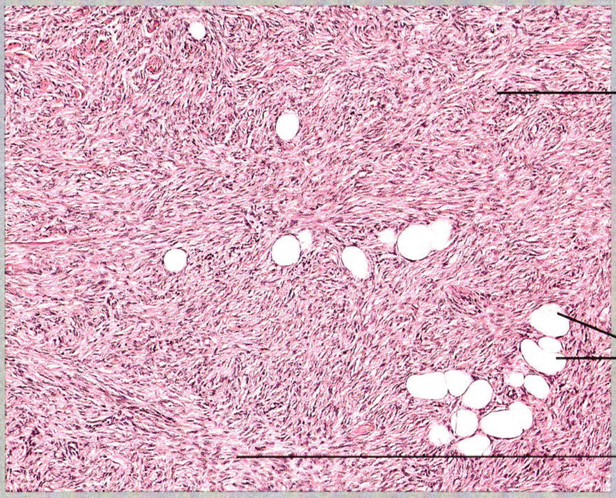

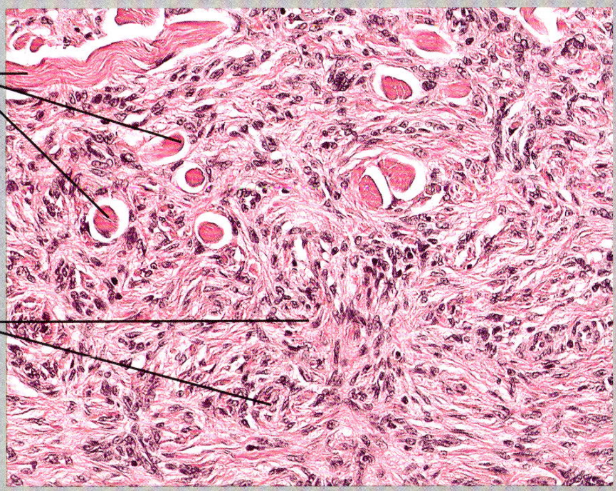

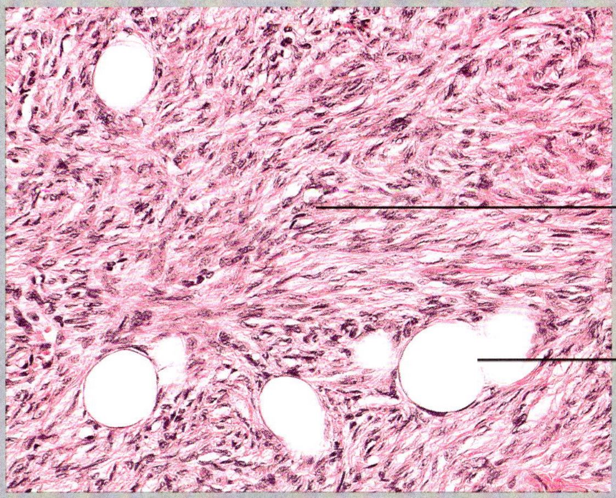

DERMATOFIBROMA and dermatofibrosarcoma protuberans are lesions comprised of dense diffuse infiltrates of mostly oval-shaped cells that tend to occupy at least much of the thickness of the dermis. Their nuclei are not atypical as a rule, and mitotic figures are few or absent. Despite the histopathologic features in common, dermatofibroma and dermatofibrosarcoma protuberans are confused with one another mostly because their names sound so much alike and because general pathologists persist in designating dermatofibroma a tumor, i.e., a neoplasm, rather than the inflammatory process that it actually is.

Clinically, dermatofibromas appear as firm, brown, hairless papules and nodules on the extremities, especially the lower ones. They arise secondary to trauma, often in the form of puncture wounds and arthropod (especially mosquito) bites, but sometimes secondary to ruptured follicles or follicular cysts. Therefore, the term dermatofibrosis describes the lesion more aptly, conveying that it is a type of fibrosing dermatitis, rather than a neoplasm of fibrocytes.

Many synonyms have been given to dermatofibroma, depending upon clinical and histopathologic nuances and the stage in the pathologic process at which it was sampled by biopsy. Nodulus cutaneous expresses the nodularity seen clinically. Fibroma durum describes the hardness of some lesions. During the relatively early granulation tissue phase of its development, blood vessels are prominent, thus earning the appellation sclerosing hemangioma. Later, secondary to extravasation of erythrocytes, histiocytes ingest hemosiderin and lipid, and therefore the term histiocytoma is employed. When both histiocytes and fibrocytes are numerous, the lesion sometimes is called a fibrous histiocytoma. To very old lesions in which fibrocytes are decreased in number and bundles of collagen have a homogeneous appearance, the name subepidermal nodular fibrosis (sclerosis) has been applied. Irrespective of histopathologic variation, dermatofibromas behave like a fibrosing inflammatory process, i.e., they regress slowly in time, leaving a macular hypopigmented center and hyperpigmented rim as residuum.

By contrast, dermatofibrosarcoma protuberans begins clinically as a skin-colored, slightly yellowish or pink macule or patch that, in time, becomes an indurated plaque upon which firm papules, nodules, and tumors arise eventually. The lesion occurs predominantly on the trunk and proximal portions of the extremities, but may appear on other sites such as the face. Even though dermatofibrosarcoma protuberans is slow-growing, it may extend deep into the subcutaneous fat and beyond it into skeletal muscle and fascia, but metastases rarely occur and then hardly ever beyond regional lymph nodes.

The exact nosologic status of dermatofibrosarcoma protuberans is not yet established with certainty. Some authors contend that it is a fibrocytic neoplasm, whereas others argue that it is a neural one. The presence of melanocytes within some lesions of dermatofibrosarcoma protuberans, the fibrillary bundles of collagen, the S-shaped and wavy nuclei, and the abundance often of acid mucosubstances indicate that it may be a neoplasm of perineural fibrocytes.

The limited usefulness of the terms "benign" and "malignant" in the description of cutaneous neoplasms is well illustrated in the case of dermatofibrosarcoma protuberans. Is the neoplasm benign or malignant? If by malignant one means having the potential for metastasis, then dermatofibrosarcoma protuberans is malignant. But dermatofibrosarcoma protuberans, like basal-cell carcinoma, metastasizes rarely, tending instead to persist at a local site following repeated attempts at extirpation of it. In fact, most lesions of dermatofibrosarcoma protuberans, like most basal-cell carcinomas, are not threatening to the lives of patients. Nonetheless, they should be removed completely during the first procedure that is designed to do that. In order to accomplish that desideratum it is necessary for a surgeon to carry an excision considerably beyond what are thought clinically to be the lateral and deep margins of the neoplasm. If less than that is done, dermatofibrosarcoma protuberans doubtlessly will persist at the local site because some neoplastic cells are left behind during the original procedure. "Wide and deep excision" has no value for primary cutaneous malignant melanoma; only enough skin to ensure that that malignant neoplasm has been removed completely is requisite. In contrast, "wide and deep excision" *is* necessary for dermatofibrosarcoma protuberans, angiosarcoma of the scalp, and microcystic adnexal carcinoma, all of which are notorious for persistence at local sites as a consequence of insufficient margins of excision. Mohs' micrographic surgery is an alternative to generous excisions by scalpel for removal of these recalcitrant neoplasms.

44. Lichen Amyloidosis *vs.* Colloid Milium

Lichen Amyloidosis	*Colloid Milium*
1. Scalloped surface	1. Domed surface
2. Foci of compact orthokeratosis and epidermal hyperplasia overlie globules of amyloid	2. Thinned epidermis with loss of the normal pattern between epidermal rete ridges and dermal papillae above deposits of colloid
3. Individually necrotic keratinocytes in the epidermis often	3. No necrotic keratinocytes in the epidermis
4. Rete ridges form pincers around subepidermal deposits of amyloid	4. No pincers formed by rete ridges
5. Amyloid within broadened dermal papillae	5. Colloid within the upper half of the reticular dermis
6. Amyloid deposited in small globules	6. Colloid deposited in large homogeneous accumulations
7. Amyloid is amphophilic or eosinophilic in sections stained with hematoxylin and eosin	7. Colloid is amphophilic or basophilic in sections stained by hematoxylin and eosin
8. No clefts within globules of amyloid	8. Clefts within nodules of colloid
9. Stellate fibrocytes and melanophages associated intimately with globules of amyloid	9. A few thin fibrocytes associated with colloid, but no macrophages
10. Angioplasia in conjunction with amyloid	10. No angioplasia
11. No solar elastosis near amyloid	11. Solar elastosis present always at the periphery of colloid

Lichen Amyloidosus | Colloid Milium

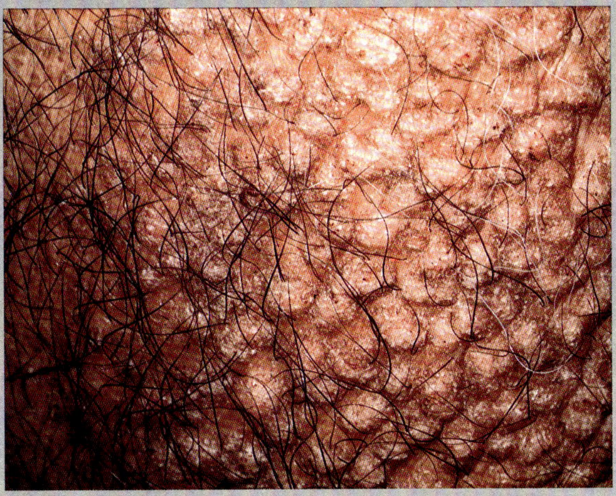

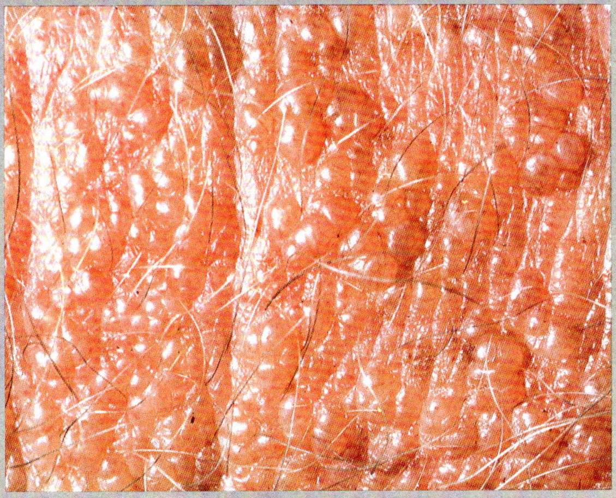

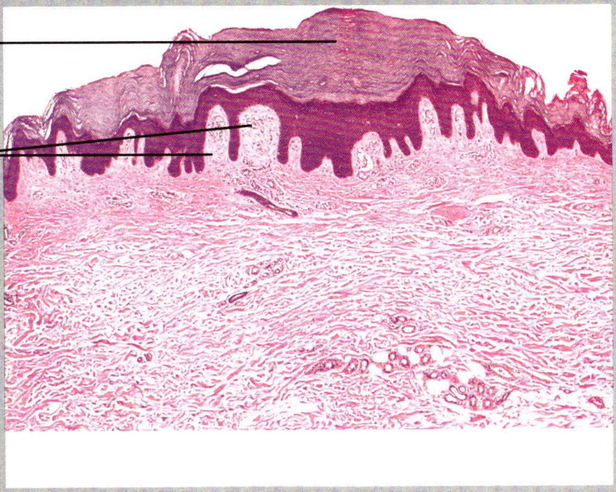

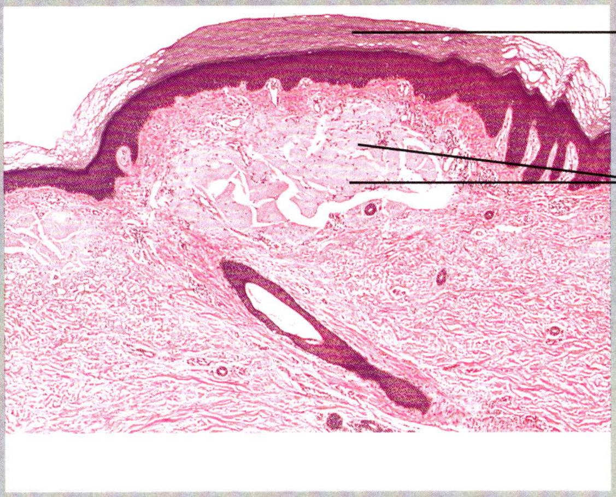

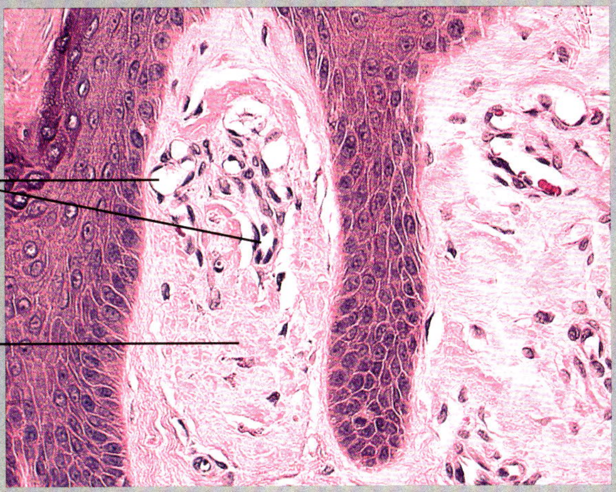

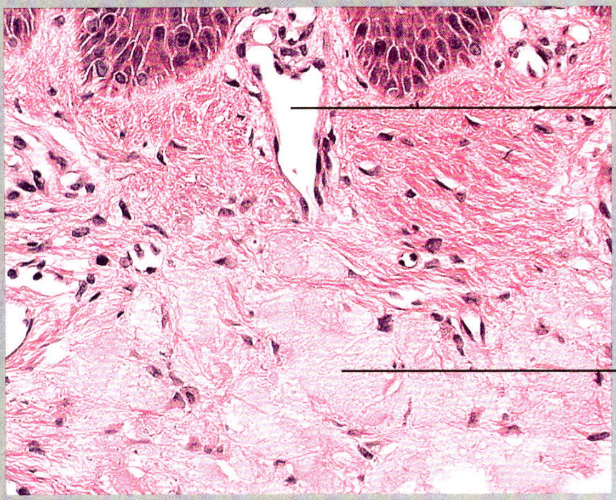

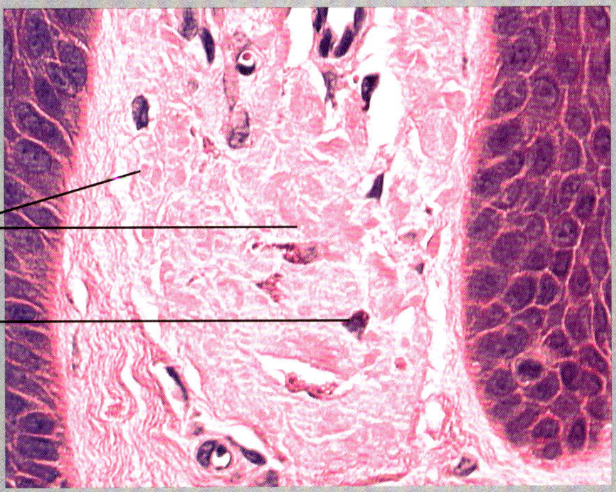

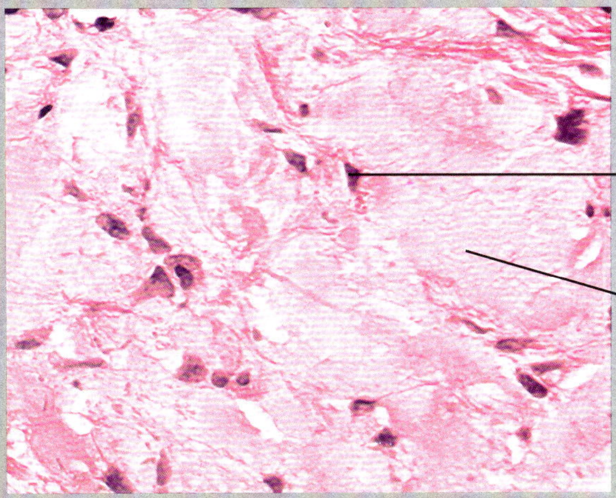

LICHEN amyloidosis and colloid milium both result from deposits of homogeneous material, but of different chemical natures, in the upper part of the dermis. In both, fibrocytes are affiliated closely with the deposits of homogeneous material. In fact, it is likely that fibrocytes are responsible for the formation of amyloid in lichen amyloidosis and colloid in colloid milium.

Because of the highly characteristic histopathologic features just listed, specialized stains need not be performed routinely to differentiate between amyloid and colloid. When necessary for academic resolution of the issue, Congo red is the most reliable stain for differentiation because it is positive by dichroism for amyloid, and negative for colloid. Crystal violet stain for amyloid is prettier and more dramatic, but less reliable.

The clinical lesion of lichen amyloidosis consists of agminated, discrete, slightly raised, brownish-red translucent papules that often are keratotic. The condition is intensely pruritic and occurs most commonly on the anterior aspects of the legs, but in some instances may be widespread. Macular amyloidosis, as the title implies, begins as flat lesions. In contrast to lichen amyloidosis, macular amyloidosis has a predilection for the interscapular region. The keratotic papules of lichen amyloidosis are consequent not only to progressive accumulations of amyloid in the papillary dermis, but to the effects of persistent rubbing as well. In short, superimposition of lichen simplex chronicus upon macular amyloidosis transforms that condition into lichen amyloidosis. The evidence for that is prominent compact orthokeratosis and hypergranulosis in virtually all lesions of lichen amyloidosis, signs of persistent, prolonged rubbing. Macular amyloidosis that has not been rubbed, and therefore not thickened by lichen simplex chronicus, remains flat, as it is stereotypically in the interscapular region. A current hypothesis about how amyloid is formed in the upper portion of the dermis in lesions of macular amyloidosis and lichen amyloidosis holds that globules of amyloid derive from necrotic keratinocytes in the epidermis and when those apoptotic bodies are acted upon by fibrocytes, amyloid is the result.

Colloid milium consists of discrete, smooth, yellowish, translucent, waxy papules on sun-exposed areas, especially the malar eminences of the face and dorsa of the hands. Sometimes the papules of colloid milium are restricted to the left side of the face and the dorsa of the left hand in persons who spend much of their time driving cars in sunny climates, such as taxi drivers. At first glance, the smooth translucent papules of colloid milium may be misinterpreted as tense vesicles or as "juicy" edematous papules of polymorphous light eruption. Histopathologically, colloid is surrounded always by copious amounts of solar elastosis, and both of them are stained bluish-gray by hematoxylin and eosin. These findings indicate that colloid and elastotic material are related closely to one another. Amyloid, by contrast, is not connected to damage by sunlight.

Whereas colloid in the skin is found only in colloid milium, amyloid is detected in a variety of circumstances other than in the macular and papular (lichenoid) forms. For example, amyloid is present around blood vessels in the skin and subcutaneous fat of patients with systemic amyloidosis, in large solitary nodules of nodular amyloidosis and, most commonly, as an incidental finding in a host of inflammatory, hamartomatous, and neoplastic conditions in the skin, especially in seborrheic keratoses, trichoepitheliomas, and basal-cell carcinomas. These are conditions in which individual keratinocytes tend to undergo necrosis.

45. Pretibial Myxedema *vs.* Scleromyxedema

	Pretibial Myxedema		*Scleromyxedema*
1.	Epidermis slightly thickened and hyperkeratotic often	1.	Epidermis normal or only slightly hyperplastic usually
2.	Abnormalities mostly in the upper half of the dermis in fully developed lesions	2.	Abnormalities throughout the entire dermis and even into septa of the subcutaneous fat in fully developed lesions
3.	Huge quantities of acid mucosubstances distributed diffusely throughout the upper half of the dermis	3.	Slight and subtle increase in acid mucosubstances within the dermis focally
4.	Very wide separation of collagen bundles by acid mucosubstances	4.	Slight separation of collagen bundles by acid mucosubstances
5.	Mast cells increased markedly in mucinous areas	5.	Mast cells increased slightly in mucinous foci
6.	Fibrocytes increased slightly and scattered as solitary units within the mucin-rich stroma, mostly in the upper half of the dermis	6.	Fibrocytes increased markedly with their long axes parallel to the epidermis; some fibrocytes aggregated into fascicles within the subtly mucinous stroma throughout the entire dermis
7.	Fibrocytes oval, spindle-shaped, and stellate	7.	Fibrocytes oval and spindle-shaped; not stellate
8.	No apparent increase in amount of collagen	8.	Increased amount of basophilic-staining collagen
9.	Hair follicles spared by the process	9.	Hair follicles destroyed by the process
10.	No perivascular infiltrate of inflammatory cells	10.	Sparse infiltrate of inflammatory cells around an increased number of dilated blood vessels

Pretibial Myxedema

Scleromyxedema

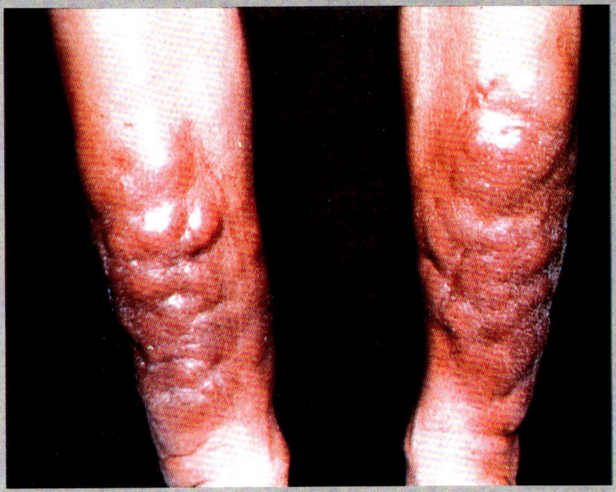

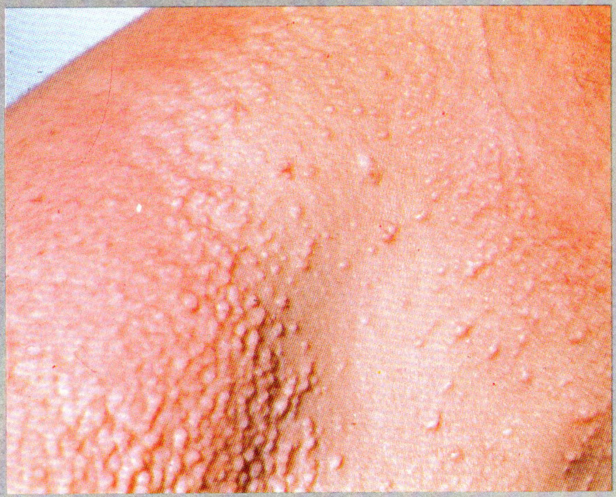

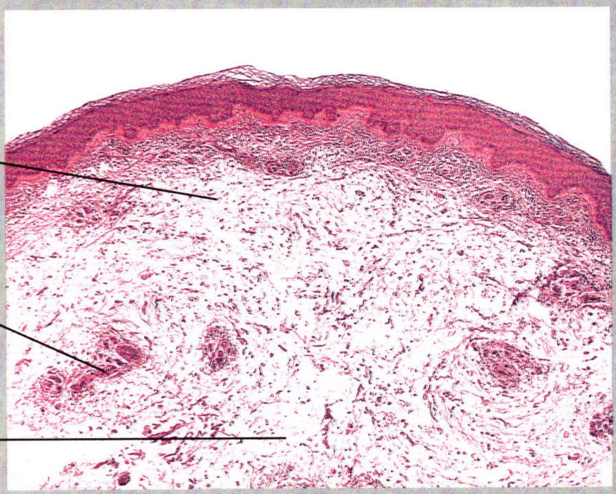

abundant mucin in the reticular dermis

proliferation of blood vessels

lake of mucin

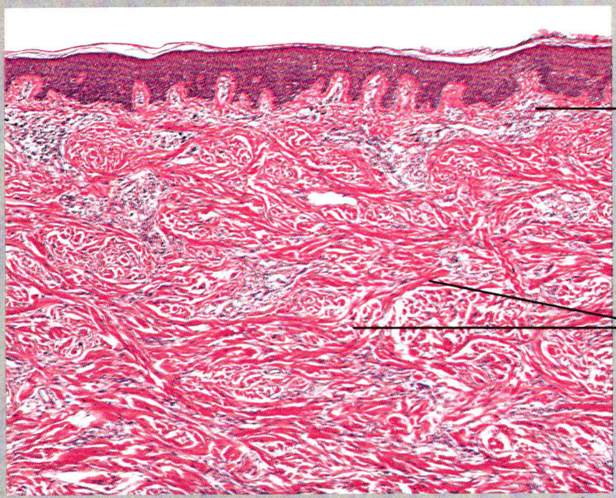

sparse infiltrate of lymphocytes

bundles of collagen in haphazard array

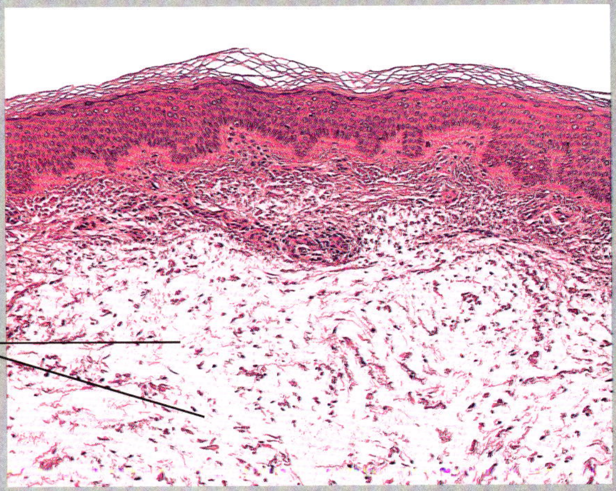

abundant mucin

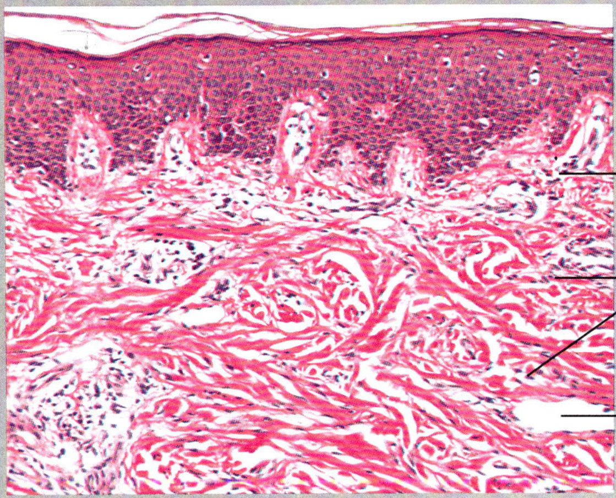

slight perivascular infiltrate

increased number of fibrocytes

dilated blood vessel

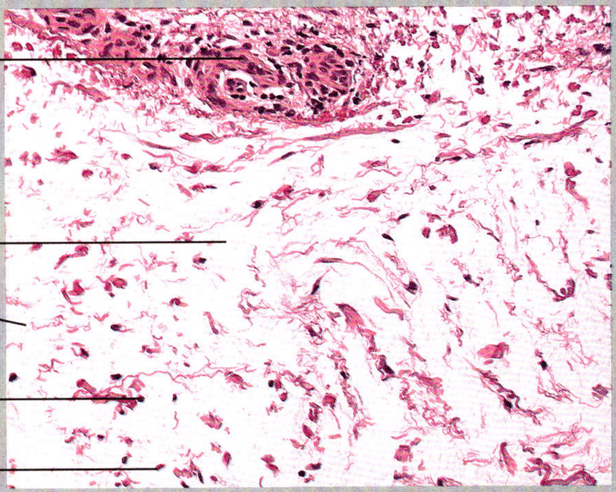

proliferation of blood vessels

mucin

wisp of collagen

mast cell

fibrocyte

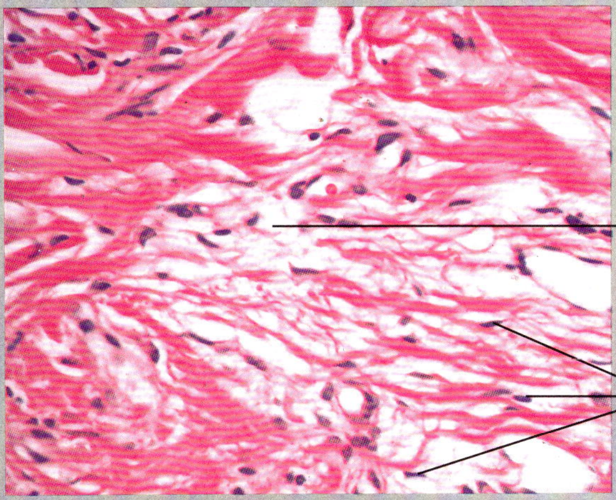

mucin slight

increased number of fibrocytes

PRETIBIAL myxedema and scleromyxedema are more alike in name than they are in histopathologic findings. In a sense, both are cutaneous mucinoses in which there is an increased number of fibrocytes and mast cells in zones of acid mucosubstances.

Pretibial myxedema may develop occasionally in patients who are euthyroid, but commonly it is a manifestation of hyperthyroidism. Clinically, the lesions appear on anterior aspects of the lower extremities and consist of firm, raised, yellow-tan plaques and nodules. Signs of thyrotoxicosis concurrent with pretibial myxedema are exophthalmos and acropathy. The causative factor of this triad is thought to be long-acting thyroid stimulator, an immunoglobulin of the IgG class. Not uncommonly, pretibial myxedema develops after therapy for thyrotoxicosis.

Papular mucinosis and lichen myxedematosus are synonyms for scleromyxedema. Clinically, the disease, when florid, consists of diffuse induration topped by small reddish papules. When the face is involved markedly, as it usually is, the clinical differential diagnosis is the acrosclerotic form of scleroderma. Other features of scleromyxedema are light-chain immunoglobulinopathy that involves IgG, and association with multiple myeloma.

The mucin in both pretibial myxedema and scleromyxedema is hyaluronic acid because it is stained by colloidal iron and alcian blue at pH 2.5 and, metachromatically, by toluidine blue at pH 3.0. Histopathologically, in sections stained by hematoxylin and eosin, mucin appears as basophilic, granular, and stringy material.

At scanning magnification, scleromyxedema is a kind of fibroplasia, whereas pretibial myxedema is a mucinosis. Strictly speaking, scleromyxedema is no more a "mucinosis" than is granuloma annulare. The latter is a granulomatous disease with deposits of mucin focally, and the former is a fibrosing process with deposits of mucin focally. These deposits are most impressive at an early stage in the evolution of the process.

Scleromyxedema sometimes must be differentiated histopathologically from the interstitial type of granuloma annulare in which epithelioid histiocytes may be confused for fibrocytes and in which mucin may be deposited in foci. The histopathologic differential diagnosis of pretibial myxedema includes widespread myxedema and focal mucinosis. The mucin in widespread myxedema is not as massive as in pretibial myxedema, and in focal mucinosis is not as diffuse (i.e., it is discrete and well circumscribed) as in pretibial myxedema.

The hardness of the skin in scleromyxedema results from formation of new collagen, whereas the firmness of pretibial myxedema is consequent to extraordinarily large deposits of mucin.

Glossary

abscess refers to a collection of neutrophils that may form within the epidermis, hair follicles, dermis, and subcutaneous fat, or in any site in any organ. When the neutrophils undergo degeneration, lipid accumulates in their cytoplasm; it is this fat that gives pus its yellow appearance.

acantholysis describes the process by which acantholytic cells come into being, namely, by dissolution of intercellular bridges and subsequently becoming round.

acantholytic cell refers to an epithelial cell that has separated from another epithelial cell, and consequently has become round. Cells in the spinous, granular, and cornified layers may undergo acantholysis.

acid mucosubstance is a histochemical term for a polymer of glucose and amino groups (mucopolysaccharides, glycosaminoglycans) that takes a stain in an acid medium.

acinar means, literally, pertaining to a bunch of grapes; figuratively, in pathology, it refers to spaces lined by epithelium, especially to gland-like or duct-like structures.

acral parts of the skin refers to the distal parts, especially the skin of the fingers and toes, but also of the nose and ears.

active junctional nevus is a term that should never be used because it has not been defined in a standard way, and because no nevus fixed in formalin can be active. Allen, who used it first, intended it as a synonym for "melanocarcinoma in situ."

amphophilic means having both basophilic and eosinophilic staining qualities.

anagen indicates that part of the follicular cycle during which hairs grow and the inferior segment of a hair follicle is marked by a fully developed bulb with a matrix and a papilla that contains abundant mucin, an outer sheath replete with glycogen, and an inner sheath.

apoptosis refers to a kind of necrosis of keratinocytes in which the necrotic cells are phagocytized.

arborization describes a tree-like shape that is a result of inward turning of epithelial structures of adnexa at the periphery of a structure such as a common wart, a seborrheic keratosis, or a pyogenic granuloma around which it sometimes is called, inaccurately, an "epidermal collarette." In truth, the elongated collars of epithelium are eccrine ducts and hair follicles, not epidermal rete ridges.

atopy is applied to a genetic disposition to development of allergic rhinitis allergic asthma, atopic dermatitis, and allergic urticaria.

atrophy refers to a decrease in the amount of tissue. Clinically, "superficial atrophy" describes thinning of the skin, shininess, loss of the skin markings, telangiectases, and pigmentary changes that, in sum, correspond histopathologically to sclerosis of the papillary dermis with obliteration of discrete papillae, a thinned epidermis, and therefore, pronounced loss of the normal undulating pattern between rete ridges and dermal papillae. An example of superficial atrophy is the changes that occur following application of high-potency corticosteroids under occlusion. Mid-atrophy presents itself clinically as an out-pouching of skin known as anetoderma. The process affects the mid-reticular dermis where there is loss of collagen bundles and elastic fibers. An example of mid-atrophy is "macular" atrophy that follows extensive suppurative folliculitis of acne vulgaris. Deep atrophy is seen clinically as a gully and results from loss of subcutaneous fat. A stereotypical example is lipodystrophy.

atypia is applied to nuclei that are large, hyperchromatic, variable in size and shape, and associated with prominent nucleoli. It should be employed only to describe nuclei and to neither cytoplasm nor architectural pattern.

ballooning describes intracellular edema, recognizable by swollen, pale cytoplasm of affected keratinocytes.

basal-cell proliferation refers to an increased number of basal cells as occurs sometimes in focal acantholytic dyskeratosis and in the epidermis above dermatofibromas.

basaloid means resembling the cells of the basal layer of the epidermis, such as those that make up much of seborrheic keratoses and all of basal-cell carcinomas, the latter being like germinative cells in an embryo.

basement membrane of the epidermis denotes an anatomic zone defined by an undulating line, when viewed by conventional microscopy, between the epidermis and the dermis that takes the PAS stain. It is composed of type IV collagen.

basket-weave pattern of the stratum corneum describes the normal appearance of the cornified layer (except for that on palms and soles) in sections of skin viewed by conventional microscopy.

benign is a word that characterizes the behavior of a neoplasm, namely, one that does not have the potential to cause death by local destruction or by metastases. That behavior is reflected in the silhouette of a neoplasm as it is viewed at scanning magnification. It should not be used to describe cytologic characteristics that are properly designated "typical" or "atypical" nuclei.

bulbous refers to a shape that resembles a bulb, like the bulb of a light, a flower, an onion, or normal follicular papillae and abnormal dermal papillae like those in lichen amyloidosus.

catagen designates the involutional stage of the follicular cycle in which the inferior segment of a hair follicle is characterized by necrotic (apoptotic) keratinocytes, a shrunken appearance, and a thickened, corrugated, glassy membrane.

cholesterol clefts are elongated spaces with pointed ends that presumably represent sites from which crystals of cholesterol have been removed from tissue by agents used in processing specimens of tissue for histologic examination.

Civatte bodies are necrotic keratinocytes, also termed colloid bodies, hyaline bodies, and apoptotic bodies.

cleft specifies a narow space that usually is an artifact of histologic preparation (e.g., in basal-cell carcinomas, Spitz's nevi, and focal acantholytic dyskeratosis); it is differentiated from a blister by absence of plasma within the space.

coarse bundles of collagen in vertical streaks refers to a diagnostic sign of persistent rubbing of skin in lichen simplex chronicus and its variants prurigo nodularis and picker's nodule; coarse collagen bundles in a thickened papillary dermis are oriented parallel to one another and to the rete ridges and perpendicular to the skin surface.

collarette of epithelium alludes to the inward bowing of epithelial structures of adnexa that surround a pyogenic granuloma, verruca, seborrheic keratosis, and so forth.

colloid bodies are necrotic keratinocytes, also termed Civatte bodies, hyaline bodies, and apoptotic bodies.

column refers to epithelial cells in a row greater than two.

compact orthokeratosis designates the normal configuration of the stratum corneum on palms and soles and in some pathologic conditions, such as lichen simplex chronicus, where cornified cells are packed together.

concentric fibroplasia refers to wiry bundles of collagen that are parallel to one another and also to elongated rete ridges and dermal papillae beneath a proliferation of melanocytes at the dermo-epidermal junction. The finding is usually mentioned in the context of lamellar fibroplasia with which it is reported to differ, the latter consisting of wiry bundles of collagen parallel to one another at bases of rete ridges that harbor nests of melanocytes. In actuality, concentric and lamellar fibroplasia are continuous with one another and are simply different orientations of a single pathologic process that is a nonspecific response to benign and malignant proliferations of melanocytes.

connective tissue nevus denotes a hamartoma of the fat (nevus lipomatosus) or of the dermis, either the papillary dermis (where it may resemble numerous contiguous skin tags) or the reticular dermis (where it involves collagen, elastic tissue, or both).

cord refers to epithelial cells in a row of two.

cornoid lamellation designates a column of parakeratosis that extends above the viable epidermis and into it, where vacuolated and dyskeratotic cells are accompaniments; it is requisite for the histopathologic diagnosis of porokeratosis in any of its several forms.

crust denotes a collection of plasma that contains white blood cells, red blood cells, or both.

cyst signifies an epithelium-lined sac. In skin, a cyst is lined almost always by epithelium of an adnexal structure and houses its product. For example, an infundibular cyst (also termed "epidermoid cyst") is lined by epithelium that resembles the upper portion of a hair follicle and contains cornified cells in basket-weave or laminated pattern. An isthmus-catagen cyst is lined by epithelium that resembles the isthmic portion of the outer sheath and the outer sheath at the base of a hair follicle in catagen. It contains cornified cells that are arranged compactly and tend to calcify. An apocrine gland cyst (also termed "apocrine hidrocystoma") is lined by epithelium that shows "decapitation" secretion and contains apocrine secretion.

degeneration, in classic pathology, refers to alterations in the cytoplasm of cells and in intercellular materials, e.g., fatty degeneration and degeneration of collagen, that are reflected in quality of staining.

degeneration of collagen describes loss of the normal structure of collagen bundles usually as a result of anoxemia or the action of lysosomal enzymes from leukocytes. It is seen as granular basophilia of bundles of collagen in sections stained by hematoxylin and eosin. It should not be referred to as "necrosis of collagen" because collagen is a fiber and therefore cannot undergo necrosis.

deposit is the accumulation of a substance such as mucin, amyloid, or urate not normally present in quantity in the skin.

desmoplasia designates fibroplasia that develops in response to certain epithelial neoplasms such as malignant melanoma.

differentiation refers to the relative capability of a neoplasm to resemble a normal structure; when successful, neoplasms are designated well differentiated, and if unsuccessful, they are termed undifferentiated.

digitated refers to one type of papillation, namely, finger-like projections above the skin surface, as in verruca vulgaris; synonymous with verrucous.

DOPA is an acronym for dihydroxyphenylalanine which is oxidized by dopa-oxidase in a positive DOPA reaction, i.e., one in which melanogenesis occurs.

dyskeratotic cell is one that has cornified prematurely with a pyknotic nucleus and brightly eosinophilic cytoplasm, as in focal acantholytic dyskeratosis or in squamous-cell carcinoma in situ.

ecchymosis is a purpuric patch that results from bleeding into the upper part of the dermis.

eddies of squamous cells describes whorls of spinous cells that seem to form around intra-epithelial sebaceous ducts that spiral through zones of infundibular hyperplasia, especially in seborrheic keratoses and warts that have been irritated. They usually signal biologic benignancy.

elastotic material is synonymous with solar elastosis, i.e., the altered spaghetti-like basophilic connective tissue produced by fibrocytes that have been exposed for many years to the damaging effects of ultraviolet light.

endophytic means growing inward from the skin surface like a resolving verruca vulgaris.

epidermal hyperplasia refers to increased numbers of spinous cells in the epidermis. We use it as a synonym for acanthosis.

epidermal nevus denotes a hamartoma characterized by more cells than is normal for epidermis and by hyperkeratotic papillations and/or digitations as is seen in bullous congenital ichthyosiform erythroderma.

epidermopoiesis means the making of epidermis i.e., the process of maturation of epidermal basal cells into cornified cells.

epithelial structures of adnexa designates derivatives of the embryonal ectoderm such as hair follicles, sebaceous glands and ducts, apocrine glands and ducts, and eccrine glands and ducts.

epithelioid refers to the cohesive arrangement of non-epithelial in a manner like epithelial cells, e.g., epithelioid histiocytes in sarcoidosis and epithelioid melanocytes in Spitz's nevi. Epithelioid cells have oval nuclei and pink cytoplasm when stained by hematoxylin and eosin.

epithelioid tubercle describes a collection of epithelioid histiocytes. When not surrounded by lymphocytes they are termed "naked tubercles," a characteristic feature of sarcoidal granulomas; when surrounded by lymphocytes, they form tuberculoid granulomas.

erosion signifies loss of part or all of the epidermis without loss of any dermal tissue.

exo-endophytic means growing outward and inward from the skin surface like a fully developed verruca vulgaris.

exophytic means growing outward from the skin surface like an acrochordon.

fascicle designates an elongated collection of spindle- or oval-shaped cells that tends to intersect with similar bunches of cells as in dermatofibrosarcoma protuberans.

fibrillar denotes arrangement in fibrils, i.e., delicate slender strands of connective tissue as in the collagen bundles that constitute a neurofibroma.

fibrotic tracts are linear bands of fibrosis that form at sites of permanently extinct hair follicles such as those of lichen planopilaris.

fibrous tracts are linear bands of fibrous tissue that form normally behind hair follicles that have retracted in catagen and telogen.

figurate means to represent by a figure, outline, or visible shape and is usually applied to figurate erythemas like erythema annulare centrifugum. Figurate presentations also are associated with inflammatory diseases like the urticarial stage of bullous pemphigoid, erythema multiforme, and Lyme disease, and with the neoplastic disease mycosis fungoides in the plaque stage. "Figurate" is a better term for these erythemas than "gyrate," which means to move in a spiral.

focal acantholytic dyskeratosis describes a focus of suprabasal cleft above which there are acantholytic and dyskeratotic cells in the spinous and granular zones and, above them, parakeratosis. These changes are seen stereotypically in Darier's disease, but also in Grover's disease, one manifestation of an epidermal nevus, a type of solitary keratosis, and a specific kind of infundibular cyst known incorrectly as "warty dyskeratoma," as well as a histopathological finding incidental to diseases of various kinds and even to sections of seemingly normal skin.

follicular mucinosis refers to the presence of abnormal collections of acid mucosubstances within the epithelium of hair follicles and sebaceous lobules, either as a process sui generis (i.e., alopecia mucinosa) or secondary to other conditions such as mycosis fungoides, other cutaneous lymphomas, and angiolymphoid hyperplasia with eosinophilia.

frond-like means leaf-like.

germinal center designates a zone within a lymphoid follicle constituted of B-lymphocytes at different stages of maturation, namely, small round, small cleaved, and large cleaved immunoblasts and plasma cells, as well as dendritic reticular cells and macrophages, some of which may contain tingible bodies. Germinal centers are found normally in lymph nodes and other lymphoid tissues, and abnormally in other organs such as the skin, e.g., in various inflammatory diseases such as pseudolymphomas, and in concert with certain neoplastic diseases such as basal-cell carcinomas rarely. Simulators of germinal centers appear in one type of B-cell lymphoma, to wit, follicular lymphoma.

germinative cells, as their name implies, are reproductive cells and, in particular those of embryonic buds of future hair follicles, sebaceous units, and apocrine units. These buds, which take origin from surface ectoderm, are known as "follicular germs." A benign neoplasm constituted mostly of follicular germinative cells is termed "trichoblastoma."

glassy membrane is a synonym for the PAS-positive basement membrane that surrounds the inferior segment of a hair follicle.

granulation tissue describes highly vascular, edematous connective tissue that contains a mixed-cell infiltrate and forms in response to certain traumas to skin such as incisions, punctures, and the extraction, suddenly, of a "hang nail."

granuloma is a collection of inflammatory cells most of which are epithelioid histiocytes.

granulomatous dermatitis designates inflammatory infiltrates in the skin in which histiocytes predominate, at least focally. It may be divided morphologically by conventional microscopy into nodular and diffuse types, and the nodular type may be subdivided as tuberculoid, sarcoidal, palisaded, suppurative, and foreign body.

guttate means drop-sized and -shaped and usually is applied to eruptive lesions of psoriasis and to a distinctive type of parapsoriasis that probably represents macular, and sometimes patch, lesions of mycosis fungoides.

hematoma is a nodule formed by bleeding into the reticular dermis and/or the subcutaneous fat.

homogenization of collagen refers to a uniform appearance of collagen as a consequence of amalgamation of bundles with loss of the distinctive orthogonal pattern of them. The term is inaccurate because collagen cannot become homogenized. There can be sclerosis, as in late lesions of necrobiosis lipoidica, or packing of bundles of collagen as in fully developed lesions of scleroderma.

horn pseudocysts are whorls of delicate, laminated orthokeratotic cells that represent sections cut at a tangent through tunnels of infundibular epithelium such as those that occur within some seborrheic keratoses and trichoepitheliomas.

hyaline bodies are necrotic keratinocytes, also termed colloid bodies, Civatte bodies, and apoptotic bodies.

hyperchromasia means "over coloration" as in increased intensity of nuclear staining in atypical nuclei.

hypergranulosis means an increased thickness of the stratum granulosum like that in lichen planus and lichen simplex chronicus. The change is most notable in follicular infundibula.

ichthyosis is a skin condition characterized by fish-like scales, e.g., ichthyosis vulgaris, X-linked ichthyosis, lamellar ichthyosis, and acquired ichthyosis. Bullous congenital ichthyosiform erythroderma and ichthyosis hystrix are not ichthyoses because they are devoid of fish-like scales. They are one variant of epidermal nevus, i.e., the epidermolytic hyperkeratotic type.

"id" reaction" conveys the sense of papules, papulovesicles, and vesicles that develop at a distant site, presumably because of a hypersensitivity reaction of tissue to fungal or other antigens at another site. The process is fundamentally a spongiotic one.

"Indian-file" arrangement of neoplastic cells describes atypical epithelial cells arranged as single cells, i.e., strands between collagen bundles. The pattern is especially common in metastatic carcinoma, but is not exclusive to it. The term "strands" is preferable to "Indian-file."

"infiltrating" margins refers to the interposition of neoplastic cells between collagen bundles particularly at the periphery of a lesion. A better morphologic description is "poor circumscription" of a neoplasm.

infundibulum of a hair follicle specifies the upper funnel-shaped portion bounded by the ostium above and the duct of a sebaceous gland below.

intradermal nevus refers to a condition that consists of nests, cords, and strands of melanocytes within the dermis.

invasion is a term that is defined imprecisely in general pathology and, in our opinion, is reserved best for militarists. If melanoma is "invasive," so, too, are all compound nevi; if basal-cell carcinoma is "invasive," so, too, is trichoepithelioma.

"irregularly" psoriasiform denotes elongated rete ridges of uneven lengths, but with preservation of the normal undulating pattern between rete ridges and dermal papillae, as is seen in lichen simplex chronicus.

isthmic portion of a hair follicle designates the uppermost portion of the outer sheath bounded by the duct of the sebaceous gland above and the site of attachment of the muscle of hair erection below.

junctional activity is a term that should never be used because it has not been defined in a standard way and, furthermore, once fixed in formalin, cells are no longer active.

junctional nevus refers to a condition composed of nests of melanocytes that are confined to the epidermis, usually at the dermo-epidermal junction.

lamellar fibroplasia describes collagen bundles (and fibrocytes) in the papillary dermis arranged in parallel to one another and seated beneath nests of melanocytes at the dermo-epidermal junction. The finding is nonspecific and may be observed in association with any proliferation of melanocytes, typical or atypical, at the dermo-epidermal junction, e.g., simple lentigines, junctional and compound nevi, melanomas in situ, and melanomas unmodified. Lamellar fibroplasia is purported to contrast with concentric fibroplasia, but the two are merely different names for a continuous pathologic condition viewed from different perspectives.

laminated orthokeratosis refers to the configuration of the stratum corneum in some pathologic states such as icthyosis vulgaris and X-linked ichthyosis, wherein the cornified cells are arranged in plate-like fashion.

Langer's lines refers to lines along which surgical excisions gape or fall together depending upon whether they are made across or parallel to them. These lines were charted by Langer, who pierced the skin of cadavers with an awl.

leukocytoclasis refers to the breaking up of leukocytes (karyorrhexis) resulting in nuclear "dust," usually made up of the fragments of the nuclei of polymorphonuclear leukocytes as in leukocytoclastic (allergic) vasculitis. Nuclear "dust" may also result from fragmentation of lymphocytes, such as in lupus erythematosus profundus.

lichenification denotes thickening of the skin characterized clinically by induration, hyperpigmentation, and accentuation of normal skin markings. Histopathologically, the epidermis is hyperplastic and the papillary dermis is thickened by coarse bundles of collagen arranged in vertical streaks.

lichenoid means resembling lichen planus clinically, i.e., flat-topped papules, and histopathologically, i.e., a band-like infiltrate in a thickened papillary dermis that usually obscures the dermo-epidermal junction along which there are vacuolar alteration and necrotic keratinocytes.

lobular panniculitis refers to an inflammatory process in the panniculus adiposus in which the inflammatory-cell infiltrate, when viewed with scanning magnification, is situated mostly in fat lobules, such as pancreatic panniculitis and lupus erythematosus profundus.

lymphoid follicle refers to a circumscribed collection of mostly small round lymphocytes within which a germinal center may form.

macule refers to a small, flat nonpalpable spot on the skin, up to 1 cm in size and of different color than that of the surrounding normal skin.

malignant is a word that describes the behavior of a neoplasm, namely, one that has the potential to cause death by local destruction or by metastases. That behavior is reflected in the silhouette of a neoplasm as it is viewed at scanning magnification. It does not pertain to cytologic characteristics that are properly described as having typical or atypical nuclei.

maturation designates the end stage of development of a cell, e.g., cornified cells for basal cells and smaller nuclei of melanocytes at the base of a compound or intradermal nevus, in contrast to the situation with melanocytes of melanoma, which usually do not become smaller with progressive descent.

melanophage refers to a macrophage that has ingested melanin.

metastasis means "out of place," i.e., the spread by blood or lymph vessels of neoplastic cells from a primary neoplasm to distant sites. Metastases usually cause death.

mixed inflammatory-cell infiltrate describes an infiltrate composed of different types of inflammatory cells, i.e., more than simply lymphocytes and histiocytes, but also neutrophils, eosinophils, or plasma cells.

Munro's microabscess signifies a small collection of neutrophils within the epidermis (spinous and granular zone, and cornified layer) of psoriasis.

necrotic cell is one that has died and is characterized by a nucleus that shows signs of pyknosis, karyorrhexis, or karyolysis, and cytoplasm that is brightly eosinophilic. Keratinocytes may undergo necrosis suddenly as in erythema multiforme, fixed drug eruptions, and burns of different kinds. Keratinocytes do not cornify when they die rapidly because time does not permit it. Keratinocytes do cornify, however, when they die slowly, and for that reason they are named "dyskeratotic" cells, as are found in lichen planus, the verrucous stage of incontinentia pigmenti, and Bowen's disease. Cytologically, a keratinocyte with a pyknotic nucleus that died rapidly cannot be differentiated from one that died slowly. The differentiation requires visualization of the cornified layer to see if it is normal (as is the case when keratinocytes die rapidly) or parakeratotic or compactly orthokeratotic (when they die slowly).

necrotizing vasculitis is an inaccurate term for small-vessel vasculitis because the only viable cells in those vessels are endothelial cells and they do not undergo necrosis in the process. At times, degeneration of collagen may be observed in some small-vessel vasculitides, but that is very different from necrosis. In short, small-vessel vasculitides should be named specifically, e.g., leukocytoclastic vasculitis, septic vasculitis, livedo vasculitis, or Degos' disease, and not be misnamed "necrotizing."

nests are roundish collections of cells, such as melanocytes in melanocytic nevi and atypical lymphocytes in mycosis fungoides.

nevoid means like a hamartoma or a malformation.

nevus is a word that must be modified always, e.g., a hamartoma in the sense of an organoid nevus such as nevus sebaceus of Jadassohn, and a neoplasm in the sense of a proliferation of melanocytes in an acquired melanocytic nevus.

nevus cell is a misnomer for a melanocyte in the dermis of a compound or intradermal type of melanocytic nevus. There are no nevus cells, nevocytes, or nevomelanocytes; all cells reputed to be them are melanocytes.

nodule is a dome-shaped solid lesion formed of cells, deposits, or elements of connective tissue.

orthokeratosis, more accurately termed orthohyperkeratosis, designates hyperkeratosis in which nuclei are not retained in the cells of the cornified layer. It may be subclassified as compact, laminated, or basket-weave in appearance.

Paget cell refers to a neoplastic cell that is found in the adenocarcinomas of mammary and extramammary Paget's disease. It is characterized by a large, round, or oval nucleus and abundant pale-staining cytoplasm that in extramammary Paget's disease, especially, contains mucosubstances demonstrable by staining with hematoxylin and eosin, and more vividly, with specialized stains. As a consequence, signet-ring cells are common in extramammary Paget's disease, but not in mammary Paget's disease.

pagetoid cell resembles the cells of mammary and, especially, extramammary Paget's disease by having a large round or oval nucleus and abundant pale-staining cytoplasm as occurs, for example, in Bowen's disease and in pagetoid malignant melanoma. Pagetoid cells do not usually house mucosubstances in their cytoplasm in contrast to the neoplastic cells of extramammary Paget's disease.

pagetoid pattern describes the scatter, like bird shot or buck shot, of Paget or pagetoid cells throughout an epithelium as is the pattern in mammary and extramammary Paget's disease on the one hand, and Bowen's disease and malignant melanoma on the other.

papillated describes nipple-shaped elevations above the skin surface and is synonymous with mamillated. The term is used to designate by conventional microscopy the surface of conditions like acanthosis nigricans and nevus sebaceus.

papillomatosis describes the projection of dermal papillae slightly or markedly above the skin surface, such as in acanthosis nigricans and some connective tissue nevi. The epidermis overlying the elongated papillae may not necessarily be thickened.

papillomatous is synonymous with papillated.

papulovesicle describes a combination of a papule (i.e., a small slightly elevated solid lesion) and a vesicle (i.e., a small slightly elevated fluid-containing lesion) as is seen in insect bites, Grover's disease, and Gianotti-Crosti disease.

parakeratosis is applied to retention of nuclei in the cells of the cornified layer. This usually is the result of accelerated epidermopoiesis as in psoriasis or faulty epidermopoiesis as in Bowen's disease.

parapsoriasis en plaques is a synonym for one expression of the early patch stage of mycosis fungoides.

patch refers to a broad flat lesion.

Pautrier's microabscess denotes a collection of atypical lymphocytes within the epidermis of lesions of mycosis fungoides. The term is a misnomer because abscess specifies a collection of neutrophils, not lymphocytes.

pedunculated refers to a polypoid excrescence, i.e., attached to the skin by a stalk such as an acrochordon.

petechia denotes a pinpoint punctum of extravasated red blood cells in the upper part of the dermis as occurs in Schamberg's disease.

plaque refers to an elevated broad lesion, often formed by coalescence of papules, as occurs in lichen amyloidosis.

pleomorphism indicates variation in size and shape of nuclei as usually occurs in a malignant neoplastic process. Pleomorphism of nuclei may be noted episodically in nuclei of benign neoplasms, e.g., Spitz's nevus, and even of inflammatory diseases, e.g., in keratinocytes within the epidermis of lesions induced by the drug busulfan.

poikiloderma vasculare atrophicans is a synonym for the late patch stage of mycosis fungoides, i.e., what originally was a plaque of mycosis fungoides that has undergone regression with residual features of poikiloderma, namely, atrophy, telangiectases, hyperpigmentation, and hypopigmentation.

polymorphic eruption means having more than one type of primary and/or secondary skin lesion, i.e., a combination of macules, papules, vesicles, and so on, as in Mucha-Habermann disease.

polypoid means like a polyp, i.e., an excrescence above the skin surface that has a narrow base and a stalk like an acrochordon.

proliferation of atypical melanocytes describes an increased number of melanocytes with atypical nuclei within and sometimes above the basal layer of the epidermis and epithelial structures of adnexa. It is descriptive and not specifically diagnostic. For example, it is not synonymous with melanoma in situ because such a proliferation may also occur in junctional Spitz's nevi and several other simulators of melanoma.

pseudoglandular describes a structure that resembles an authentic gland as may form in certain squamous-cell carcinomas characterized by suprabasal clefts and acantholytic, dyskeratotic cells.

psoriasiform means resembling psoriasis clinically as reddish plaques covered by scales, and histopathologically as elongated, often thin rete ridges of approximately equal lengths with preservation of the normal undulating pattern between rete ridges and dermal papillae.

purpura refers to the purple color caused by visible hemorrhage in skin and can be subclassified as petechiae, ecchymoses, and hematomas.

"pushing" margins is a term applied to the smooth rounded borders of a neoplasm that appears to grow centrifugally. A more precise morphologic designation is a well-circumscribed neoplasm.

reticulum-cell sarcoma is an antiquated term for nodular lesions of mycosis fungoides and large-cell lymphomas in the skin whose cells resemble histiocytes, but are actually atypical T-lymphocytes. Newer terms for reticulum-cell sarcoma include histiocytic, centroblastic, lymphoblastic, and immunoblastic lymphomas.

satellitosis signifies nearby metastasis, i.e., within 5.0 cm of the primary malignant neoplasm, and sometimes may be apparent in the same tissue specimen as the primary neoplasm.

scale designates a collection of orthokeratotic cells, parakeratotic cells, or both.

scale-crust describes a combination of a scale (cornified cells) and a crust (plasma that contains blood cells).

sclerosis refers to a type of fibrosis characterized by a uniform appearance of collagen bundles, colloquially designated "homogenization," and associated with a decreased number of fibrocytes.

sebaceous follicle refers to a vellus-hair follicle on a face characterized by a prominent infundibulum, a puny inferior segment, and one or more large sebaceous glands.

sebaceous secretion is holocrine secretion of over-mature sebaceous cells that represent the end product of maturation of sebocytes.

sebum is composed mostly of sebaceous secretion and other materials that are carried with it in its journey through a sebaceous duct and follicular infundibulum to the skin surface, namely, squames, *Pityrosporum ovale* and *orbiculare*, *Staphylococcus epidermidis*, *Propionibacterium acnes*, and *Demodex*.

septal panniculitis refers to an inflammatory process in the panniculus adiposus in which the infiltrate of inflammatory cells is situated mostly in the septa, rather than mostly in the lobules, as viewed with scanning magnification. In actuality, there is no pure septal panniculitis or lobular panniculitis; some overlap is inevitable, but erythema nodosum remains the stereotype of septal panniculitis.

sessile means seated, i.e., a broad-based excrescence above the skin surface such as some keratoacanthomas.

siderophage refers to a macrophage that has ingested iron.

solar elastosis is synonymous with elastotic material, i.e., the altered spaghetti-like basophilic connective tissue, presumably collagen coated by elastin, produced by fibrocytes that long have been affected by sunlight.

spongiform pustule describes a collection of neutrophils in the spinous and granular zones of the epidermis where remnants of cell membranes give the pustule a sponge-like appearance. A spongiform pustule is not specific for any one disease, but may be seen in such disparate conditions as pustular psoriasis and its many synonyms, halogenodermas, and pyoderma gangrenosum.

spongiosis refers to intercellular edema recognizable by widened intercellular spaces across which intercellular bridges are stretched and thereby appear elongated. Spongiosis always is mediated by cells, usually inflammatory ones such as lymphocytes and eosinophils in allergic contact dermatitis, for example, but also by neoplastic cells such as lymphocytes of mycosis fungoides.

spongiotic psoriasiform dermatitis signifies intercellular edema in a hyperplastic epidermis in which the pattern of epidermal rete ridges and dermal papillae is preserved, as is seen in fully developed lesions of allergic contact and nummular dermatitis.

spontaneous means self-generated, which is incompatible with biologic processes. Therefore, all so-called spontaneous phenomena like spontaneous keloids and spontaneous regression of melanoma are not spontaneous at all. The former results from external trauma and the latter from the effects of lymphocytes.

squamoid means resembling the cells of the spinous zone of the epidermis, like those cells that make up a verruca or a verrucous squamous-cell carcinoma.

strand refers to epithelial cells in single file.

subcorneal pustule describes a collection of neutrophils situated immediately beneath the cornified layer of the epidermis.

supra-papillary plate refers to the portion of the epidermis situated immediately above the summit of a dermal papilla.

telangiectasis signifies a dilated end-vessel, usually a dilated capillary and venule.

telogen refers to the resting stage of the follicular cycle in which the inferior segment of a hair follicle has retracted to the level of the site of attachment of a muscle of hair erection; the infundibulum and isthmus are uninvolved during the stages of the follicular cycle.

trabecula is a synonym for a septum, as in a fibrous trabecula in the subcutaneous fat.

tricholemmal sheath describes the external or outer sheath of a hair follicle, which in anagen contains abundant glycogen.

trichomalacia means literally "softening of hair," but refers histopathologically to pleated hair shafts that contain clumps of melanin as a result of twisting hairs to and fro in trichotillomania. The hairs in that condition are normal, not soft. The abnormality is psychological.

tubercle is a term in gross pathology for potato-like structures that, on histopathologic examination, are seen to consist mostly of epithelioid histiocytes.

tuberculoid, in general pathology, refers to histopathologic findings that resemble those of tuberculosis and, in cutaneous pathology, of lupus vulgaris in particular. Tuberculoid granulomas also occur, for example, in tuberculoid leprosy, the recidivans expression of leishmaniasis, infections by atypical mycobacteria and, uncommonly, in sarcoidosis.

tumor means a swelling. This term should not be used synonymously with neoplasm or to modify cells as in "tumor cell(s)." Neoplasm and neoplastic cells are more precise and, therefore, preferable terms.

ulcer indicates loss of the entire epidermis and at least some of the dermis.

vacuolar alteration describes tiny spaces on either side of the basement membrane at the dermo-epidermal junction; *liquefaction degeneration* is synonymous.

vasculitis means an inflammatory process associated with characteristic morphologic changes in the walls and lumens of blood vessels, namely, for small-vessel vasculitis fibrin in the walls of venules and/or thrombi within lumens of venules, and for large-vessel vasculitis inflammatory cells within the walls of arteries and veins. The most common vasculitis in skin is leukocytoclastic vasculitis.

vegetation describes a heaped-up collection of scale-crusts, sometimes hemorrhagic, often purulent, as is seen in pemphigus vegetans.

vellus is applied to the fine delicate hairs found on much of the body, e.g., the face, arms, and trunk, in contrast to terminal hairs, which are broader, longer, and darker, and which are found on the scalp, in the axillae, and in the pubic region. Hair follicles that produce vellus hairs are known as vellus follicles and those that manufacture terminal hairs are designated terminal follicles.

verrucous means like a verruca, e.g., clinically a rough, finger-shaped lesion and one characterized histopathologically by digitated epidermal hyperplasia or neoplasia; digitated is synonymous.

vesiculopustule applies to a lesion that has features of both a small blister that contains plasma and a pustule that contains numerous neutrophils.

villous describes papillated projections that resemble intestinal villi, such as the appearance of dermal papillae in pemphigus vulgaris.